There are few academic books that a reader finds simultaneously insigh[t]
Beach's insights into how hope is constructed and functions will serve
for all future writing on this topic. It is this focus on hope that makes
experience in the academy.

Teresa L. Thompson is Professor in the Department of Communication, Dayton University, and Editor of *Health Communication*

Never before has such a record of family talk about death been analyzed in anything approaching such detail, and with such a respectful yet sophisticated analytic apparatus. An absorbing catalogue of the ways in which the family makes its 'cancer journey' in talk: how delicate matters are broached, how the unsayable is said, and how mundane reality is talked into being in the cross-fire of calls to institutions intruding into the scene. The result is unique. It is both a contribution to our technical understanding of talk as a medium of social action, and a humane testament to the power of social science to illuminate hopeful conduct as well as darker reaches of the human journey.

Charles Antaki is Professor of Language and Social Psychology, Loughborough University, England, and Editor of *Research on Language and Social Interaction*

This research, funded early on by the American Cancer Society, has great potential to improve the quality of life for cancer patients and their families. When cancer touches a person's life, the shock wave reverberates throughout the family and extended family. Professor Beach's research provides groundbreaking insights into that effect and how families cope throughout their cancer experience. Health Care professionals who want to understand family dynamics, outside of the examinations and treatment rooms, will find this book fascinating and inspiring.

Lynda Barbour is Health Promotion Director, Border Sierra Region, American Cancer Society, San Diego

A Natural History of Family Cancer is a powerful book on the human response to illness. It breaks new ground in the field of health communication by delving deep into the world of one family as its members cope with a cancer diagnosis and the progression of the illness over more than a year. By showing how key social activities are achieved on a moment-by-moment basis, and by revealing the details of their organization, Beach preserves and respects the texture of the family members' experiences. The result is a profoundly intimate, humane example of scholarship. Given its scope, one could design an entire course around this book or use it alongside others in communication, sociology, linguistics, anthropology, and a wide variety of courses in medically related professions.

Virginia Teas Gill is Associate Professor, Department of Sociology and Anthropology, Illinois State University, and author of numerous articles on communication during medical interviewing.

Professor Beach makes clear how fundamental practices of everyday conversation—such as news delivery, storytelling, use of figurative expressions, and assessments—are primary resources utilized by family members to manage crisis and disruptions, create shared realities, but also negotiate and defend their positions regarding what each family claims rights to know and experience. . . . A valuable contribution to the social and medical sciences that is equally important to read for scholars of interaction, medical sociologists, medical psychologists, and medical practitioners.

Anssi Peräkylä is Professor in the Department of Sociology, University of Helsinki, and author of *Aids Counseling: Institutional Interaction and Clinical Practice*

A compelling report from unique and amazing materials . . . Wayne Beach identifies exciting intellectual challenges for conversation analysis and interactional linguistics, while simultaneously maintaining a rare humanity in his treatment of these unique materials from critical moments in the life of a family.

Cecilia E. Ford is Professor of English Language and Linguistics/Rhetoric and Composition, University of Wisconsin–Madison, and (among others books) is author of *Women Speaking Up: Getting and Using Turns in Workplace Meetings* (2008)

A patient suffering from cancer sounds a call of conscience in desperate need of heartfelt acknowledgment. Beach offers a finally tuned assessment of this call and the discourse that it provokes.

Michael J. Hyde is University Distinguished Professor of Communication Ethics & Fellow, W. K. Kellogg Foundation, Department of Communication, Program in Bioethics, Health, and Society, School of Medicine, Wake Forest University, and author of *The Call of Conscience: Heidegger and Levinas, Rhetoric and the Euthanasia Debate*.

Cancer does inhabit individual bodies, but its *meaning* is absolutely worked out between and among us. We cannot overlook the social and communicative aspects of health, life, death, and identity. This extraordinary book provides a way into these issues, even though there is nothing particularly exotic, famous, evil, heroic, or sensational about these people and their communication. And that is part of the beauty and power of how, through their communication, ordinary people make sense of and manage their all-too-ordinary, difficult circumstances. Professor Beach has spent more than a decade working with these materials, and this book shows the fruits of that extended labor . . .

> **Phillip Glenn** is Professor, Department of Communication Studies, Emerson College, and author of *Laughter in Interaction*

With surgical and delicate precision, Beach opens up everyday conversations about illness to show us ways of coping and hoping in the face of difficulty and possible death. And with elegance, Beach maintains a balance between the scientific and humanistic aspects of illness and its treatment...an empathetic storyteller who invites us to consider the lived experience of his subjects—their personal challenges, emotional turmoil, humorous exchanges, endearing actions, and resolute efforts. *A Natural History of Family Cancer* positions him as one of the world's leading experts on communication within families working to manage the illness of a loved one

> **Curtis D. LeBaron** is Warren Jones Fellow and Associate Professor of Organizational Leadership and Strategy, Marriot School of Management, Brigham Young University, and Co-Editor of *Studies in Language and Social Interaction: In Honor of Robert Hopper*

This is a unique book . . . It offers an approach to emotion, experience and understanding which locates these psychological phenomena in their home environments—for example, as grief is expressed and shared acts of commiseration take place. Beach's technical and rigorous analysis does not detract from the book's sensitivity. Instead, with exquisite detail readers are allowed into the world of a family reeling from the original diagnosis and evolving sickness. It is at the same time a profound contribution to modern social psychology, an important new way of conducting medical sociology, and a significant addition to our understanding of contemporary family life.

> **Jonathan Potter** is Professor of Discourse Analysis at Loughborough University, England, and (among other books) is the author of *Representing Reality: Discourse, Rhetoric, and Social Construction* (1996)

Professor Beach brings us into the interactional world of family members living through the emotional and practical roller coaster of a mom's cancer diagnosis, treatment and eventual death...particular ways of talking that provide for the very constitution of knowledge, optimism, hope, despair, sympathy, comfort and practical action. Studying a family's experience of cancer in this way affords perspective and insight not ordinarily available, going well beyond what the patient and her family members may think or feel, examining not only how they construct those thoughts and feelings in interaction with one another, but also how they manage the many practical contingencies of social life inherent in the progression of illness

> **Jenny Mandelbaum** is Associate Professor, Department of Communication, Rutgers University, and Co-Editor of *Studies in Language and Social Interaction: In Honor of Robert Hopper.*

Without focusing directly on clinical communication, but family phone conversations, this book powerfully demonstrates that encounters between cancer patients and medical practitioners are merely individual moments, and threads, in the complex warp and weft of families using communication to manage cancer . . . Analysis expands our understanding of the social organization of the delivery of good and bad health news, troubles tellings, and commiseration. *A Natural History of Family Cancer* is an important contribution to the study of language and social interaction, as well as family and health communication

> **Jeffrey D. Robinson** is Associate Professor, Department of Communication, Rutgers University, and author of numerous articles on conversational interaction and medical interviewing.

A Natural History of Family Cancer

Interactional Resources for Managing Illness

Hampton Press Communication Series
HEALTH COMMUNICATION
Gary L. Kreps, *series editor*

A Natural History of Family Cancer: Interactional Resources for Managing Illness
Wayne A. Beach

Communication in Recovery: Perspectives on Twelve-Step Groups
Lynette S. Eastland, Sandra L. Herndon, & Jeanine R. Barr (eds.)

Communicating in the Clinic: Negotiating Frontstage and Backstage Teamwork
Laura L. Ellingson

Media-Mediated Aids
Linda K. Fuller (ed.)

Cancer-Related Information Seeking
J. David Johnson

Changing the Culture of College Drinking: A Socially Situated
    Health Communication Campaign
Linda C. Lederman & Lea P. Stewart

Handbook of Communication and Cancer Care
Dan O'Hair, Gary L. Kreps, & Lisa Sparks, (eds.)

Crisis Communication and the Public Health
Matthew Seeger and Timothy Sellnow (eds.)

Cancer, Communication and Aging
Lisa Sparks, Dan O'Hair, & Gary L. Kreps (eds.)

Cancer and Death: A Love Story in two Voices
Leah Vande Berg & Nick Trujillo

Communicating Spirituality in Health Care
Margaret A. Wills (ed.)

A Natural History of Family Cancer

Interactional Resources for Managing Illness

Wayne A. Beach

San Diego State University

HAMPTON PRESS, INC.
CRESSKILL, NEW JERSEY

Printed in the United States of America

Library of Congress Cataloging-in-Publication Data

Beach, Wayne A.
  A natural history of family cancer : interactional resources for managing
illness / Wayne A. Beach.
     p. ; cm. -- (Health communication)
  Includes bibliographical references and indexes.
  ISBN 978-1-57273-690-0 (hardbound) -- ISBN 978-1-57273-691-7 (paperbound)
  1. Cancer--Patients--Family relationships. 2. Communication in medicine. I.
Title. II. Series: Health communication (Cresskill, N.J.)
  [DNLM: 1. Neoplasms--psychology. 2. Adaptation, Psychological. 3.
Communication. 4. Family--psychology. 5. Social Support. QZ 200 B365n 2009]
  RC262.B336 2009
  362.196'994--dc22
                                   2009011210

Cover designed by Wendy Shapiro

Hampton Press, Inc.
23 Broadway
Cresskill, NJ 07626

To my children, Brandon & Dylan,
whose love, patience, and insights edify me daily

And for all cancer patients, family members, & friends
Lay and professional caregivers alike
Journeying through diagnosis, treatment, & prognosis
Bound together by communication
Shaping the lives we know

CONTENTS

~ III ~
MANAGING LIFE IN TIMES OF UNCERTAINTY AND CRISIS

~ IV ~
REPORTING ON AND ASSESSING MEDICAL CARE

~ VI ~
PAST, PRESENT, AND FUTURE PERSPECTIVES

FOREWORD

Douglas W. Maynard

University of Wisconsin, Madison

This book deals with the so-called *cancer journey*. It is an examination of recorded telephone calls from the moment a patient is diagnosed with cancer to the time over a year later when she dies. The conversations take place among this cancer patient, her husband, her son (who made the recordings), her sister, her mother, and between the son and various others.

The cancer journey: This is a phrase that seems to have entered the English lexicon as a ubiquitous metaphor for what happens to diagnosed oncology patients along with their families, friends, and health care providers. The phrase draws on the notion of travel from one place to another and suggests many possibilities. Maybe having cancer involves an expedition to unknown lands, a voyage across uncharted and choppy waters, a flight through stormy weather, or—in less charitable terms—a tour of hell. On the other hand, some narrators equate the cancer journey to an enlightening mission of discovery, whether it regards the self, social relations with others, or the very meaning of life itself.

Even Susan Sontag, otherwise critical of using metaphors to describe illness,[1] famously draws on the journey when she proposes that we all belong to two kingdoms—that of the well and that of the sick. Although we prefer the "passport" situating us in the wellness kingdom, from time to time we must "emigrate" to the realm of illness. Cancer journey as metaphor also brings to mind the need for narratives of illness that Arthur Frank describes,[2] for the metaphor encompasses the concept of "wreckage" as the patient loses a map and destination and must find new goals or end points by drawing a fresh chart and using stories about restitution and repair, interruption and chaos, or quest and heroism.

Of course there is not a single cancer journey or only a few types of travel through oncology, even metaphorically speaking. Instead, there are many, many different kinds of expeditions depending on the type of cancer, the person, the family, the health professionals, the place where the illness is diagnosed, and a plenitude of other contingencies. Within this plenitude, the metaphor, as it describes an individual's experience, provides for a more general understanding. We may not have had cancer, or we may not have had the cancer that another has had. Or we may be the one who has had cancer whereas others have not. However, because we all know in some degree what journeys, expeditions, voyages, flights, tours, or missions entail, by way of the metaphor we can make sense of others' or they can make sense of our own involvement with cancer as a form of illness.

Such mutual understanding cannot be complete, however, because metaphors also hide aspects of the experiential phenomenon they attempt to describe.[3] That is, in translating one experience in terms of another, they necessarily eviscerate aspects of the original occurrence. Another shortcoming of the metaphor is that it glosses what actually happens in experience. One value of this exceptional book is that by focusing squarely on communication in everyday life, the shortcomings of "metaphor" are replaced with a close look at how family members actually talk about and manage the difficulties that cancer occasions for them. Its author, Wayne Beach, knows about "the cancer journey" not because he has been diagnosed with cancer, but because of the empirical data at the core of this book, his own mother's illness, and his extensive dialogue with friends and colleagues (and their significant others) who have suffered with cancer. And, drawing on Packer,[4] he makes a fine distinction, also in journey-metaphorical terms, between persons from a balcony as they watch travelers go by on the road and the travelers themselves. The "balconeers" have one version of what the trek is like, an abstracted and distanced one, whereas the travelers, through confronting the minutiae of actual journeying, know that trek in a concrete and detailed way. In these terms, and unlike writings that use narrative, metaphor, anecdote and other literary forms to capture what having cancer or being close to someone with the disease entails, this book provides an in-depth view of what a cancer journey really is in the everyday, everynight, real-time courses of actions and interactions that encompass patients and their significant personal and professional others.

That *A Natural History of Family Cancer* provides this view is due to the remarkable nature of these phone calls and the kind of analysis brought to bear on their interactional organization. I first came in contact with the data because of an interest in "bad news", when Professor Beach (in the mid-1990s) generously shared with me a piece of his recent collection for my own study.[5] At the time, he told me about the 61 telephone calls and the 13-month period of time in which they were recorded. So I knew there was more but could barely imagine what the rest of the collection would look like, even after he published several papers using the data. Now the corpus has been analyzed in its entirety, and we readers are made privy to a variegated and otherwise elusive set of communicative events surrounding one person's cancer.

But we as readers are not mere balconeers and we do not have to rely on metaphors and stories to grasp the cancer journey. Professor Beach employs the powerful tools of conversation analysis to bring us close to these events and examine them in their detail. It is not only that this book is, as the title suggests, a "natural history", which reveals interactions in which participants ongoingly deal with the cancer news, cars, dogs, food, airlines, their relationships, and a myriad of quotidian concerns related and unrelated to the cancer. It is also an inquiry into "naturally occurring interaction", preserving the talk and interactions among participants according to their own orientations. This kind of inquiry requires an interest beyond what participants say. It means paying attention to silences, overlapping talk, sound stretches, breathing, laughter, words, utterances, sequences, and numerous other features recruited to achieve social actions. Rather than relying on the abstractions of metaphor or narrative or anecdote, conversation analysts suggest that it is in original talk—with all its seeming perturbations—that order, organization, and participants' sense-making are to be discovered.

The analytic revelation of sense making in the situation derives from a preoccupation with the question of how participants talk to one another. The idea is that social actions and activities constructed through conversation are methodical. Accordingly, by examining talk closely we can develop knowledge about the tacit methods through which participants assemble their actions and activities. By explicating the "how", we paradoxically become privy to both the fine-grained detail of the social world and the general features such as dealing with its changing configurations or showing particular emotional states that figure in the human experience of that world. This is because as participants attend, moment by moment, to the "how" of their talk and social interaction, they are "doing" or accomplishing the visibility of the objective-seeming world that they know in common and take for granted. Moreover, they are using tools that transcend the particular situation in which they are embedded. With this kind of analytic sensibility, chapter by chapter Professor Beach shows us (among other matters):

- How dad initially tells son about mom's cancer, and how Son receives this news such that it has a given texture just for them;
- How mom and son especially (but also others), both earlier and later in the course of the disease, discuss the cancer and come to display collaboratively and publicly in their interaction (and not just cognitively) intense forms of affect surrounding the cancer experiences;
- How family members deploy "figurative expressions" to act with resolve, readiness, and restraint in relation to pain, being together, and confronting finality;
- How they relate to one another and to doctors in terms of differing states of knowledge about the cancer;
- How son, dad and mom's sister handle the delicate topic of mom's longtime smoking habit and how it figures (or does not) in the course of her illness;
- How, in the face of extreme circumstances, family members use expressions of humor and of hope in regulated ways to manage these circumstances.

Investigating how participants engage in all these and other activities involves a concern with conversational practices. The book thereby contributes to the burgeoning field of conversation analysis, showing, for example, the overall sequential environment for the sharing of what Professor Beach calls "commiserative and epistemic space" (see Chapter 10). Some, but not all, attempts at this sharing are successful, and to view the moments when one party takes a particular affective stance and the other aligns with or refrains from endorsing that stance is to appreciate just how delicate these moments are because of the ways that the sequencing of talk works. This monograph, while thoroughly embedded in the conversation analytic enterprise, also is an utterly unique form of that enterprise: In addition to examining the moments or *episodes* of interaction, it is a kind of *longitudinal* inquiry as it traces the family interactions–serially, chronologically, and cumulatively–over time.[6]

To read this book, therefore, is an informative and dramatic journey in itself. But let me return to the "cancer journey" metaphor as Professor Beach addresses it (page 547):

> One grounded and relevant way to describe a "cancer journey" . . . is to begin noticing how those involved report that they were, are and will be preoccupied with what is essentially an expedition through illness. . . . The more serious the prognosis, the more incessant the work required to monitor, manage, and report on not just what is happening, but how best to cope with and survive many undulating passages.

The "incessant work" to which Professor Beach refers includes the methods and practices by which this patient and her others come to learn about what the cancer is for her, themselves, and for their shared future. Carefully, the book grounds itself in the talk and actions of this one patient and, more often, of those in her social surroundings. To switch metaphors, it probes a concrete network of practices that tie a family, a community, and health care practitioners together in an intricate web. This web is unique to this family, community, and set of practitioners, and it consequently has a specific warp and weft. Yet the practices whereby participants assemble it will have relevance for understanding other settings involving cancer or illness. Accordingly, the findings in *A Natural History of Family Cancer* are applicable to a variety of lay and professional audiences who, from a variety of perspectives, may be interested in any or all parts of the web. Readers, I suspect, can absorb chapters selectively or the book as a whole and will be rewarded with a metaphoric journey, to be sure, but also something deeper than that—something that is as close as analytically possible to being there.

NOTES

1. Susan Sontag, *Illness as Metaphor* (New York: Farrar, Straus, Giroux, 1977).
2. Arthur W. Frank, *The Wounded Storyteller: Body, Illness, and Ethics* (Chicago: University of Chicago Press, 1995).
3. See, for example, George Lakoff and Mark Johnson, *Metaphors We Live By* (Chicago: University of Chicago Press, 1980).
4. Packer, J.I. (1973). *Knowing God.* (Downers Grove, IL: Intervarsity Press).
5. Douglas W. Maynard, *Bad News, Good News: Conversational Order in Everyday Talk and Clinical Settings* (Chicago: University of Chicago Press, 2003).
6. I have discussed the distinction between episodic and longitudinal conversation analysis in *Bad News, Good News*, pp. 78–9.

ACKNOWLEDGMENTS

Any project extending over a decade has been influenced by seemingly countless discussions and written exchanges with others. This volume is certainly no exception. I am deeply indebted to all who have triggered thoughts that would not have otherwise existed, provided constructive feedback for refining coarse insights, and offered ongoing encouragement to pursue fundamental understandings about how family members talk through cancer on the telephone. As a result of others' involvements, what was once an amazingly rich but unwieldy corpus of phone calls became, over time, a manageable resource for excavating primary social activities comprising family cancer journeys.

It is, of course, impossible to mention all friends, colleagues, undergraduate and graduate students, cancer patients and survivors, family members, physicians, nurses, therapists, clergy and others who have, knowingly or not, contributed to shaping the following chapters. In particular, it is important to acknowledge the hundreds, if not thousands of individuals who have participated in data/listening sessions. In classroom environments, during conference meetings, in unison with lectures at other universities, and across numerous community venues I have been fortunate to collaborate in sessions where a fascinating array of embryonic, at times penetrating discussions emerged in response to the "Malignancy" audio recordings and transcriptions. While the analytic limitations of the findings in this volume are entirely my own, your interest in and involvement with these materials is not taken for granted.

A brief history of this project is provided in the Introduction (Chapter 1), including how timely it was to receive a grant from the American Cancer Society (ACS) in 1998, which "officially" launched this project. What is not mentioned is that during that same year, I began lecturing on these materials through invitations from other universities. Initial talks were hosted by Phil Glenn at Southern Illinois University, Doug Maynard at Indiana University, Robert Hopper at the University of Texas, and Char Jones for the Myhre Lecture Series at Carroll College. Subsequent lectures have occurred at the University of California, Santa Barbara, repeated visits to the Medical Centers at the University of California in San Diego and Irvine, the UCLA Center on Everyday Lives of Families (CELF), and during a University Symposium lecture series at Rutgers University, hosted by Jenny Mandelbaum. In addition, I have been fortunate to share and discuss these materials with diverse community health care organizations.

These unique occasions have provided invaluable and cumulative learning experiences—enriching opportunities to talk through work-in-progress, brainstorm possibilities, and gain a fuller appreciation for interrelationships among interaction, health, communication, families, and cancer.

Over the course of this project, the scholarship and support of David Buller, Mary Buller, Greg Desilet, Paul Drew, Rich Frankel, Phil Glenn, John Heritage, Robert Hopper, Gail Jefferson, Leslie Jarmon, Char Jones, Curt LeBaron, Wendy Leeds-Hurwitz, Jenny

Mandelbaum, Doug Maynard, Anita Pomerantz, Anssi Peräkylä, Jeff Robinson, Manny Schegloff, and Tanya Stivers—to name only a few—have also significantly influenced this undertaking.

Many others have also generously given of their time and energy: During their tenure as graduate students, Rebecca Meyer assisted in producing initial transcriptions, Jen Anderson, Lanie Lockwood, and Jeff Good worked with me as co-authors on earlier papers, and both Elisa Pigeron and Alison Crase helped to move these materials forward; Dave Dunning invested a portion of his sabbatical to visit with me in San Diego, offer comments on drafts of chapters, and envision how basic research findings might be transformed into innovative curriculum packages; Ongoing discussions with Preston Ribnick and Lilly Green, of PRG Solutions, Inc., have opened my eyes to new horizons for disseminating these basic research findings across cancer centers, medical groups, schools of medicine, and numerous disciplines examining health, communication, family life, and medical care; Donna Albert has been a great resource for resolving textual problems; and Linda Barbour (ACS) has offered helpful collaborations.

I am fortunate to have received continual support from colleagues at SDSU in the School of Communication, especially Jan Andersen (now at Emerson College), Peter Andersen, Dave Dozier, and Brian Spitzberg who have all had more conversations with me about this work than any of us can remember.

Various grants-in-aid from SDSU have facilitated my research efforts. And the adaptation of these materials into a theatrical production would not have been possible without the instrumental efforts by Dean Joyce Gattas and Michele Schlecht, the Dean's Excellence Fund in the College of Professional Studies and Fine Arts, and an award from the President's Leadership Fund (PLF). The Arthur & Rise Johnson Foundation, and the Salah Hassein family have also made it possible for this and related projects to become refined and connected.

In 2002 I directed a master's thesis by Lanie Lockwood, who began to explore the possibility of adapting the transcriptions—a naturally occurring corpus with considerable dramatic potential—into a script to be employed for a theatrical (and everyday life) performance. An agreement was made then, and continues, that no dialogue would be added that was not initially uttered during family members' actual phone conversations. Thanks to theatre professionals Paula Kalustian, Patricia Loughrey, Marybeth Bielawski-DeLeo, and Carla Nell for helping to adapt these materials into preliminary workshop readings and nearly sold-out performances at SDSU's Experimental Theatre. Thanks also to Bill Trumpfhheller and his public relations staff at Nuffer, Smith, & Tucker for their generous support. Over one thousand audience members have now heard and reacted to the lives of these family members as they navigated through their cancer journey together—in their own words and enacted through actual, detailed conversation analytic transcriptions—and new efforts are currently underway to write a new script and disseminate these materials nationwide. Though I am by no means a theatre expert, I am gradually learning about how to function as an Executive Producer. I've come to realize that this is a worthwhile effort since I have observed first hand, through "talk-back" sessions following performances, just how these materials can touch the hearts and lives of so many audience members who were drawn to hear and respond to these family conversations. I am now more convinced than ever that how cancer gets talked out during interactions among family, friends, and care providers strikes a critically important and resonant chord with countless individuals, families, and medical experts world-wide.

With humble acknowledgment, these performances were dedicated to "the family" that donated these recorded phone calls. That recognition carries over to this volume. As I note in the Introduction, the family's rationale for providing these recordings for my analysis is both courageous and inspiring. What a difference it makes to have access to routine yet extraordinary conversations.

A few years back, I met initially with Barbara Bernstein about publishing two lengthy books with Hampton Press—one on communication among family members facing cancer, and the other about patient-provider interactions in the clinic. My rationale was straightforward: Because we live our lives in home and related environments, and routinely rely on clinical visitations to manage illness, each should be investigated in unison with the other. This was a vision that Barbara shared, and her support and patience throughout these related projects has been deeply appreciated. So too has Gary Kreps, Hampton Press editor for the series on health communication, been a great resource who not only understands what I am trying to accomplish, but can situate and eloquently speak for this work across the larger framework of research on health and illness. The editing provided by Elaine Bernstein and Mariann Hutlak was also extremely helpful. Taken together, those working with Hampton Press are extremely skilled yet personable, and I am glad to be collaborating with them. Discussions with graphic artist Wendy Shapiro, who designed the "cancer cell" and other features on the front/back cover, have been creative and visually alluring.

My MBS and members of LJCC have been a wellspring of heartfelt encouragement and inspiration. Thanks for reminding me that our largest projects are barely footnotes on the text of divine order.

As we all know only too well, writing gets accomplished on a day-to-day basis and accumulates slowly. My son Brandon and daughter Dylan have made countless visits to "your study" over the years, at times to just have a chat and see how I was doing but, even more frequently, to persuade me to "quit working" so that we might move onto more important agendas like playing, exercising, eating, shopping, and other basics of everyday living. I cannot thank them enough for their persistence, endurance, and unconditional love. Though Brandon and Dylan did not get to know my mother because her life was taken by cancer at an early age of seventy, they did realize that she had something to do with why I was writing this volume. And for them that was a good enough reason to explain the time I was investing—though it often did little, and understandably so, to curtail their impatience! As yet more time passes, it is my hope that each will better grasp the relevance of what has been undertaken and the joy they continue to provide during each phase of the journey.

INTRODUCTION

A family.
A phone call.
A diagnosis . . .
One family's journey through cancer.[1]

In 1988, a graduate student attached a recording device on his telephone to begin studying naturally occurring conversations. During the first recorded call to his dad, son was informed that his mom had been diagnosed with cancer. The next morning, son called his mom to discuss her reactions to the bad news. Over the next 13 months and 61 phone calls, from diagnosis until only hours before the death of his mom, son continued to record conversations that occurred with family members, friends, and service providers.

Within one year following his mother's death, the family donated the recordings to me with the hope that they might be analyzed for two primary and related reasons: to advance understandings of how everyday conversations get organized and eventually, if possible, to rely on this knowledge to assist other families and medical experts as they communicate throughout cancer journeys.

This volume takes the first essential step by offering a close examination of the interactional organization of routine phone calls among family members, and others, over the course of a naturally occurring journey through cancer. Throughout these calls, family members rely on talk when attempting to understand complex and often uncertain matters comprising cancer diagnosis, treatment, prognosis, and related key social activities. Their interactions reveal no small measures of personal challenges, emotional turmoil, humorous exchanges, endearing actions, and resolute efforts to remain hopeful in the progressive face of terminal cancer.

In just the ways those involved in the phone calls made available their concerns and priorities to one another, they are preserved in the calls for repeated hearings and inspection. Because family members first treated an array of matters as significant *for them*, the chapters herein examine how such activities are achieved interactionally. The time, attention, and detail invested by family members to address emerging and changing cancer circumstances made it possible to pursue a research agenda anchored in ordinary conversational involvements. Whatever efforts I have invested in analyzing these phone conversations, however, simply pale in comparison to how this family (and any family encountering cancer) relies

1

on communication daily when updating news, making decisions, arranging plans, envisioning the future, commiserating, managing conflicts, and caring for one another in often subtle yet remarkable ways.

I once read the following depiction of "balconeers vs. travellers" that speaks directly
to the studies offered in this volume:

> [picture] persons sitting on the high front balcony of a Spanish house watching travellers
> go by on the road below. The "balconeers" can overhear the traveller's talk and chat with
> them; they may comment critically on the way that the travelers walk; or they may dis-
> cuss questions about the road, how it can exist at all or lead anywhere, what might be
> seen from different points along it, and so forth; but they are onlookers, and their prob-
> lems are theoretical only. The travellers, by contrast, face problems which, though they
> have their theoretical angle, are essentially practical—problems of the "which-way-to-
> go" and "how-to-make-it" type, problems which call not merely for comprehension but
> for decision and action too. Balconeers and travelers may think over the same area, yet
> their problems differ. . . . Now this is a book for travellers, and it is with traveller's ques-
> tions that it deals. (Packer, 1973, pp. 5-6)

When studying family members' audio recorded phone calls, it becomes necessary to lay
bare problems encountered by "travellers", not "balconeers". It is "travellers" who face
practical, on-the-road circumstances. Their decisions and actions are tailored to contingent
problems, events requiring solutions that "onlookers" may theoretically envision, yet ultimately fail to grasp and comprehend.

This volume, however, is not designed exclusively for those having experienced cancer
directly, as a cancer patient, or indirectly but consequentially as a family member, friend,
or significant other. Rather, it is about the primal nature of our shared and inevitable journeys through time and illness together: Altogether common, inherently social and thus
interactional events comprising daily living when matters of illness, disease, life, and death
move to the forefront and require our attention. But the materials herein are not limited to
such primordial features of daily existence, that is, living in and with ailing bodies triggering a vast array of ordinary conversations. In addition, analysts of human interaction may
well find the materials herein to be useful as exemplars of particular kinds of interactional
practices, of interest apart from (but not insensitive to) how speakers talk about and
through cancer journeys. In the ways moments herein might compliment the making of
collections, and thus the identification of distinct patterns of human conduct-in-interac-
tion, these data will serve related and important heuristic functions.

The second request made by the family donating these phone calls—that such knowledge might be employed to aid patients, family members, and medical experts to improve
communication throughout cancer journeys—is a mountain requiring an altogether different kind of expedition. It is a laudable goal to rely on emerging findings in order to provide enhanced educational opportunities for cancer patients, family members, and various
medical professionals involved in cancer care. But this goal is only beginning to be realized,
a delay that has been purposeful. A fundamental empirical foundation must first exist if,
and when, grounded curricula might be developed and utilized to make clear the alternatives for communicating in the midst of cancer. Any attempts to shape communication
toward more efficient and effective techniques must arise from a unique blending of
resources: the descriptive identification of patterns comprising interaction, personal experience, medical expertise, and a model for designing, facilitating, and implementing innovative educational programs for diverse individuals, families, and provider teams involved
throughout cancer journeys. These possibilities are overviewed in the final chapter of this
volume.

At the outset, it must also be emphasized that whatever insights and findings might eventually emerge from this investigation and however they might be adapted in the future for educational and training purposes, are made possible because of one family's courageous efforts. Without the son's recording efforts, and the family's willingness to allow for such undertakings following mom's death, it would not be possible to even initiate this tip-of-the-iceberg investigation.

BACKGROUND FOR THE STUDY: AN UNMOTIVATED AND INAUSPICIOUS BEGINNING

The following chapters represent a culmination of a decade of research on how ordinary phone interactions are primary resources for navigating through social, emotional, technical, and biomedical concerns associated with cancer. This extended research project, however, had an entirely unmotivated and inauspicious beginning. When I received these recordings in the early 1990s, it was by no means a result of strategic planning and efforts to carefully design and enact a long-term research protocol. Rather, the materials came my way unexpected and without fanfare. The son, representing the family, simply provided me with a box of audio recordings. It was the family's request that I delay working on the interactions "for a few years" and then, if I pursued them for research and educational purposes, guarantee the family anonymity. It turned out that their request to "delay" was not a problem. It was some five years later before I produced even an initial transcription of the two-minute opening of just the first phone call (between dad and son, analyzed in Chapter 3). In retrospect, I became intrigued when using this excerpt for very preliminary listening and data sessions with students. Even though I did have a rough sense of the contents and trajectory of this phone call corpus, I had not listened systematically to anything more than portions of the first call. Apparently, I lacked any particular interest in or motivation to pursue the full range of these materials, especially at the expense of other research involvements. The remainder of the recordings were simply put aside in favor of other (and competing) research interests emerging at that time, including a related project published in 1996 as *Conversations about Illness: Family Preoccupations with Bulimia*. In my final chapter for that book, addressing future implications for studying interaction and social problems, I wrote an initial preview of how it might become possible to begin investigating "the routine nature of making sense of, and dealing with "problems" associated with, terminal cancer" (p. 110). For the first time, I attempted to describe some of the basic observations drawn from what I referred to as the "Malignancy" phone calls:

> Certain kinds of "problems" have arisen, including: how the original malignancy diagnosis was delivered by the father and receipted as "news" by the son; how this "news" was both passed on to others and continually updated and revised; and how "bad news" gave rise to a preference for "good news" as the illness progressed. And there are other emergent features to consider when conversations about illness are examined . . . inherent difficulties with describing and understanding complex medical terminology, and in so doing constructing versions of what doctors have told participants about the illness and, relatedly, lay versions of how and why doctors and medical staff are proceeding with treatments; the curious interplay between biomedical descriptions of an illness (e.g., talking about body parts such as "adrenal gland" and "tumors") and emotions displayed about the illness process (e.g., frustrations in having to wait for "results" or "tests", having little or no control over processes you don't really understand); and ways in which commiseration, comfort, confusion, or anger are initially worked through and are, in these ways, made available for repeated inspection as sequentially organized achievements. (p. 110)

A Chance Occurrence?

In 1998 I received a long-distance phone call from my mother (in Iowa). She informed me that she had been diagnosed with lung cancer. During the next several months I was involved in many calls with family members, doctors, and friends. Attempts were made to understand the nature of my mom's diagnosis, her prescribed medications and treatments, and of course if her prognosis was terminal (and if so, just how long she might have to live). Considerable time was also invested talking about how mom and other family members were coping and feeling, how we could best work as a team to manage mom's progressive illness, and how to coordinate other practical matters such as finances, travel plans, and caregiving visits. In a very short period of time, these topics and concerns became altogether normal features of our daily social and family lives.

Over time, and during many of these calls, it did not go unnoticed that I was now a son (sibling and friend) in the midst of my/our own cancer journey. No longer a communication researcher who had the option and privilege to study one set of materials or the next, I was relying heavily on phone calls to update, assess, and simply deal with the apparent inevitability of my own mother's failing health. Being intimately involved in a family cancer journey was not my/our choice. But communication about cancer quickly became my/our preoccupation, immediately following mom's diagnosis.

At the same time I realized that as life moved forward, the world did not come to a halt simply because we were facing cancer together as a family. It became clear (at least to me) that it was perhaps not a coincidence that another family, who had earlier donated what I had come to refer to as "those family cancer calls", had also navigated their way through cancer. As each day and week passed I began to more fully realize that, and how, all cancer patients and family members must get caught up in what became routine, often uncertain, and at times delicate telephone conversations about "cancer". In some unknown ways, and for reasons we could not fully understand, cancer had found its way into the life of my/our family. And *somehow* we were getting through it . . . managing . . . just. But *how* so?

My mom died only four months following her initial diagnosis. Only months later, I applied for and received a grant from the American Cancer Society (ACS: #ROG-98-172-01) to generate full (anonymous) transcriptions from the 61 donated calls,[2] initiate an extended literature review on communication, families, and cancer, and to produce initial manuscripts identifying communication activities involved in how family members talk about, and through, cancer on the telephone. Not surprisingly, materials I had basically ignored for years were now heard and understood to be extremely rich and timely "data"!

Repeated listening and data sessions were (and remain) entirely engrossing. As my research proceeded by reading hundreds of scholarly papers and speaking initially with dozens (and now hundreds) of cancer and health experts, it became clear that these family cancer recordings represented the *first natural history* of a family talking through cancer on the telephone. Materials of this kind were nowhere to be found in the published social and medical sciences. Although other recorded collections may exist elsewhere, such as those possibly gathered and "owned" by particular families and their members, I remain unaware of such materials.

The Phone Calls

In a written reflection, ten years following his mother's death, the son reflects on calling his dad on the phone and being informed, for the first time, that "mother had cancer":

> My father answered. I remembered thinking almost immediately that something seemed wrong. Then he told me that my mother had cancer. . . .When the call ended, my mind was reeling. . . . I looked around the room for something to focus on. My eyes fell on the recorder. I realized it had been on the whole time. . . . I decided to leave the recording device on that telephone, and there it stayed until my mother died. (1997)

The description "something seemed wrong" recalls a hint of trouble at the outset of the call, and "my mind was reeling" begins to reveal the impact of having heard and attempted to assimilate such bad news following the call's completion. Equally striking are the son's realization that the initial conversation had unknowingly been recorded, and his decision to continue recording phone conversations "until my mother died".

A similar "reeling" experience was reported by Byock:

> I was the first person to know that my father was dying. I realized it during a phone call eighteen months before he would die. . . . My mind was reeling. I leaned against the dresser in our bedroom, the phone to my ear, my forehead in my hand. He was dying. (1997, pp. 1-2)

In neither of the two phone calls described above, involving sons talking with their dad/father, do the sons write that they were *explicitly* informed that their loved ones were "dying". Rather, in the first instance the son reports being staggered by news about his mother's cancer diagnosis (which, it turns out, was described by dad in Call #1 as being located in several parts of mom's body, a serious diagnosis confirmed and elaborated by mom in Call #2). And in the second description above, the son (a physician) reports his ability to draw conclusions from his father's listing of symptoms to surmise that the disease was terminal. Only in retrospect can it now be determined that son's mom died *13 months* following a formal cancer diagnosis (see Timeline in Chapter 2), and in the second case that son's father would live another *18 months* before his life would end. Each reporting and realization of problems occurred at the *outset* of extended illness journeys, leading in each instance to death.

But what happens *between* diagnosis and death? The details of even these initial phone calls are not accessible through sons' written reflections. Nor are the subsequent, and no doubt frequent and varied phone calls between family members, addressed through their writing. In contrast, the "Malignancy" phone calls allow access to interactional details that written reflections (nor reported memories, as in Chapter 15) cannot capture. Recordings make available how family members enact an amazing array of social activities, collaborations tailored to and reflecting the natural emergence of events triggered by a serious disease. The phone calls also allow for an exploration of family life, often assumed to be known yet taken-for-granted, and therefore an opportunity to ground traditional conceptions of health and illness as inherently social, communicative problems in contemporary society.

Though these are lofty priorities, one way to frame the work in this volume is to understand that no matter how detailed the following analyses might be, they are only a preliminary attempt to make some headway toward understanding the complexities of routine family life, especially (but by no means exclusively) surrounding cancer as an illness.

Preview of the Chapters

The volume begins with an overview of what is known and methodological alternatives for advancing understandings about communication, interaction, and family cancer. In

Chapter 1, an extensive literature review reveals that because the impacts of cancer extend well beyond patients' experiences, primary importance needs to be given to the critical roles of communication throughout "family cancer journeys". Yet the predominant empirical focus has been on individuals' reported experiences, not on actual real-time communication events. The omnipresence of talk-in-interaction thus remains, essentially, an unexplored area of cancer, health, and illness.

As research on family members' conversations is in its infancy, Chapter 2 proposes that Conversation Analysis (CA) is a viable methodological alternative for closely examining how speakers achieve social interaction. Throughout the volume, the analysis of single moments is complemented with collections of similar kinds of activities. Because the "Malignancy" corpus is comprised of a series of phone calls occurring over a period of 13 months, contrasts are offered between "episodic" and "longitudinal" approaches to data analysis. These calls provide rare opportunities to understand the sustained and managed relevance of multiple interactions, within and across phone calls, as family members navigate their ways through events over time. In order to provide readers with a grounded chronology of activities, the chapter concludes with a time-line of the 61 phone calls and a discussion of how these recordings are unique when compared with other *natural history* investigations.

Data analysis begins with case studies of Calls #1 and #2 when, as noted previously, initial conversations about mom's diagnosis occur between dad-son and mom-son. In Chapter 3, it is shown that as news deliverer, dad exhibits and claims knowledge that son does not possess. An extended phone opening reveals delay and resistance to announcing and receiving "bad news" directly. So doing allows dad and son the opportunity to forecast and anticipate the "valence" of news before it has been articulated. Also apparent were biomedical and stoic orientations to mom's dilemma. In the ways personal and emotional reactions by dad and son were initially minimized (even though they gradually became more apparent as Call #1 unfolded), additional evidence is provided that stoic demeanors are normalized resources for managing and coping with the onset of dreaded news events.

In Chapter 4, a series of excerpts are examined from Call #2 as son speaks with mom, the morning following Call #1 with dad, about her cancer diagnosis. At the outset of the call mom forecasts her troubled health condition and, throughout, is shown to enact the voice of a "wounded body". Speaking as a cancer patient, she offers blunt and authoritative descriptions about the extremity of her "verdict". These orientations create problems not only for son's response, but eventually for mom and son not knowing what or how to respond to such "bad news". In the midst of these difficult moments, mom demonstrates the right and ability to "know" about her experiences and condition in ways that son, as news-recipient and non-cancer patient, can only "guess". Noticeable shifts occur between "despair" and "hope", and each apologizes to the other for having to deal with uncertain and dreaded cancer circumstances that they did not ask for, but must inevitably deal with.

How do family members interactionally manage their lives during periods of uncertainty and potential crisis? Chapters 5-7 address this question in three related ways. First, Chapter 5 begins with how son's discussions with mom and dad result in a decision to travel home before mom dies. Repeated calls to different airlines are examined to discover how son "makes his case" for receiving discounted "compassion" fares to be with his family. These calls with airline representatives are shown to be highly organized. Across a series of calls, son's "problem narratives" become streamlined as deliberate efforts are enacted (though unsuccessfully) to received discounted fares. At times, son also pursues special understandings from call-takers who, in turn, withhold providing the compassion son was pursuing. These encounters make clear that talking with strangers, such as bureaucratic representatives, is normal but trying business when life and death converge in daily life.

In Chapter 6, excerpts from four calls within two days (#11-12 and #17-18) evidence how problems with travel and scheduling continue following son's calls to the airlines.

Each set of moments is intertwined with inherent ambiguities associated with mom's changing health status: Is mom dying and if so, when? Has her condition stabilized? Should son's travel home occur immediately or in the near future—and (again) when might that be? Living in flux with mom's volatile cancer is shown to be uncertain and frustrating for family members in the face of changing news across calls. Family members must rely on their own lay diagnoses about cancer, while also orienting to a possible future they neither fully understand nor control. Once again, however, these ambiguities are balanced with glimpses of hope that mom may soon be able to come home from the hospital.

Among other important features, Calls #3-18 are marked by a *state of readiness*. In Chapter 7, family members are shown to work together to maintain emergency preparedness and a chronic sense of urgency tied to mom's imminent yet unpredictable death. One primary resource for organizing these interactions are *figurative expressions* (or *figures of speech*), including repeated references to activities such as *keeping one's bags packed*, *lesson plans current*, *lists up to date*, and *staying by the phone*. Twenty-six of these expressions are analyzed to reveal the interactional work involved in achieving social actions such as readiness, resolve, and references to cancer impacts. This collection of moments unequivocally supports prior research on sequential environments involving topical transition and closure, but also extends understandings of speakers' diverse methods for organizing moments involving disagreement, disaffiliation, and lack of alignment.

The "Malignancy" corpus is fraught with activities in which family members report on and assess medical care. Doctors' opinions, strategies for treatment, and hopes for the future are shown to be critically important as family members seek to understand mom's condition. How do family members describe medical experts' explanations of biomedical procedures? In Chapter 8, a collection of their commonsense (lay) versions of doctors' reportings (and others' summaries of what doctors told them) are examined. Specific features of their "lay" status are identified, including searching and producing dysfluencies prior to stating biomedical terms (e.g., "needle biopsy results"), and glossing key details (e.g., "the thyroid *stuff*"). When referencing nonpresent and often anonymous persons (e.g., with "they" and "the doctor"), family members also subordinate themselves to doctors' authority. Yet, in turn, they reenact doctors' authoritative stance when updating others (e.g., as serious and unemotional). Indeed, speakers exhibited being more knowledgeable when reporting what doctors told them than when offering their own opinions about events surrounding mom's care.

At times family members produce positive and negative assessments about care provided by both doctors and hospitals, supporting and displaying frustration with those responsible for mom's care. Chapter 9 focuses on the interactions comprising these assessments, including praises and complaints about doctors, medical staff, and provided care. Central to this chapter are not only how and why family members critique and praise medical experts, but how speakers invoke primary knowledge as a basis for their assessments. Matters of *social epistemics*—or claiming superior rights to assess, know, defend, take responsibility for, and act upon circumstances—have been repeatedly addressed in prior chapters (particularly 3 & 4). These moments are often delicately constructed, because family members are vying to determine who has the right to act authoritatively on matters relevant to mom's cancer care. Almost ironically, ensuring the best quality care for mom requires close attention to interactional matters such as agreeing and disagreeing about key decisions. By advancing and defending positions anchored in contrasting knowledge and opinions about mom's health, family members work their way through practical circumstances in the course of caring for mom.

The next four chapters (10–13) address a variety of *enduring* and *endearing* interactions across the phone call corpus. Chapter 10 extends the ongoing discussion of "social epistemics" threaded throughout this volume. An examination is offered of how family members rely on few words, and have little else to say, about being entangled within perplexing cancer circumstances (e.g., "pt Sh:i:t. hh…Yeah $I know.$"). These brief but complex and significant social actions occur within particular sequential environments: Following the delivery and reception of news, and elaboration, as speakers work toward closing down difficult topics—about which there is much to say, but few words are needed or available to express individual and shared experiences. These exchanges demonstrate *shared commiserative space* as speakers exhibit understanding, identification with, and appreciation for what each other is experiencing: being in, and affected by, the realities of cancer they are constructing together. However, during such joint commiseration, family members also stake out territory involving (a) who knows and experiences what, and more, about cancer experiences, and (b) who is consequently in a primary position to report on, and best care for, mom and other family members. Family members are shown to move in and out of these commiserative yet territorial moments, topic transitions recurrently marked by shifts to "hopeful, bright side" sequences. These shifts counter (at least for the moment) cancer-related and (possible) relational difficulties inherent to negotiating rights and claims for action.

Family members tell and retell a number of stories as mom's cancer progresses. Chapter 11 analyzes the interactional organization of stories-in-a-series involving "cigarettes", "devastation", and "mom's hair". The complexities of these activities are revealed when considering the breadth and depth of examined social actions: Exhibiting entitlements to report on experiences; reported speech and action (i.e., taking on the voice and evaluating another's actions); venting frustration; inviting and declining potentially derogatory collaborations; avoiding conflicts about, and building, family alliances; during retellings, deleting and embellishing another's prior telling; the moral contamination of "gossip"; how potentially serious topics get transformed into humorous and playful collaborations; ways that residing together, in imaginary and fleeting worlds, offer a respite to what repeatedly becomes the next business-at-hand—returning to talk about the practical tasks and stark realities associated with mom's dying.

When overviewing prior chapters, references have been made to "hope", or "being hopeful", as though speakers have resources allowing them to counter despair and better cope with the seemingly countless challenges of cancer. Indeed they do. The next two chapters address hope (and optimism), not only as what people experience individually but as recognizable, social activities people collaborate in producing through interaction. Chapter 12 provides a review of secular, spiritual, and social scientific conceptions of hope to clarify how, and what, people have put their faith in that allows them to be hopeful (or not). Seven initial instances are previewed, from Calls #1 & #2, to exemplify that managing hope (and optimism) is a practical matter for family members while working through troubling illness circumstances. Before providing a more extended analysis (in Chapter 13), however, an "experiment" on hope is offered by first examining basic, traditional secular and spiritual conceptions of hope in society. A description of social scientific research efforts (both quantitative and qualitative) is also offered, studies that have been designed to reveal whether (or not) hope makes a practical difference in persons' daily lives (and if so, how). A comparison of these diverse perspectives provides a clear distinction between secular, spiritual, and social scientific orientations to hope, and alternatively, how hope might begin to be understood as interactional achievements.

In the following Chapter 13, the initially identified seven instances in Calls #1 & #2 are analyzed in more detail. From a collection of nearly 50 additional moments identified throughout the Malignancy corpus, a sampling of 25 instances are selected. The case is advanced that family members' "hopeful" orientations are frequently employed, and thus critical resources, for coping with mom's ongoing cancer problems. Activities such as buffering impacts on the family, warding off depression and despair, edifying one another, and co-constructing joy—even in the midst of displayed anguish, anxiety, and suffering—are primal aspects of this family's journey through cancer. In practical and interactionally distinct ways, family members demonstrate that there are indeed delicate relationships between "hope" and a host of activities: Ongoing uncertainty, shifts from bad to good news, choice, reasons to "keep fighting" and "fight the battle together", and emphasizing a positive future. A summary of explicit and implicit references to hope and hopeful possibilities is provided to characterize the interactional work involved when addressing burdens arising from the often harsh and restrictive impositions of illness. As life moves forward in times of crisis, routine worldly problems arise in which various secular, spiritual, and social scientific conceptions of hope get implemented and shaped into social action.

This volume closes with two final chapters. In Chapter 14, an epilogue is provided addressing how previous chapters reframe what is known and understood about family cancer journeys. Implications for future research on ordinary conversations and family cancer interactions are described, as are possibilities for adapting this research for innovative educational programs.

And finally, in Chapter 15, a retrospective interview with the son, dad, and aunt—18 years following mom's diagnosis—is provided. This interview reveals family members' reflections on critical issues across a wide range of topics such as: alternative styles and challenges for coping with the diagnosis, treatment, and prognosis of terminal cancer; the fallacy of "control"; managing the "roller-coaster" of cancer; reflections about particular phone calls; the importance of play and humor; and survivors' advice for others experiencing cancer (and related health issues). These discussions reveal important perspectives on family members' experiences. And though not utilized herein to reveal marked contrasts between information retrievable from interviews and empirical findings that can only be generated from close analysis of recorded and transcribed conversations, implications for such differences and similarities are apparent.

BELUGA WHALES IN HUMAN FORM

Recently, while watching a program on *The Travel Channel* entitled *Alaska's Arctic Wildlife*, the narrator commented that "The social structure of the Beluga whale is little understood. It is only now beginning to be studied". Equally unexplored is the social organization of how family members talk about and through cancer (and indeed, all illnesses). The communicative consequences of cancer diagnosis, treatment, and prognosis are obviously enormous yet little understood as interactional achievements.

We are like Beluga whales in human form, a known but minimally understood social species.

I am continually reminded of this kinship when visiting San Diego's SeaWorld with my two children. As our faces get pressed onto massive water-filled tanks, inhabited and navigated so effortlessly by Belugas and other mammals, thoughts are drawn into a mysterious and puzzling underwater world: Why do these aqua environments somehow appear normal and coherent, despite our inability to fully recognize how and why these beautiful creatures think, feel, communicate, and simply do what they do together every day?

Human illness journeys are also routinely familiar and thus highly patterned. Yet the moments we collaborate in producing are only vaguely transparent. The family recordings examined herein are rare yet critically important—extraordinary yet mundane and routine, foreign yet strikingly familiar to all who have encountered them. Though only a single family's conversations are studied in this volume, these are universal circumstances and therefore primal exemplars of the human social condition. It is clear that families confronting cancer are constantly involved in seeking interactional solutions to medical problems. But, again, *how* so?

It has been my good fortune to work with this collection of phone calls, an experience similar to harvesting grain from remarkably fertile fields that I did not plant. In the ways this volume provides an empirical and theoretical foundation for understanding these common yet opaque social activities, progress will have been made to clarify the murky waters of how family members rely on communication when journeying through illness together. This study is only a partial down payment on a project of mammoth proportions: Gaining an enhanced appreciation for human interaction as the primary social resource for managing the trials, tribulations, hopes and triumphs of cancer.

NOTES

1. This basic description was utilized in a recent theatrical production focusing on how family members talk through cancer on the telephone. This production was based on actual dialogue of family members in the "Malignancy" phone call series. Implications for this and related work are addressed in Chapter 14.
2. Prior to my application, The American Cancer Society (ACS) had not funded such a research opportunity—that is, to investigate how family members' conversations about cancer on the telephone—in part because they were not aware that (a) such materials existed, and (b) if so, they could be systematically and rigorously investigated. When these possibilities were confirmed by reviewers, the grant was awarded and the investigation moved forward.

I

COMMUNICATION, INTERACTION, AND FAMILY CANCER

1

COMMUNICATION AND FAMILY CANCER JOURNEYS

It is widely recognized that cancer is the most ubiquitous deadly disease in the world today and the second leading cause of death in America (American Cancer Society, 2006; Kumar & Clark, 1990). Three out of four families in the Western world are somehow impacted (Siegel, Sales, & Schulz, 1991; Lichtman & Taylor, 1986), just as three quarters of American families are at some time affected by cancer (Bloom, 2000). The American Cancer Society (2006) estimates that nearly 1.4 million Americans will be diagnosed with cancer this year alone, resulting in more than one-half million deaths. Men have an approximate 50% and women a 33% lifetime risk of being diagnosed with cancer, and greater than 50% of all cancer patients cannot be cured (MacDonald, 1996). If rates of incidence remain stable, the total number of cancer cases is expected to double by 2050 (Edwards et al., 2002).

These are striking and humbling statistics. Each year, in San Diego County alone (a population of 3 million), approximately 11,600 persons are diagnosed with cancer—an average of 31 daily "malignant" diagnoses. In the state of California (a population of 36 million) the 2007 cancer statistics reveal approximately 133,000 new cancer diagnoses, an average of 15 new cases every hour, every day (see http://www.ccrcal.org/PDF/ACS2007.pdf). And Californians are not more likely to be diagnosed with cancer than other Americans.

The critical importance of communication for managing cancer diagnosis, treatment, and care is indisputable. When considering only San Diego and regional California areas as case studies, how many phone calls and face-to-face interactions (in home, work, and clinical environments) occurred in which talk about cancer occurred before, and following, the receipt of news about "benign" or "malignant" biopsy results? Every month, how many thousands of additional patients receive "benign" news about biopsies taken because cancer may have been suspected, but not confirmed? How many additional phone calls get initiated following "positive" diagnoses, throughout indefinite periods of time, as patients' cancer gets treated and enters remission (or not)? The sheer mass of these calls in San Diego and California, let alone the nation and world, makes patently clear that although the family interactions studied herein are distinctive and certainly *one of a kind*, they represent an incalculable number of daily conversations focused upon describing, explaining, and keeping others informed about the impacts of cancer on health and well being.

A vast number of encounters also occur with medical experts, bureaucratic and institutional representatives, during clinical interviews and consultations (e.g., see Beach, 2009; Heritage & Maynard, 2006). The phone calls examined herein, however, reveal that family members are narrators of their own experiences and observations about cancer diagnosis, treatment, and quality of living. Although family members function as conduits for what doctors have informed them, they also invest considerable time attempting to make sense of technical matters and simply cope with inherently uncertain, often foreign and complex details about something called "cancer". But how do family members work together and rely on one another when navigating their way through cancer journeys?

COMMUNICATION AS CENTRAL FOR CANCER CARE?

This chapter summarizes an extensive review of "communication" within a vast body of literature comprising a field of inquiry commonly referred to as "psychosocial oncology". At the outset, several primary and related conclusions can be drawn and summarized as follows:

- Understanding how families communicate about and talk through cancer is an omnipresent, yet generally unexplored, area of health and illness.
- There exists a *noticeable absence* of interactional research focusing on communicative activities throughout cancer journeys.
- A basic inconsistency is noted: As communication processes are increasingly theorized as central to psycho-oncological research, empirical verification of interactional patterns is limited. Grounded knowledge about how participants rely on communication to organize cancer-related care and treatment is thus underspecified.

With few exceptions (e.g., see Beach, Easter, Good, & Pigeron, 2004; Lutfey & Maynard, 1998; Maynard & Frankel, 2006), grounded understandings of the interactional organization of social activities associated with cancer are not available within the social and medical sciences. Cumulative knowledge about communication and cancer-related incidents is theoretically rich, but empirically underdeveloped: Little is known about how cancer patients, family members, and health professionals organize their interactions when talking through a host of illness predicaments. Although it has been repeatedly noted that a cancer diagnosis significantly alters social relationships (Gotcher, 1993; Freeman, 1996; Kristjanson & Ashcroft, 1994; Maynard, 1996, 1997, 2003; *USA Today*, 1994), research on how families actually interact throughout cancer diagnosis, treatment, coping, and care is in its infancy.

Related studies focusing on communication and illness reveal similar findings (see Babrow & Kline, 2000; Babrow, Hines, & Kasch, 2000). In Beach's (1996) examination of how family members talk through problems with *bulimia*, for example, a review of nearly 300 research studies revealed that although *family communication* was the single best predictor of eating disorders and caregiving problems, "not a single study was found that directly examined interactions between either family members expressing bulimic concerns or grandparent-grandchildren conversations on any set of health-care topics". (p. 19). Similar conclusions are drawn by Lutfey and Maynard (1998) in their analysis of how a physician delivers bad news in an oncology setting: Prior research on illness, death, and dying "emphasizes abstract, internal experiences of individuals who confront mortal or chronic illness . . . typifications and generalizations" (p. 1) that essentially overlook how illness is communicatively managed.

Moving Away from Patient's Isolated Experiences?

Although a general research trend promotes the critical importance of communication in cancer care, and thus a movement away from cancer as "an isolated experience of the patient" (Baider, Cooper, & De-Nour, 1986, p. xvii; Veach, Nicholas, & Barton, 2002; Naber, Halstead, Broome, & Rehwalt, 1995), there exists a predominant focus on individuals' experiences accessed through self-report and anecdotal data in psycho-oncological investigations. By utilizing survey research methods, questionnaires, interviews, and direct observation (reconstructed through note-taking and diaries) rich insights are offered about individuals' perceptions of, and reported experiences about, relationships and coping mechanisms.

Extant research on communication and cancer thus reveals a proclivity of theoretical explanations generated from empirical data grounded in individuals' self-reports. Valuable as individuals' self-reports about cancer journeys might be, however, they provide only indirect and general assessments of omnipresent interactional engagements. Questions remain, therefore, as to whether and how perceptual orientations adequately capture family members' procedures for co-authoring and socially constructing versions of cancer events over time. Self-report data should not be treated as synonymous with "real time" examinations of actual communication events: observations anchored in audio recordings of telephone calls, and/or video recordings of face-to-face interactions, in unison with carefully produced transcriptions facilitating close analysis of communication activities comprising cancer journeys. What individuals say about communication often stands in marked contrast to how interactions reported on actually get *done*, in part because self-reports offer only general depictions of detailed and contingently organized interactional involvements (Atkinson & Heritage, 1984).

Increasing Attention Given to Communication and Cancer

In contrast to considerable attention given to examining phone conversations for organizing and making sense of everyday life activities and events (see, e.g., Hopper, 1992; Schegloff 1968, 1986), it is notable that phone calls per se have not been utilized for closely inspecting diverse and complex interactions addressing cancer. Yet historically and with increasing regularity, more general concerns with *communication* have emerged as primary concerns for researchers focusing on cancer diagnosis, treatment, coping and care (e.g., see Kreps & Kunimoto, 1994; O'Hair, Kreps, & Sparks, 2007). And for good reason:

- Family members who communicate psychosocial support promote enduring family relationships, function as more effective caregivers, and experience less stress (Leiber, Plumb, Gerstenzang, & Holland, 1976; Litman, 1974; Rose, 1990; Rowland, 1990a, 1990b).
- Open, honest, and frequent communication is essential for ensuring that patients' and family members' wishes are heard and attended to when facilitating decision making regarding care options (Bloom, 1996; Hilton, 1994; Keller, Henrich, Sellschopp, & Beutel, 1996; Northouse & Northouse, 1987; Stevenson, 1985).
- Communication is directly associated with quality of care and life in terminal cancer (Engle, Fox-Hill, & Graney, 1998; Gotcher, 1993; Heusinkveld, 1972; Shields, 1984).
- Throughout uncertain and often troubling cancer journeys, a vast amount of time and effort is invested by cancer patients, family members, and health professionals as they attempt to manage understandings, relationships, and healing outcomes (e.g., see Benjamin, 1987; Bloom, 1996; Dunkel-Schetter & Wortman, 1982; Hilton, 1994; Keller et al., 1996; Kristjanson & Ashcroft, 1994; Northouse & Northouse, 1987; Zerwekh, 1984).

The primacy of communication has been evident for at least 20 years, when cancer became associated with various "interpersonal dynamics" contributing to dysfunctional communication barriers in social relationships (Dunkel-Schetter & Wortman, 1982)— including the family, which "constitutes perhaps the most important social context within which illness occurs" (Litman, 1974, p. 495). Because "the family must somehow endure" (Rait & Lederberg, 1990, p. 586) throughout changes and problems associated with cancer, communication is perhaps best understood as fundamental for quality of life and survival of the family unit. Diverse research has targeted basic needs for:

- Clinicians and caregivers to assist in facilitating and improving communication between patients and family members (Epstein & Street, 2007; Glimeus, Birgegard, Hoffman & Kvale, 1995; Lewis, Pearson, Corcoran-Perry, & Narayan, 1997; Skorupka & Bohnet, 1982).
- Providing advice to practitioners on how to better communicate with cancer patients and their families (see Bennett & Alison, 1995; Bertolone & Scott, 1990; Cournos, 1990; Epstein & Street, 2007; Foley, 1993; Lomax, 1997; Pace, 1993; Parle, Maguire, & Heaven, 1997; Rittenberg, 1996; Sullivan, 1990; Weissman, 1997; Westman, Lewandowski, & Procter 1993).
- Utilizing support groups as a forum for sharing experiences (Epstein & Street, 2007; McGuire & Kantor, 1987; Mulcahey & Young, 1995).

Taken together, these targeted areas testify to the broad importance of enhancing communication between individuals whose lives have somehow been impacted by cancer.

Yet surprisingly little knowledge has been generated about *how* cancer patients, family members, and health professionals actually talk through diverse illness predicaments — including distinctive patterns through which communication troubles arise, get resolved, and/or perpetuated. For example, no studies were reviewed that carefully examine how families *interactionally* accomplish such work as "open and frequent communication", "supporting" (but see Pistrang, Barker, & Rutter, 1997), or "coping". An empirical foundation for understanding ordinary social, and thus communicative activities of cancer journeys, remains to be constructed.

This chapter is organized into three sections. First, a more detailed discussion is offered of *how* communication has been identified as central to family relationships, yet accessed through individuals' reportings. Specific examples, drawn from both qualitative and quantitative research methods, are provided to illustrate the predominance and limitations of self-reports for studying communication and psychosocial oncology. Second, an overview is provided of how communication has been directly investigated in related medical encounters and family interactions. Primary attention given to provider-patient interactions makes clear the need to also understand how family members work through illness journeys. Finally, the potential for converging communication research on ordinary interactions, with alternative approaches to psychosocial oncology, is addressed.

PREDOMINANCE AND LIMITATIONS
OF SELF-REPORTS IN PSYCHOSOCIAL ONCOLOGY

Communication among cancer patients, family members, and health professionals is enormously important for cancer patients and caregivers' lives. A comprehensive review of the *Journal of Psychosocial Oncology* revealed that attention has been given to an array of topics critical to communication—coping and adjustment before and after a parent's death (Mireault & Compas, 1996), social support from family, friends, and health professionals

(Ma, 1996; Wortman & Dunkel-Schetter, 1979), quality of life (Fuller & Swensen, 1992; Yancik, Edwards, & Yates, 1989), overcoming the challenges of long-term illness (Benjamin, 1987), facilitating hopefulness (Bunston, Mings, Mackie, & Jones, 1995), and the need for qualitative methods (Waxler-Morrison, Doll, & Hislop, 1995). Across these articles, and a broader review of psycho-oncological studies discussed below, the vast majority of investigations are rooted in "reported", "perceived", and/or "experienced" information when generating observations about communication events.

Cancer, Communication, and Family Relationships

Diverse psychosocial reviews of cancer and families (Blanchard, Ruckdeschel, & Albrecht, 1996; Crosson, 1998; Heath, 1996a, 1996b) confirm the long-standing and unequivocal importance attributed to "communication" and "relationships" (see Blitzer et al., 1990; Butow et al., 1996; Chesler & Barbarin, 1987; Conrad, 1987; Eden, Black, & Emery, 1993; Finlay, Stott, & Kinnersley, 1995; Foley, 1993; Friedenbergs et al., 1982; Friedman & DiMatteo, 1982; Keitel, Cramer, & Zevon, 1990; Lichter, 1987; Montazeri, Milroy, Gillis, & McEwen, 1996; Mulcahey & Young, 1995; Northouse & Northouse, 1987; Pace, 1993; Paternoster, 1990; Ptacek & Eberhardt, 1996; Rittenberg, 1996; Scherz, Edwards, & Kallail, 1995; Stuber, 1995; Watson, 1994; Wortman & Dunkel-Schetter, 1979). Understanding comprehensive psychosocial support for cancer and the improvement of "quality of life" requires careful attention to communication (Razavi & Delvaux, 1995). Even when "communication" is not specifically mentioned, social support, relationships, and social networks are hailed as essential and beneficial to patients coping with cancer (see Bloom, Kang, & Romano, 1991; Creagan, 1993; Davis, 1963; Kutner, 1987; Lyons & Meade, 1995).

Across these and related communication studies, numerous and important findings have been repeatedly observed and verified.

Open and frequent communication between patients and their families, when working through the anguish and uncertainty of cancer (Bloom, 1996; Hilton, 1994; Keller et al., 1996; Northouse & Northouse, 1987) and when communicating about illness within the family, has been associated with "positive rehabilitation outcomes" (Mesters et al., 1997, p. 269). Although families may be expected to feel comfortable when discussing cancer, enacting "normal" conversations and interactions with the patient (Benjamin, 1987), much of the literature suggests that cancer leads to difficult and inconsistent patterns of communication (Dunkel-Schetter & Wortman, 1982).

It is curious, but not surprising, that open and frequent communication regarding cancer has been described as rare among family members (Gotcher, 1995; Heinrich, Schag, & Ganz, 1984). Because cancer is often viewed as an intruder in the family (Farrow, Cash, & Simmons, 1990), families are confronted with numerous dilemmas throughout their cancer experiences (Fitzgerald, 1994; Fitzsimmons, 1994; Seaburn, Lorenz, Campbell, & Winfield, 1996). Indeed, the discussion of unpleasant cancer issues may disrupt and violate traditional communication patterns (Gotcher, 1995), what Maynard (1996, 1997, 2003) has described as a "rupture" of everyday experience. Problems in communication routinely arise as families learn to cope with their evolving cancer situations (Hinds, 1992; Lichter, 1987). For example, over time family members may experience difficulty determining their "job" within the family system, simply because cancer arises from unknown origins and possesses an uncertain future (Comaroff & Maguire, 1986; Karp, 1992; Stewart & Sullivan, 1982).

Perhaps one of the most difficult and ongoing tasks, especially in cases involving terminal cancer diagnoses, is the routine management of interpersonal relationships (Calman, 1987; *USA Today*, 1994). A major stressor for patients is "altered interpersonal relationships" (Rowland, 1990a, p. 26), and the majority of cancer patients report moderate to severe problems in family relationships (Dunkel-Schetter & Wortman, 1982; Gotay, 1984;

Heinrich et al., 1984; Rowland, 1990b). It has repeatedly been argued that interpersonal problems affect the quality of life of both patients and family caregivers (Leiber et al., 1976; Rowland, 1990a, 1990b).

Interpersonal crises are normal as cancer patients and loved ones cope with the disruptive nature of cancer. Family caregivers play a vital role in terminal patients' social lives, functioning as mediators between the patient and the outside world. In Addington-Hall and McCarthy's (1995) study of over 2,000 terminal cancer patients, more than 80% of the primary caregivers were family members. Three additional and significant findings support continued focus on patient-family communication: (a) Terminal cancer patients communicate predominantly with family caregivers (rather than others) about their physical and emotional condition (Hinton, 1998); (b) Patient-family communication predicts patient level of adjustment to cancer (Gotcher, 1993); and (c) The family "tends to be involved in the decision-making and therapeutic process at every stage of a member's illness" (Litman, 1974, p. 501).

In a related review of 200 research articles focusing on the family's "journey" through cancer, Kristjanson and Ashcroft (1994) identified four themes emerging from the literature: (a) *Developmental stage of the family*—problems and concerns faced by families, taking into account the ages and relationships of the patient and family members; (b) *Cancer illness trajectory*—family's experience over time as the illness progresses, characterized by preventive, diagnostic, acute care, remission, rehabilitation and possible recurrence and terminal stages; (c) *Family responses to cancer*—family's needs, demands, role changes, communication, and health; and (d) *Health-care provider behaviors*—helpful/caring behaviors involving health-care provider communication with families. Throughout Kristjanson and Ashcroft's (1994) exhaustive review, complex roles of "communication"—both within the family and with health professionals—are repeatedly characterized as a central factor in the family process (e.g., in providing social support). However, as previewed at the outset of this chapter, access to communication patterns and coping mechanisms are gained through interviews, questionnaires/surveys, and theoretical speculation; individuals' self-reported experiences have been emphasized to generate insights about communication and relationships.

This emphasis on self-report data can be contrasted with Gubrium and Holstein's (1990) observation that constructing and maintaining a family is inherently a social, interactional process: Families derive their distinctive character not from a setting or societal label, but through the interactional achievement of a wide spectrum of family involvements as traditions, ideologies, and problems are shared and confronted over time. Through close examination of members' communication activities, grounded understandings of what families "do" and "are" can be generated.

For example, communication activities comprising "caregiving", "emotional support", "healing", and "grieving" remain to be examined interactionally. Similarly, work on cancer and emotion makes reference to such problems as "communication barriers", but leaves unspecified how such communication gets achieved (Barraclough, 1994). These empirical and theoretical tendencies are further exemplified in *Communication with the Cancer Patient* (Surbone & Zwitter, 1997), an edited volume providing rich, valuable, and alternative overviews of communication pervasiveness and impact, but limited "communication data" made available for readers' inspections.

Analyses of recorded and transcribed *interactions*, though rare in psychosocial research, offer an alternative to relying exclusively on self-reported information about the complex roles of communication throughout cancer journeys. In these cases, readers are provided with excerpts drawn from real-time communication events. One alternative is to emphasize content-analytic observations about individuals' comments during key moments, as with the following:

> In a study of audio-recorded informal conversations between nurses and terminally ill patients, one nurse eased a patient's relative by saying, "you are not holding us up. My time is your time love, ok . . . and don't ever worry about whether you should . . ". when the relative indicated that the nurse had spent a great deal of time tending to the family. (Hunt, 1991)

Notice, however, that examining the social action of "easing" a relative is accomplished through quoting of an isolated utterance emphasizing the nurse's individual actions. What is not made clear is how the speakers worked *together* to enact this episode: How was nurse's utterance designed as *responsive* to some prior turns-at-talk and the actions they were understood by the nurse to be displaying? How was nurse's "easing" itself consequential for ensuing talk, that is, as the relative heard and responded (or not) to nurse's apparent offering of assurance? Without closely examining the *interactional* environment within which such "easing" is claimed to have occurred, the focus remains on individuals' contributions (in this instance, only the nurse) rather than on emergent communication patterns co-enacted by speakers. Further, little progress can be made toward describing and explaining basic communication patterns: How do nurses and relatives collaborate in managing what appears to be, but can not be communicatively substantiated as, a potentially delicate moment of cancer *caregiving*?

And as noted, few studies have attempted to examine interactions through which patients and families express needs and accomplish such work as "supporting or coping" (Surbone & Switter, 1997). One such study (Pistrang, Barker, & Rutter, 1997), however, revealed that tape-assisted recalls of breast cancer patients' interactions with their partners yielded insights into how support attempts are delivered effectively and why those attempts sometimes fail. Researchers found that patients perceived the most unhelpful messages as lacking empathy and changing the focus of a conversation concerning the illness. Although the investigators employed tape recordings as the foundation for investigating support in cancer care, the data provided were reconstructed versions of prescribed conversations, not naturally occurring interactions among patients and their partners.

Three Types of Self-Reportings

Selected studies are briefly summarized below to demonstrate what typically counts as self-reported "data", and thus to clarify how empirical and theoretical claims about communication and psychosocial oncology are typically advanced.

Anecdotal and Narrative Experiences

The first set of examples involves *anecdotal* and *narrative* data, representing individuals' summarized versions of personal experiences with cancer events.

- In a case study of a man with small-cell lung cancer, "Jack" reported that his wife created an emotional scene upon learning of his condition, but eventually the couple was able to talk to each other much more easily (Barraclough, 1994).
- A study of family communication patterns in coping with breast cancer indicated that "talkers" (people who discussed the illness often) shared their concerns and fears and were open to listening with one another more often than "nontalkers" (people who rarely discussed the illness), although "talkers" had been talkers even prior to diagnosis (Hilton, 1994).

With the cases above, readers do not have direct access to activities reported—that is, being able to talk to each other much more easily, how talkers and non-talkers share their concerns and fears about breast cancer—but rather must rely upon reportings about such phenomena as evidence for communication scenes and patterns.

Although these data are generated from subjects' and/or researchers' subjective experiences, such qualitative studies of personal narratives provide extremely rich and deeply moving stories of cancer experiences for researchers, practitioners, and family members. For example, attention is given to a wide array of narrations central to patients' experiences and survival (Frank, 1991, 1995; Gabb, 1996; Goodell, 1992; Komp, 1992; Meyer & Rao, 1997; Mott, 1996; Surbone, 1996; Ott, 1999), family members helping each other cope (Broccolo, 1997; Hensel, 1997), living with a cancer patient (Joseph, 1992; Spears, 1990), experiences of those who suffer from deaths of loved ones (Brookes, 1997; Byock, 1997; Ellis, 1993; Haber, 1995; Milton, 1996), nurses' experiences (Iocovozzi, 1991; Parisi, 1996; Renz, 1994; Spears, 1990), and diverse family survival guides for coping with cancer (Benjamin, 1987; Hermann, Wojtkowiak, Houts, & Kahn, 1988; Kowalczyk, 1995; Quill, 1991).

Interviews

The second source of self-reported data involve *interviews*. Typically, actual quotes are utilized from interviewees' reported experiences about communication events and activities:

- During ten interviews with family caregivers, one woman indicated that to fulfill caregiver responsibilities, "you stop thinking about yourself. You spend your time thinking of the other person and what they need. You learn to fetch and carry a lot" (D. Beach, 1993, p. 39).
- In a study identity in cancer survivorship, one participant reported that during chemotherapy, "many family members called a lot, some too much. It was too hard to repeat the story over and over again" (Ott, 1999, p. 109).
- A study of communication with parents of children with cancer found that all 23 sets of parents interviewed reported deep shock and devastation upon learning of the illness, though 19 of the families "did not in retrospect wish that the information had been given in any different way (Eden, Black, & MacKinlay, 1994, p. 108).
- In a discussion with a clinical social worker, a cancer patient said, "'I'm not very well educated and I don't understand some of the language used by my doctor when describing my cancer and treatment. I'm afraid to ask'"(Farrow, Cash & Simmons, 1990, p. 4).

These reportings are responsive to interviewers' solicitations of information via diverse question formats. Findings are also shaped by interviewers' analysis of key moments within these reportings, resulting in a reconstructed sense of social order based on multiple informants' experiences. A focus on caregiving, for example, may emphasize what a caregiver is "thinking" rather than how he or she relies upon communication when enacting caregiving tasks. Similarly, attention can be given to parents' retrospective wishes about receiving bad news about their childrens' cancer and not the interactions comprising these news informings. Or, a patient's being "afraid to ask" about a doctor's language, rather than actual moments in medical interviews in which doctors employ technical language and patients may (or may not) seek clarification.

An abundance of research relying on interview data exists where researchers solicit and individuals respond to selected cancer-related topics. These studies provide insight into issues such as attitudes toward medical decision making (Blackhall et al., 1995), the psychological aspects of caring for family members with cancer (Williamson & Schulz, 1995), suffering of family caregivers (Hinds, 1992), aspects of psychological coping (Wellisch, Hoffman, & Gritz, 1996), distress within families experiencing cancer (Schulz, Schulz, Schulz, & von Kerekjarto, 1996), "remodeling" of relationships after diagnosis of serious illness (Lyons & Meade, 1995), changes in families and coping after the cancer death of a child (Martinson, McClowry, Davies, & Kuhlenkamp, 1994), and social work as a support system (Barnhart et al., 1994). In one interview study, Robinson (1993) found that "normalization", or treating the patient as normal, is a strong reported theme and preference among patients and families coping with a chronic condition. Normalization processes involve the construction of life stories, which are inevitably socially and thus interactionally enacted (see also Capps & Ochs, 1995), though they may be (and usually are) examined apart from the interactional environments in which they initially occurred.

In a unique application of participant observation, Peräkylä (1991) provides rich insights into "hope work" within a hospital setting (see Chapters 12 & 13). Over time, as people were observed going about their business in hospital wards, copious field notes were generated and thorough descriptions of how people go about "conveying hope" are offered. In his reflexive conclusions, however, Peräkylä emphasizes that "hope work" is accomplished exclusively in and through conversation (see Chapter 12). Such interactional involvements are described as best accessed by examinations of actual recordings, not sole reliance upon researcher's observations, perceptions, and memories about the complexities of communication events.

In contrast, across numerous studies, interview and other field data are often mistaken for actual communication. What people "report" about reconstructed and/or imagined interactions is treated as synonymous with real time communication events. Within the communication discipline, Gotcher and Edwards (1990) describe their investigation as a study of "actual interaction", yet data are acquired not through recordings of people interacting. Rather, a survey and interviews revealing selected memories about interactions are employed. Implications about interactions can be drawn from analyzing interview data, of course, without examining the interactions themselves. For example, Gotcher (1993) interviewed breast and prostate cancer patients and concluded that

> "emotional support" was determined to be "highly valued" by families and most likely to decrease anxiety, guilt, hostility, and depression which are primary factors that compromise psychological distress. . . . If patient-family interactions can facilitate emotional support, and thereby decrease psychological problems, then patient-family interactions could enhance prognosis and ultimate survival. (p. 185)

Other research regarding interaction within families with a cancer patient has also relied upon interview data, followed by coding and/or quantification (Bailey, 1985; Eden, Black, & MacKinaly, 1994; Gotcher, 1993; Northouse, 1994) designed to better understand content and themes but not distinct interactional patterns. A partial exception is a study done by Weihs and Reiss (1996) as they examined transcripts of a family conversing about the stresses they faced with cancer. However, as the recordings were made while a researcher was present, the resulting discourse was produced as an upshot of specific questions asked by the interviewer. Content-analytic findings, such as "security of attachment" and "insecure relational processes", raise key implications for understanding family interactions but are not to be mistaken for patterns co-enacted by family members outside of an interview format.

Surveys

A third source of predominantly employed data involves *surveys* of participants (e.g., cancer patients and caregivers). Participants respond to varying measurement scales (e.g., paper and pencil) and/or phone interviews shaped by predetermined questionnaire formats, which trigger recallings of prior communication scenes and patterns:

- In a survey of cancer patients at a major cancer treatment center in the South, 48 patients reported having imagined interactions with doctors, spouses, and family members (Gotcher & Edwards, 1990).
- In a survey of 102 cancer patients receiving radiation therapy, patients who effectively adjusted to their illness in seven areas (including areas such as domestic environment, family relationships, social environment, and psychological distress) communicated more frequently and reported receiving more emotional support than did patients who did not adjust well to their illness (Gotcher, 1995).
- In a survey of communication between cancer patients and their spouses, approximately two-thirds of patients and their spouses reported talking about the illness "very often", and only 22% of spouses and 11% of the patients reported difficulty in candidly discussing the illness (Keller et al., 1996).

Through surveys, then, these instances reveal how patients (and their spouses) reported "having imagined interactions", "communicated more frequently and reported receiving more emotional support", and "reported talking about the illness" in various ways. In each instance, access is (once again) not gained to the events being reported on, but rather triggered recollections about those activities.

A considerable corpus of quantitative, variable-analytic research has focused on cancer and families, relying predominantly on self-report data generated from measurement scaling instruments. These quantitative studies have examined illness-related demands impacting such variables as maternal depressive mood and opinions about marital quality (Lewis & Hammond, 1996), coping among parents of pediatric cancer patients (Shapiro & Shumaker, 1987), behavioral problems of siblings of children who have cancer (Sloper & While, 1996), and "family functioning" as a "resource variable" (Fobair & Zabora, 1995). Attention has also been given to assessing adult cancer patients' orientations to support from family, friends, and health professionals (Rose, 1990), examining coping variables within families (Edwards et al., 1002; Friedrich, Jowarski, Copeland, & Pendergrass, 1994; Hilton, 1994; Walsh-Burke, 1990), effects on rehabilitation of openness regarding illness within families (Mesters et al., 1997), "supportive communication as uncertainty management" (Ford, Babrow, & Stohl, 1996), family communication patterns and a child's adjustment to cancer (Jospe, 1989), and adjustments among couples (Hoskins, 1995; Keller et al., 1996; Vess, Moreland, & Schwebel, 1985). Several researchers (e.g., Jospe, 1989; Martinson et al., 1994; Miller, 1988; Seale, 1991; Walsh-Burke, 1990) have also integrated methods (e.g., interview and questionnaire data) to solicit individuals' views from multiple perspectives.

Taken together, these studies reconfirm that communication is considered one of the fundamental needs of patients and families facing cancer (Shields et al., 1995). Similarly, within the communication discipline, scales and questionnaires have been employed to conclude that matters of frequency, honesty, encouragement, and handling troubling topics were central communicative issues (Gotcher, 1995), and that interaction with family members is central in "determining whether a patient had adjusted effectively" (Gotcher, 1992, p. 21). In these and related variable-analytic studies, communication is posited as centrally important for achieving such actions as moods, opinions, marital satisfaction, cohesiveness, expressiveness, and support. Overwhelmingly, communication is accessed through subjects' self-reported reactions and experiences, not by analyzing how family members coordinate their interactions in real time.

From the contrasting yet similar cancer experiences only sketched above, communication is unequivocally the most important social resource when dealing with difficult cancer predicaments. However suggestive and heuristic these self-reported findings might be, *communication activities per se remain predominantly anecdotal, hypothetical, self-descriptive and expressive, and/or reconstructed.* Reported interactions reveal important potential, including the ability to "facilitate emotional support" and thus "enhance prognosis and ultimate survival" (Gotcher, 1993, p. 185). Yet family members' interactions, so fundamental to naturally occurring events, remain to be systematically explored.

COMMUNICATION, CANCER, AND FAMILY INTERACTIONS

As discussed more fully in Chapter 2, Conversation Analysis (CA) is a viable methodological alternative for closely examining the detailed and patterned organization of interactions in natural settings, including involvements in both clinical and home environments. What follows is a summary of how research has tended to examine clinical encounters rather than family conversations in home environments. A glimpse is also provided of popular culture: cartoonists' drawings, designed to capture their own and others' cancer journeys, including family members diagnosed with terminal cancer.

The Tendency and Limitations of Studying Communication in Clinical Encounters

Conversation analytic studies of medical interactions have focused almost exclusively on clinical and institutional encounters (e.g., see Beach, 1995a, 1995b, 2009; Beach & Dixson, 2001; Frankel, 1995; Heath, 1988; Heritage & Maynard, 2006; Jones, 1997; Jones & LaBaron, 2002; Maynard, 1992; Robinson, 2001, 2003; Stivers, 2002). Considerable attention has been given to talk *within* clinical encounters involving medical interviewers, therapists, patients, and family members (e.g., see, Beach & Dixson, 2001; Beach & LeBaron, 2002; Beach & Mandelbaum, 2005; Drew & Heritage, 1992; Gill & Maynard, 1988, 1991, 1995; Heritage & Maynard, 2006; Heritage & Stivers, 1999; Kinnell & Maynard, 1996; Morris & Cheneil, 1995; Peräkylä, 1993, 1995; Stivers, 2007).

During medical interviews, recent though comparatively few studies have focused on how providers deliver, and patients respond, to both good and bad news regarding cancer (see Lutfey & Maynard, 1998; Maynard & Frankel, 2006). Limited attention has also been given to how cancer patients provide explanations (Gill & Maynard, 2006), and solicit diagnostic information (Jones & Beach, 2005), from doctors who (in various ways) tend to resist patients' voluntary contributions.

Lutfey and Maynard (1998), for example, analyze how the same physician delivers bad news (allusively and indirectly) to three different patients in an oncology setting. Of relevance to the prior discussion of the predominance of self-reports, they frame their inquiry by observing how prior research on illness, death, and dying "emphasizes abstract, internal experiences of individuals who confront mortal or chronic illness . . . typifications and generalizations" (p. 1) that fall short of exposing communication problems emerging from allusive and indirect approaches to delivering bad news. The implications of their discussion emphasizes a recurrent theme: how treating individuals as units of analysis essentially overlooks how illness processes get socially organized and embedded within communicative contexts.

Research on medical encounters, only briefly alluded to here, provides considerable insight into the construction and preservation of professional-lay relationships, most notably the asymmetries that distinctly characterize them. Such inquiries are, unequivocally, of central importance to comprehending illness management as a communicative achievement. Examining how lay persons communicate about health and illness in no way diminishes the need for researching clinical encounters throughout health prevention and management (e.g., see, Rootman & Hershfield, 1994). On the contrary, considerable attention has been and needs to be given to talk *within* clinical encounters involving doctors, therapists, patients, family members and significant others (e.g., see, Beach, 2009; Drew & Heritage, 1992; Heritage & Maynard, 2006; Morris & Cheneil, 1995; Peräkylä, 1995). Studies of clinical encounters provide considerable insight into the construction and preservation of professional-lay relationships (e.g., see Gill, Halkowski, & Roberts, 2001; Heritage & Stivers, 1999; Robinson, 2001; Stivers & Heritage, 2001). Indeed, the delivery and receipt of diagnostic news has most commonly been associated with practitioner-patient communication in clinical encounters (Frankel, 1995; Heath, 1992; Maynard, 1992). Critical issues have been addressed, such as how "dreaded issues" get raised and addressed in AIDS counseling (Peräkylä, 1993, 1995), practices through which distinct phases of medical interviews get accomplished (see Heritage & Maynard, 2006), patients' narratives and explanations regarding clinical visits (Gill, 1998; Gill & Maynard, 2006; Halkowski, 2006), relationships among *lay diagnosis* and how patients navigate their ways through medical encounters (Beach, 2001).

However as Ira Byock, past president of the American Academy of Hospice and Palliative Medicine, observed: "Dying cannot be reduced to a collection of diagnoses. For the individual and the family, the enormity and depth of this final transition dwarfs the myriad medical problems" (1997, p. 35; see also Glaser & Strauss, 1965). Selected studies of interactions among family members addressing health issues do exist. Attention has been given to problems associated with the pursuit and avoidance of bulimia (Beach, 1996), death announcements among friends and acquaintances (Holt, 1993), and dilemmas involved in giving and receiving unsolicited advice (Heritage & Lindstrom, 1998; Heritage & Sefi, 1992; Heritage & Sorjonen, 1994) between British home health care nurses and first-time mothers.

Cartoon Portrayals of Real Life Cancer Journeys

A series of insightful and creative books have been published by cancer patients, writers, reporters, and/or artists who have directly experienced their own or others' cancer (e.g., see, Ackerman & Ackerman, 2002; Acocella Marchetto, 2006; Blachman, 2006; Brabner, Perkar, & Stack, 1994; Clifford & Palmer, 2002; Di Giacomo, 2003; Engelberg, 1995; Fies, 2006). In the preface to *Mom's Cancer*, for example, Fies (2006) describes himself as engaging in a form of "underground journalism: dispatches from the front lines of a battle into which my family stumbled unprepared". His cartoons serially trace his mom's and family's fight with metastatic lung cancer, from biopsy through remission. Though the family recognizes that vigilance is always needed and "cure" can only be hoped for, Fies provides an "honest, earnest effort to turn something bad into something good". The captions in Figure 1.1 reconstruct a family meeting called by mom.

When family members attempt to deliver news to mom about her cancer diagnosis, mom displays an inability to grasp the seriousness of her condition. Notice that Fies' reconstructions of the family conversation also include his private thoughts (in boxes with "Geez" and "Why isn't mom getting any of this?"). Readers, then, have access to Fies' memories of the interaction (though he reports "that my family members remember some of these events very differently") and to otherwise inaccessible thoughts and feelings he had when reacting to particular exchanges and events.

An earlier cartoon series was produced by Engelberg (1995) when, at 43 years of age and mother of a 4-year-old son, she was diagnosed with breast cancer. A prior interest in "autobiographical comics" (pp. x-xii) was relied on as she "created the first cartoon while waiting for the biopsy, before I knew for sure that the tumor was malignant". A rendering of her biopsy experience appears in Figure 1.2.

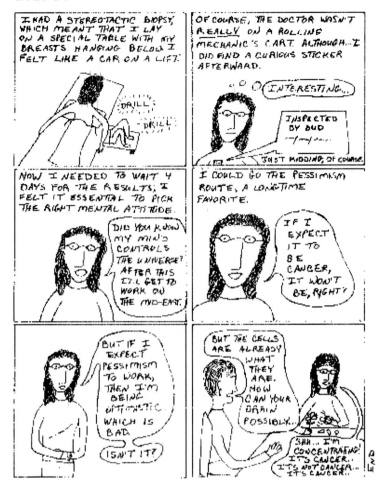

Figure 1.1. *A Humorous Graphic Memoir About Breast Cancer*

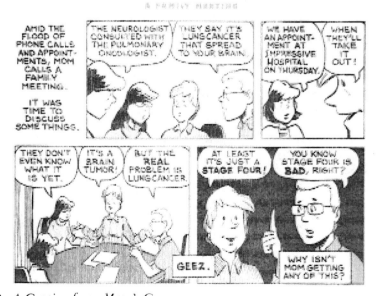

Figure 1.2. *A Caption from Mom's Cancer*

The self-reflective narrative she provides is revealing and humorous. As with Fies'
Mom's Cancer, readers are offered access to her private thoughts as she remembered them.
And in the last caption, a reconstructed (or possibly imagined conversation) with an
unidentified person is provided, who questions her ability to deny cancer diagnosis. In
response, Engelberg states "SHH . . . I'm concentrating!" and then proceeds to pluck ped-
als from a flower to determine whether she has cancer or not.

I find the comics by Fies, Engelberg, and others to be penetrating and discerning. Their
unique portrayals have universal appeal to all who undergo cancer journeys. A resonant
chord is struck with readers drawn to discover whether, and how, others working through
cancer have had similar thoughts, feelings, and interactions. As Fies states, "You are not
alone".

In many ways these graphic cartoons have gotten closer to revealing human experiences, and especially the organization of everyday interactions, than a massive amount of
social scientific literature designed to expose relationships between communication and
cancer. As writers and artists, these authors make actual circumstances available for others'
inspection and reflection. Of course, readers are reliant on authors' memories and reconstructed sense of social order (e.g., see, Coulter, 1979). There are no real-time recordings,
nor transcriptions, of naturally occurring settings and the interactions comprising daily life.
Nor can the details of their depictions be authenticated by others' inspection of "independent" or more "objective" materials. But that is not the goal for these authors, who have
developed their own valuable techniques for capturing how cancer impacts all persons
involved in diagnosis, treatment, and prognosis.

MOVING TOWARD ANALYSIS OF INTERACTIONAL DATA

In this initial chapter, a review of the history of psycho-oncological research makes clear
that researchers have tended to examine social activities by investigating individuals' perceived, interpreted, and/or reconstructed experiences. Though only briefly addressed, so
too have cartoonists relied on their individual abilities to reconstruct and graphically visualize actual cancer experiences and events. With the "Malignancy" phone calls, a unique
opportunity now exists to directly examine recordings and transcriptions of naturally
occurring events throughout a family cancer journey. It becomes possible to address empirically how interaction is a primary resource for family members during the onset, advance-
ment, and overall interactional management of cancer.

From the literature reviewed in this chapter, a wide array of interrelated communication involvements remain to be investigated. What *social* activities comprise supporting,
loving, being open and honest versus withholding and deceptive, caregiving, describing
alternative treatment options, explaining biomedical and related technical procedures,
managing uncertain and dreaded futures, assuaging others' fears, giving and receiving
advice, talking about pain and comfort, articulating complex relationships between living
and dying? It remains to be seen how, or if, such social activities—and other features of
family life not yet articulated in prior literature—are achieved through interactions comprising the collection of "Malignancy" phone calls.

2

THE "MALIGNANCY" PHONE CALL CORPUS

Analyzing Episodic and Longitudinal Interactions

The "Malignancy" corpus consists of 61 recorded phone calls occurring over a period of 13 months.[1] Primary calls occur between five family members: son, dad, mom, aunt, and grandmother. The son is involved in each call because he recorded all phone conversations at two residences.[2] A total of 26 interactional participants participate in these 61 calls, including an assortment of other conversations between the son and representatives from various airlines, his separated/ex-wife, her brother, receptionists at an academic counseling office and an animal boarding kennel, a woman the son had begun dating, an old friend from the midwest, a graduate student who covered the son's classes during travel, and a variety of other calls involving routine daily occurrences (e.g., the payment of bills, leaving messages on phone answering machines).

INDEX, TIMELINE, AND CHRONOLOGY OF PHONE CALLS

An Index of the "Malignancy" calls appears in Figure 2.1. The length, speakers involved, and vernacular titles are listed for each of the 61 calls. Titles were drawn from speakers' utterances reflecting (as best possible) the interactional focus of each phone call. Also included is a summary of the overall size and length of the collection.

By reading through the vernacular titles in Figure 2.1, it is possible to gain a sense of *what* and *how* speakers' concerns evolved over time, beginning with mom's diagnosis (Call #1) until only hours before she passed away (Call #61).

Complete transcriptions of the phone calls have been generated, employing a transcription system created and refined by Gail Jefferson (Figure 2.2). Notation symbols capture voice delivery, emphasis, intonation, pace, laughter, pauses within and between utterances, latching of contiguous utterances, speech overlap, and scenic details (e.g., music in the background, coughing, voice breaks).

An abbreviated timeline of mom's life, and a more specific chronology of the calls, appears in Figure 2.3.

CALL#	LENGTH	SPEAKER	VERNACULAR TITLE
1	22:11	Son & Dad	"it is malignant"
2	8:21	Son, Mom, & Dad	"the verdict"
3	10:16	Son, Mom, & Dad	"no life support...I just want to get there"
4	4:11	Son & American Airline	"apparently my mother's going to die"
5	4:06	Son & Continental Airlines	"our agents are temporarily busy"
6	00:16	Son & PAN AM Airlines	"you don't go where I'm trying to go"
7	00:46	Son & USAIR	"my mother's about to die"
8	4:07	Son & Continental Airlines	"I just found out my mother's going to die"
9	3:33	Son & Southwest Airlines	"looks like my mother's going to die"
10	15:25	Son & Aunt	"mom's in a lot of pain"
11	9:22	Son & Gina	"you can come lean on me"
12	7:24	Son & Dad	"stay there...this is weird...insanity"
13	6:13	Son & Gina	"very likely gonna be too late"
14	1:03	Son & Answering Machine	"I'm not coming...at least not quite yet"
15	2:52	Son & Counseling Services	"something has gone away now...put it back"
16	2:05	Son & Dog Kennel	"we've got a very temporary reprieve"
17	6:56	Son & Aunt	"it's all part of the game"
18	10:59	Son & Gina	"I don't need to show up quite yet"
19	17:35	Son & Dad	"mom's in the hospital...it's bad very bad"
20	13:17	Son & Dad	"It's a hard time"
21	1:45	Son & Gina	"I'm so excited we get it tomorrow"
22	1:09	Son & Answering Machine	"I'm real sorry I wasn't here when she called"
23	1:43	Son & Answering Machine	"I'm here and was just wondering what's going on"
24	2:46	Son & MCI	"I just recently got divorced"
25	14:58	Son & Dad	"she does have several tumors in the spine now"
26	1:37	Son & Receptionist	"figure out how to spell the child's name"
27	00:17	Son & Answering Machine	"I thought I'd call you and say hello"
28	4:58	Son & Mom	"It's kinda drizzly today"
29	00:16	Son & Answering Machine	"I was trying to get back in touch"
30	9:42	Son & Dad	"she'd be delighted to talk to ya"
31	3:37	Son & Gina	"sliding downhill again"
32	6:04	Son & Mom	"I really don't envy where you're at mom"
33	8:50	Son & Gina	"I'm so angry"

Figure 2.1. Index of the "Malignancy" Phone Call Corpus

CALL#	LENGTH	SPEAKER	VERNACULAR TITLE
34	15:18	Son & Gina	"Old habits die hard"
35	00:10	Son & Anonymous Caller	"I'm sorry I got the wrong number"
36	00:05	Son & Gina	"collect call"
37	00:20	Son & Landlord	"what's your mailing address?"
38	00:44	Son & Answering Machine	"Hola, Jean"
39	8:33	Son & Dad	"things are relatively status quo"
40	18:55	Son & Gramma	"it's a big world...a screwy confusing one"
41	39:15	Son, Dad, & Mom	"so she's not thinkin real straight...it's nuts"
42	11:24	Son & Dad	"talking to mom yesterday was a shock"
43	18:00	Son & Dad	"time is just taking its toll"
44	14:16	Son, Gina, & Mark	"cancer is not a happy disease to have"
45	21:05	Son & Dad	"tell her I'm doing more socializing"
46	7:23	Son & Gina	"Mom's just goin downhill"
47	00:06	Son & Recorded Voice	"please hang up and dial a one"
48	00:18	Son & Operator	"Southwestern Bell...area code"
49	00:20	Son & Operator	"Looking for a company named Broaderband"
50	1:09	Son & Broaderband	"ya need to actually call technical support"
51	1:30	Son & & Broaderband	"I have a copy of Printshop"
52	29:26	Son & Gramma	"she was vomiting all the time"
53	00:18	Son & Gina	"Hi there"...(phone cuts off)
54	1:49	Son & Southwest Airlines	"they don't think that my mother is going to live"
55	00:30	Son & Service Department	"customer service department is now closed"
56	2:18	Son & Sharon	"Packing?...Oh no"
57	3:44	Son & Dad	"Hold together...I love ya pop"
58	1:38	Son & Counseling Receptionist	"my mother is going to pass away"
59	1:30	Son & Gary	"good luck...let's hope we all get through this"
60	1:50	Sharon & Jean	"I don't think she's gonna make it"
61	2:39	Son & Sharon	"boy, she's terrible"

Approximate Length of Phone Call Corpus:	7 hours
Number of Transcribed Pages (Double-Spaced):	420
Shortest Call:	00:05 ((cut-off call))
Longest Call:	39:15
Approximate Average Call Length:	7:00

Figure 2.1. *Index of the "Malignancy" Phone Call Corpus* (continued)

In data headings",SDCL" stands for "San Diego Conversation Library", a collection of recordings and transcriptions of naturally occurring interactions; "Malignancy #1:2" represents the title and number of call in the data corpus, and page numbers from which data excerpts are drawn. The transcription notation system employed for data segments is an adaptation of Gail Jefferson's work (see Atkinson & Heritage [Eds.], 1984, pp. ix-xvi). The symbols may be described as follows:

:	**Colon(s):** Extended or stretched sound, syllable, or word.
–	**Underlining:** Vocalic emphasis.
(.)	**Micropause:** Brief pause of less than (0.2).
(1.2)	**Timed Pause:** Intervals occurring within and between same or different speaker's utterance.
(( ))	**Double Parentheses:** Scenic details.
( )	**Single Parentheses:** Transcriptionist doubt.
.	**Period:** Falling vocal pitch.
?	**Question Marks:** Rising vocal pitch.
↑ ↓	**Arrows:** Pitch resets; marked rising and falling shifts in intonation.
° °	**Degree Signs:** A passage of talk noticeably softer than surrounding talk.
=	**Equal Signs:** Latching of contiguous utterances, with no interval or overlap.
[ ]	**Brackets:** Speech overlap.
[[	**Double Brackets:** Simultaneous speech orientations to prior turn.
!	**Exclamation Points:** Animated speech tone.
-	**Hyphens:** Halting, abrupt cut off of sound or word.
> <	**Less Than/Greater Than Signs:** Portions of an utterance delivered at a pace noticeably quicker than surrounding talk.
OKAY	**CAPS:** Extreme loudness compared with surrounding talk.
hhh .hhh	**H's:** Audible outbreaths, possibly laughter. The more h's, the longer the aspiration. Aspirations with periods indicate audible inbreaths (e.g., .hhh). H's within parentheses (e.g., ye(hh)s) mark within-speech aspirations, possible laughter.
pt	**Lip Smack:** Often preceding an inbreath.
hah	**Laugh Syllable:** Relative closed or open position of laughter
heh	
hoh	

Figure 2.2. *Transcription Symbols*

1938	Mom Born
1940	U.V. Treatments
1952-56	High School
1958	Married
1962	Son Born
1963	First Cancer/Shunt Inserted
1969	Daughter Born
1986	Dental Implants/Cancer Undetected

DAY 1		
SEPT 1988	*After* *7 pm*	#1 Son & Dad "It is malignant"

DAY 2

	Morning	#2 Son & Mom "The verdict"

DAY 1

OCT 1989	*After* *5 pm*	#3 Son, Mom, & Dad "No life support...I just want to get there"
		#4 Son & American Airlines "Apparently my mother's going to die"
		#5 Son & Continental Airlines "Our agents are temporarily busy"
		#6 Son & PAN AM Airlines "You don't know where I'm trying to go"
		#7 Son & US AIR "My mother's about to die"
		#8 Son & Continental Airlines "I just found out my mother's going to die"
		#9 Son & Southwest Airlines "Looks like my mother's going to die"
		#10 Son & Aunt "Mom's in a lot of pain"

DAY 2

		#11 Son & Gina "you can come lean on me"
		#12 Son & Dad "stay there...this is weird...insanity"
		#13 Son & Gina "very likely gonna be too late"
		#14 Son & Answering Machine "I'm not coming...at least not yet"
		#15 Son & Counseling Services "Something has gone away...put it back"
		#16 Son & Dog Kennel "we've got a very temporary reprieve"
		#17 Son & Aunt "it's all part of the game"

DAY 3

	Night	#18 Son & Gina "I don't need to show up quite yet"
	Evening	#19 Son & Dad "mom's in the hospital... it's very bad"

DAY 4

	Morning	#20 Son & Dad "It's a hard time"
		#21 Son & Gina "I'm so excited we get it tomorrow"
		#22 Son & Answering Machine "I'm real sorry I wasn't here when she called"
		#23 Son & Answering Machine "I'm here and was just wondering what's going on"
		#24 Son & MCI "I just recently got divorced"

DAY 5

		#25 Son & Dad "she does have several tumors in the spine now"

Figure 2.3. *Abbreviated Timeline for Mom's Life (1938-1989) and Chronology of Phone Calls #1-61.*

31

OCT 1989 (*continued*)	*Daytime*	#26 Son & Receptionist "figure out how to spell the child's name" #27 Son & Answering Machine "I thought I'd call you and say hello" #28 Son & Mom "It's kinda drizzly today" #29 Son & Answering Machine "I was trying to get back in touch"

		DAY 6
	Morning	#30 Son & Dad "she'd be delighted to talk to ya"
	Daytime	#31 Son & Gina "sliding down hill again"
		#32 Son & Mom "I really don't envy where you're at mom"
	Daytime	#33 Son & Gina "I'm so angry"
	Evening	#34 Son & Gina "Old habits die hard"
		#35 Son & Anonymous Caller "I'm sorry I got the wrong number"
		#36 Son & Gina "collect call"
		#37 Son & Landlord "What's your mailing address?"
		#38 Son & Jean "Hola, Jean"

		DAY 7
	Morning	#39 Son & Dad "things are relatively status quo"

		DAY 8
	Morning	#40 Son & Gramma "it's a big world... a screwy confusing one" #41 Son, Dad, & Mom "so she's not thinkin real straight... it's nuts"

		DAY 9
	Morning	#42 Son & Dad "talking to mom yesterday was a shock" #43 Son & Dad "time is just taking its toll"
	Late Evening	#44 Son, Gina, & Mark "cancer is not a happy disease to have" #45 Son & Dad "tell her I'm doing more socializing"

		DAY 10
		#46 Son & Gina "Mom's just going downhill"
		#47 Son & Recorded Voice "please hang up and dial a one"
	Daytime	#48 Son & Operator "Southwestern Bell...area code"
		#49 Son & Operator "Looking for a company named Broaderband"
		#50 Son & Broaderband "ya need to actually call technical support"
		#51 Son & Broaderband "I have a copy of Printshop"

		DAY 11
	Morning	#52 Son & Gramma "she was vomiting all the time"
	Early Evening	#53 Son & Gina "Hi there"...(phone cuts off)
		#54 Son & Southwest Airlines "they don't think my mother is going to live"
		#55 Son & Service Department "customer service department is now closed"
		#56 Son & Sharon "Packing?...Oh no"
		#57 Son & Dad "Hold together...I love ya pop"
		#58 Son & Counseling Receptionist "my mother is going to pass away"
		#59 Son & Gary "good luck... let's hope we all get through this"

		DAY 12
	Late Evening	#60 Sharon & Jean "I don't think she's gonna make it" #61 Son & Sharon "boy she's terrible"

NOV 1989	**Mom Dies**

Figure 2.3. *Abbreviated Timeline for Mom's Life (1938–1989) and Chronology of Phone Calls #1-61* (continued)

Inherent Limitations of the "Malignancy" Collection

This chronology reveals several identifying and significant features. It can be noted that Calls #1-2 occurred in the evening and the following morning during September, 1988. There was then a 10-month gap before recordings were once again initiated in October, 1989.[3] This period of time was consequential for the development of mom's cancer. In Call #2, mom informs son about the "verdict" they had received, and she is just beginning treatments for her diagnosed cancer. In Call #3 mom speaks openly with son about her pain and imminent death. She also informs son of her decision not to be placed on "life support".

The absence of calls mirroring these phases of the family's cancer journey, during such a critical 10 months, is an obvious limitation of this corpus and the study as a whole. Because nothing can be said about the many calls occurring during this period, the daily and weekly interactions among family members remains a matter of speculation. How many phone calls might have occurred during these ten months? How did family members mange such a period of protracted and progressive illness? What communication patterns comprise the tedious, hopeful, yet gradual recognition and displayed acceptance that cancer is terminal? These and related questions cannot be fully addressed in this investigation and remain for future research (see Chapter 14).

At the outset, it is also important to note another obvious limitation of the materials and investigation: These 61 calls by no means represent the total range and diversity of family interactions during this period of 13 months. Not only were recordings not made during a period of ten months, but no doubt many other conversations (face-to-face and on the phone) occurred among family members, friends, co-workers, acquaintances, and others — none of which were recorded, many of which could yield key insights about how "cancer" becomes a topic (and even preoccupation) of peoples' lives as they navigate their way through diagnosis, death, and living without the physical presence of a loved one. And it is also important to keep in mind that only *son's* calls were being recorded, and thus no access is provided to other family members' interactions on the telephone. And how many *clinical* interactions occurred with an array of medical experts in providers' offices and at different hospitals or care facilities? What kinds of interactions occurred in the home when hospice employees (and others) visited and cared for mom (and family members)? The inability to empirically address these questions makes clear, and unequivocally so, that the phone calls examined herein are incomplete representations of this family's cancer journey.

Perhaps the most obvious limitation, however, is that these calls represent only *one families' journey through cancer*. Though universal and thus generalizable features no doubt exist across these calls, a cross-situational analysis of multiple families' interactions cannot be offered herein. Possibilities for researching more diverse family populations, building upon the empirical foundation provided in this volume, are also raised in Chapter 14.

Analytic Possibilities

The calls that do exist and form the basis for this investigation are valuable on their own merits. Though only a partial historical record, these calls are available and highly significant pieces of a larger puzzle. They should not be prematurely discounted but appropriately understood as capturing revealing moments over time, within single and across calls (often in a series), activities allowing for enhanced understandings of how family members communicate "longitudinally" when faced with cancer (see below).

The first two calls reveal how son spoke with dad in the evening, and mom the next morning, about her initial cancer diagnosis. Ten months later, phone calls occurred across twelve different days during October and November, 1989. The number of calls ranged from one (Day 7) to 9 (Day 6) in a single day—an average of nearly six calls each day. The specific dates for these calls, and the number of days between calls, could typically not be discovered from the recordings themselves. But by relying on the recordings and transcriptions themselves, especially speakers' references to such details as times, places, and holidays, it has become possible to identify such features as the time of day (i.e., morning, daytime, evening), as well as whether a call occurred on the same or subsequent days.

Even more importantly, however, are ways that family members rely upon and weave their phone calls together into an ongoing fabric of updated, revised, and constantly emerging news; anticipate, address, and reflect on troubles; and work together to make decisions, construct plans, and seek solutions for seemingly omnipresent problems.

For now, a single example will suffice. The decision for son to travel home in Call #3 triggered Calls #4-9 to the airlines. These calls are followed by a recapitulation of his prior calls (and mom's health) with his aunt in Call #10—all in the same day. Further, these interactions directly shaped many of the topics and concerns expressed in subsequent Calls #11-17, the next day, when son is shown to first speculate about his travel and mom's condition, then deal with the consequences of being told by dad to "stay there" and not travel—despite son's concerted efforts to arrange being with mom and family, and in the continued face of ambiguity about a dreaded yet inherently unknowable future.

Each chapter in this volume, whether the focus is on a single case (e.g., Chapters 3 & 4) or varying sizes of collections across similar moments as with Chapters 5-13, is designed to examine fundamental patterns of interactional conduct by family members facing cancer. But each data excerpt is also situated within a grounded chronology, mirroring how family members rely on communication to shape responses to the shifting developments encompassing a cancer journey. Many conversations are shown to be multifaceted in the ways they are temporally linked together: As progressively constructed from prior interactions, and as primary resources for organizing and resolving here-and-now problems that are consequential for shaping upcoming calls in a series.

CONVERSATION ANALYSIS

Conversation analytic (CA) methods are employed to closely examine the interactional organization of these phone calls (e.g., see Atkinson & Heritage 1984; Drew & Heritage, 1992; Ochs, Schegloff, & Thompson, 1996; Sacks, 1992; Schegloff, 2006). The overriding goal of CA is to identify patterned orientations to moment-by-moment contingencies of interaction comprising everyday life events. This mode of *analytic induction* is anchored in repeated listenings of recordings, in unison with systematic inspections of carefully produced transcriptions. Priority is given to locating and substantiating participants' methods for organizing and thus accomplishing social actions. It is an explicit and working feature of this research method that participants continually and instrinsically achieve, through an array of interactional practices, displayed understandings of emergent interactional circumstances. Observations raised during data/listening sessions are designed to reveal the organization of specific practices, recruited and enacted by speakers, who exhibit orderly ways of monitoring and responding to what was treated as meaningfully produced by prior speaker.

Two fundamental assumptions of CA research—data are naturally occurring, and interaction is sequentially designed—are further elaborated in Figure 2.4.

Specific verification issues comprising the validity, reliability, and generalizability of CA findings are summarized in Figure 2.5.

Data are naturally occurring talk and embodied activities	CA involves the direct examination of recordings and transcriptions of naturally occurring verbal, embodied (e.g., gaze, gesture, touch, and the use of instruments or objects), and nonvocal communication activities—interactions that would be occurring whether or not a recording device was present (Beach, 1990b). Observations about interactional phenomena are anchored in contingently organized features of diverse ordinary conversations and institutional encounters involving bureaucratic representatives (e.g., in medical, legal, educational, and corporate settings). Researchers do not prompt the commencement or content of the talk. Nor do they need to be present when interactions are being recorded. Data are not idealized or hypothetical constructions of communication, but records of actual interactional involvements (see Atkinson and Heritage, 1984, pp. 2-5; Heritage, 1984b, pp. 234-238). Systematic collection and analysis of interactional data may be complimented with intensive fieldwork, enacted to better understand how interaction is employed *in situ* as a resource for participants as they collaborate in organizing natural environments. However, researchers' field observations, notes, and/or interviews are not treated as primary data about interaction. Giving priority to recorded and interactional data is fundamental: The detailed contingencies comprising interactional events, and more generally the circumstances addressed through speakers' actions, cannot be intuited, anticipated in advance, nor fully reconstructed following the occurrence of any given interaction or series of involvements. Such embedded temporal and spatial features are impossible to capture by means of self-reported information.
Interaction is sequentially organized	During communication, participants continually reveal their orientations to and understandings of moment-by-moment interactional involvements. In the precise ways speakers construct and respond to turns-at-talk, and related embodied actions, they demonstrate first for one another (and subsequently for analysts' inspections) their real-time and practical understandings of evolving conduct-in-interaction. Exactly what gets achieved in communication is thus a result of how speakers construct and make available to one another their understandings of the local environment of which they are an integral part (see Beach, 1990a, 1990b; 1991, 1995a; Jefferson, 1981; Schegloff, 1991, 2006; Sigman, 1995; Wootton, 1988). A speaker's current turn at talk projects the relevance of a next turn, since "talk amounts to actions" and "action projects relevance" (Sachs, Schegloff, & Jefferson, 1974; Schegloff, 1991, p. 46; Schegloff, 2006). Not just any response will normally suffice, because speakers project the relevance of some (not just any) range of appropriate and next actions. The range of possible activities, accomplished by the second speaker, display variations of "responsiveness": Talk is sensitive to "recipient design" as "next" actions reveal how speakers hear, and orient to, specific and local social actions comprising prior speakers' utterances. By describing and explaining the precise ways participants organize and thereby shape their interactions, evidence is provided about the inherent consequentiality of communication. And because "context" is not treated as external to or removed from communication (see Beach, 1990b; Goodwin & Duranti, 1992; Mandelbaum, 1991; Schegloff, 1996b, 1997), but achieved through interaction, social actions are both context-shaping as speakers tailor them to prior and immediate circumstances, and context-renewing as speakers contribute to evolving and subsequent actions.

Figure 2.4. *Two Fundamental Assumptions of Conversation Analytic (CA) Research*

Validity	Recordings and carefully produced transcriptions allow for examinations of actual communication—as noted, not idealized, hypothetically derived, self-reported, and/or reconstructed choices and actions "driven" by participants' motives, needs, or other observer imposed phenomena (see Atkinson & Heritage, 1984, pp. 2-5; Heritage, 1984b, pp. 234-238). No details of interaction are prematurely dismissed as disorderly, accidental, or irrelevant (Heritage, 1984). This allows for what is commonly referred to as "unmotivated" analysis: As best possible, working to a)avoid pre-determining what is meaningful in interactional data, and b)minimize bringing social problems "to" analysis but rather allowing such problems (and their possible resolutions) to emerge from systematic inspections of speakers' practices for organizing actual communication events and activities. Thus, in the ways that empirical findings are grounded within and exemplified through close inspections of interactional materials, rather than preselected categories or abstract assumptions about communication practices, CA can be understood as a science for discovering and verifying the social organization of everyday life.
Reliability	However random naturally occurring conversations and institutional interactions might initially appear, there exists considerable evidence supporting a central tenet of social interaction studies: There is "order at all points" (Sacks, 1984a, 1992), much of which awaits examination by analysts and all of which was produced in the first instance as meaningful and thus in meaningful ways by participants. Recordings and transcriptions of these real-time communication involvements allow for repeated rehearings, reviewings, and reinspections of "actual and determinate" (Schegloff, 1986) social events and activities. Although neither recordings nor transcriptions are conversations in and of themselves (Beach, 1990a; Zimmerman, 1988), they nevertheless preserve and embody the integrity and distinctiveness of many conversational activities. Moreover, as selected fragments of transcriptions are made available for readers' critical inspections, attention is drawn to specific details of actions rather than glossed versions of what might or could have happened (i.e., idealized, intuited, and/or recollected data). It is also a central tenet of CA to make data available for public inspection, for example, to provide readers with the opportunity to agree and/or disagree with claims being advanced. Transcriptions are published with findings, and (as noted, when possible) recordings of the phenomena being investigated are disseminated for listening and inspection. Most recently, various websites can be accessed for which provide opportunities to repeatedly hear digitized interactional materials (e.g., see http://www.sscnet.ucla.edu/soc/faculty/schegloff/index.html).
Generalizability	CA inquiry beings with a single case study in order to form a grounded basis for developing generalizable descriptions of communication phenomena (Beach & Dixson, 2001; Hopper, 1989; Pomerantz, 1990; Schegloff, 1987; 2006). Once the foundation is laid with a single case, analysts employ a procedure of "constant comparison" to examine how larger collections of instances reflect generalized actions and patterns across diverse settings, speakers, topics, and cultures (e.g., see Atkinson & Drew, 1979; Haakana, 2001; Jefferson, 1980a, 1980b, 1984a, 1984b, 2004; Lerner, 2003, 2004; Mandelbaum, 1993; Maynard, 2003; Pomerantz, 1984a; Robinson, 2004, 2006; Schegloff, 1968). The recurrence of communication events, balanced with how actions are determined to be relevant and significant, can be examined to determine whether and how same, similar, or deviant patterns of interaction occur across a wide array of data (e.g., see Maynard, 2003; Schegloff, 1968). Working simultaneously with single cases, and collections, can yield warrantable claims (rather than under-specified assumptions) about social order.

Figure 2.5. Verification Procedures for Conversation Analysis (CA)

INTEGRATING EPISODIC
AND LONGITUDINAL INVESTIGATIONS

Because phone calls are so prominent in everyday life, considerable attention has been given to their interactional organization (see, e.g., Hopper, 1992; Schegloff, 1968, 1986; K. Tracy, 1997; S.J. Tracy, 2002; Tracy & Tracy, 1998). Historically, however, the analytic tendency of conversation analytic investigations has been to focus on social actions comprising the organization of "episodic" moments of ordinary and institutional interactions (e.g., see Atkinson, 1984; Drew & Heritage, 1992; Heritage & Atkinson, 1984; Maynard, 1997, 2003, Chapter 3; ten Have, 1999). Analyses of single cases, as well as collections of discrete actions, yield insights about a broad array of phenomena (e.g., telling and receiving stories, initiating repair, laughter, marking "change of state", closure of prior and movement toward next topics). As summarized in Figures 2.4 and 2.5 (above), by examining data drawn from a variety of speakers and social environments it becomes possible to reveal universal practices across settings, topics, speakers, and cultures.

As described previously, this study of family cancer relies on a variety of episodes of interactional conduct—"snapshots" excerpted from individual phone calls—but also addresses how these actions and calls routinely occur in a series, within short periods yet also linked (e.g., by topics and concerns comprising the business-at-hand) across larger spans of time.[4] By advancing reasonable descriptions, with plausible explanations made available to readers about transcribed data they are encouraged to inspect, CA identifies how speakers orient to social actions *as relevant for them* in the course of organizing interaction.[5]

Toward a 'Natural History' of Family Communication

This investigation, anchored in phone calls of everyday interactions, also represents one orientation to what has been described as *natural history approaches* to human communication (e.g., see Scheflen, 1971, 1973). When describing the work and legacy of Gregory Bateson, for example, Leeds-Hurwitz (1987, 2005) describes how early influences shaped the kinds of priorities given to actual, naturally occurring communication activities. For example, Bateson was raised by a father who was a biologist, and who emphasized direct observations of plants and animals in natural rather than laboratory settings. Priority was therefore given to describing and explaining whatever might be discovered in natural environments. Findings emerge from these grounded efforts, not from constructing and imposing categories created from existing theories (Bateson, 1971).[6]

By shifting attention from biology to anthropology, Bateson's interests focused on *system, pattern, structure, process, and relationships*—the kinds of generalizable activities most evident when observing human behavior in ordinary contexts (see Goodwin & Duranti, 1992). It was these interests that also attracted a host of prominent researchers, from diverse disciplines, to participate in a project entitled The Natural History of an Interview (NHI).[7] This pioneering effort was designed to conduct microanalysis of a single video recorded interaction between Bateson and a woman ("Doris") whose family was experiencing interpersonal conflict sufficient to seek psychiatric assistance. In his book *Interaction and Identity*, Mokros (1996) describes how it was Bateson's view that "the major advances in the behavioral sciences by the mid-twentieth century all involved a concern with communication"(p. 45). Aligned with this priority, the guiding purpose of the NHI was to generate "a statement of the mechanisms of relationships"(pp. 45, 68). By bringing together professionals interested in different kinds of communication problems, each bringing their distinct modes of observation to bear on a single interview between two participants, "a synthesis of a wide and abstract kind" (Bateson, 1996, p. 47) was attempted. This work had considerable impact on a generation of influential scholars, each utilizing alternative microanalytic approaches when attempting to lay bare the fundamental structures of human conduct in interaction. Indeed, the NHI has influenced the kinds of recorded and transcribed data analyzed, questions asked, findings generated, and overall strategies for investigation (Leeds-Hurwitz, 2005, pp. 144-145).

The natural history approach in this volume is not grounded in gaining access to, entering, and observing a natural setting. Rather, through donated audio recordings, the contexts built through family members' phone calls provide access to limited yet revealing dimensions of the daily lives of family members. These calls make clear that reliance on the telephone, to communicate with one another throughout a cancer journey, is a fundamental activity of social life and thus worthy of investigation on its own merits.

NOTES

1. Limited ethnographic background information regarding this family's cancer dilemma does exist: the son's written reconstructions of this 13-month period, a single excerpt of which appears in the Introduction, including descriptions of such matters as mom's medical history, ongoing health problems, and treatments for diagnosed cancer; and a series of informal and ongoing e-mail exchanges with the son, clarifying such details as speaker identifications, timelines and lapses between calls.
2. Formal permission to study these materials has been granted by the family, and approved through appropriate Human Subjects and Internal Review Board (IRB) Committees.
3. I was informed by the son that at the request of son's separated/ex-wife during divorce proceedings, recordings did not occur during a portion of these 10 months. Also, for a period of three months, when son visited his parents during the summer, no recordings were made.
4. Analysis does not attempt to "code" these episodic and serial instances into pre-determined and thus ungrounded categories of social action (e.g., see Beach, 2007). The goal is not simply nor primarily to identify "frequencies of occurrence". Frequencies per se are often difficult to discern: Single and even relatively "simple" instances often involve multiple discourse features, just as locating and substantiating what *counts* as a phenomenon is in all cases problematic. Although selected coding applications grounded in and emerging from "thick" CA descriptions have been effectively utilized (e.g., see Clayman & Heritage, 2002a, 2002b; Heritage & Robinson, 2006), the present investigation does not implement such a strategy when working with single or aggregate cases.
5. Whenever possible it is, of course, preferable that readers have audio and/or video access to complement their inspections of transcribed interactions. Increasingly, online access to digitized clips is available across varying researchers' websites. Another and very recent alternative appears in the special issue of the *Journal of Communication* (2002, 52/3), focusing on relationships among verbal and nonverbal communicative behaviors. A DVD accompanies this issue, containing digitized video clips of excerpts analyzed by several authors. Unfortunately, restrictions on access to the family phone calls analyzed herein do not currently allow for such innovative possibilities. However, a project is underway wherein permission is being sought to provide readers with selected and anonymous excerpts from the Malignancy corpus.
6. Years later, Kendon observed:

   The natural history approach proposed detailed description of whatever could be observed in an interaction. Since what was sought for was an understanding of the natural orderliness of interaction, observations must be in terms of what is there to be observed, not in terms of pre-established category systems. To decide what will be measured and counted before this is done will prevent the very understanding that is sought. (1990, p. 20)

7. Listed among researchers collaborating with Bateson was Ray Birdwhistell, who instructed Erving Goffman as an undergraduate, and they eventually became colleagues at the University of Pennsylvania (see Leeds-Hurwitz, 1987, 2005). A useful comparison of Erving Goffman's approach to the study of "the interaction order", with conversation analytic orientations to social interaction, can be found in Drew and Wootton (1988).

II

INITIAL CONVERSATIONS ABOUT MOM'S DIAGNOSIS

3

BETWEEN DAD AND SON

Delivering, Receiving, and Assimilating Bad Cancer News

Analysis begins at the beginning: The opening one and one-half minutes of the first call wherein dad informs son, for the first time, that "It is malignant". Occurring approximately 40 seconds into call #1, these are pivotal moments in the family's delivery and reception of bad news about mom's cancer:

1) SDCL: Malignancy #1:1

```
1    Son:    What's up.
2    Dad:    .hh The tum:or:: that is the:: uh adrenal gla:nd tumor
3            tests positive.=It is: malignant.
4    Son:    O:kay? =
```

This excerpt, and the sequential environment it is embedded within, is examined in more detail as the chapter unfolds. A few preliminary observations, however, begin to make clear that dad is responding to son's prior "What's up." as a bearer of news. Son is not fully informed about mom's diagnosis, and as will become evident (see Excerpt 8, below), dad relies on information drawn from talking directly with the doctor who initially delivered the news to dad and mom. By enacting technical language employed by medical practitioners, dad's announcement provides biomedical characterizations of this multifaceted and carefully delivered news. Following a description of the tumor testing "positive" (lines 2-3), dad's "It is: malignant". clarifies the upshot of this information for son's hearing. He also refrains (with "It") from referring to the problem as "cancer."

And by responding to dad's news with "O:kay?=", son is neither agreeing with dad nor treating his news as "good"—that is, where the literal equivalent of "okay" is synonymous with "everything is all right" (see Beach, 1993b, 1995a, 1995b; Pillet-Shore, 2003). Nor is son hearably displaying emotion or marked concern. Rather, although son acknowledges dad's prior description, he will be shown to rely on this "O:kay?=" when moving to ask a subsequent question about the location of mom's tumor.

Just as dad addresses *details and facts* about mom's diagnosis, so does son respond in kind by beginning to pursue a biomedical issue (i.e., tumor location). Readers may conclude that these are indeed *stoic* moments and as such are somewhat atypical, strange, or even indifferent: How could family members, in the midst of managing bad cancer news,

41

withhold substantial expression of personal and/or emotional reactions to mom's diagnosis? Maynard observes that the stoic response to bad news is recruited as a

> device to contain the impulse to *flood out* (Goffman, 1961, 55) or display strong affect, such as crying. That is, the stoic response is often paired with emotionality in various ways...there can be emotional "leakage" in an otherwise stoic response, which often merely delays an episode of crying. . . . Deliverers, we shall see, sometimes intentionally, often inadvertently, encourage stoicism on the part of their recipients. (1992, pp. 120-121)[1]

These observations begin to identify how speakers interactionally manage circumstances to constrain crying and emotional outbursts. In 911 emergency (see Whalen & Zimmerman, 1998) and clinical settings similar findings have been forwarded (see Beach & LeBaron, 2002; Heath, 1986, 2002).

This chapter extends Maynard's (e.g., 1996, 1997, 2003) work on News Delivery Sequences (NDS's) as a backdrop for revealing how dad, mom, son, aunt, gramma and others communicate as *primary and consequential family members.* In this and subsequent chapters, they will be shown to collaborate in enacting their familial structure as "participants in conversation produc[ing] the visibility of these relationships . . . as a new world comes into being through an episode of news, participants to the presentation ineluctably build or rebuild particular forms of affiliation with one another" (2003, pp. 121-122).

Attention is first drawn to establishing the interactional organization of NDS's. Particular and identifying features of distant to close relationships will be addressed. Distinctions will also be made between first-, second-, and third-party news—for example, how dad talks with son about non-present mom (this chapter), how mom talks with son about her illness (Chapter 4), how son talks with his ex-wife about mom (Chapter 5), and a larger collection of NDS's across the phone call corpus (e.g., see Chapter 6). In this chapter, the following social actions between dad and son, during the initial one and one-half minutes of the first call, will be examined: (a) initiating, forecasting, and working up to the bad news, (b) delivering and responding to mom's diagnosis, and (c) assimilating news about the malignancy (i.e., clarifying, receiving, and gradually realizing the consequences of such news). Specific attention will be given to social actions comprising their *stoic* responses, in part as coping devices for dealing with bad and otherwise ambiguous news about mom's cancer diagnosis.

BAD NEWS, COMMUNICATION, AND CANCER

Informing and being informed about bad news events can significantly alter how individuals experience and manage the routine affairs of everyday life. Bad news is "a rupture to the fabric of daily existence . . . a vehicle for understanding the social organization of the objective-seeming features of everyday life. Bad news can dissolve the obdurate orderliness of the social world" (Maynard, 1996, pp. 4-5).

When contrasted with bad news events among *friends and acquaintances* (see Beach, 1996; Holt, 1993; Maynard, 1996, 1997, 2003), a central question arises: What, if anything, is distinctive about how this dad and son (and family members more generally) deliver and receive bad cancer news? For example, Holt (1993) reveals patterns underlying how friends and acquaintances structure "death announcements" during routine phone calls. In occasioning and delivering such delicate news, speakers not only work to announce and receipt another's death, but eventually co-produce *bright side* sequences wherein inherently bad news is balanced with *hope* and *optimism* about the future (key actions addressed throughout this book, but especially in Chapters 12 & 13). One implication of Holt's (1993) study is the need to examine how recipients close to the news organize bad news events, interactions such as those enacted by dad-son as primary and consequential family members.[2]

In a related study, Maynard (1996) examined over 100 narratives drawn from bad news experiences generated from interviews, students' reconstructions, published stories, and journalistic accounts. Attention is given to different strategies for delivering bad news (i.e., forecasting, stalling, and being blunt), as well as impacts alternative approaches had on recipients' abilities to realize, come to grips with, and/or misapprehend the news. For example, in the ways that *forecasting* offers some warning or advance indication of bad news without keeping recipients indefinitely suspended or being too abrupt, it was found to aid recipients' realizations that their world is being fundamentally altered. Equally important is understanding how deliverers and recipients work together when handling the consequences of such bad news.

The present inquiry broadens this narrative evidence: The delivery and reception of bad news is anchored in real time contingencies of practical action between family members. Key actions, such as how various cues and clues comprise forecasting as a "relational structure of anticipation" (Maynard, 1996, p. 109), and how realization might be understood as a mutually elaborated process embedded within approaching, announcing, and assimilating bad news, can be addressed through close examination of the dad-son interaction below.

Occasioning the News

Working with a corpus of over 100 recorded and transcribed good and bad news deliveries (drawn from a wide variety of speakers, topics, settings, and predicaments), Maynard (1997, 2003) has observed that although news informings display universal features (several of which are addressed below), such features are neither dependent on the events themselves nor rigidly enacted. Rather, news deliveries and their receipts are part of a generic NDS through which participants assemble matters or events in the world as *news for them* of a particular kind. Produced contingently in real-time, NDS's get coenacted within and across turns at talk through the mutual articulation of in-course interactional adjustments.

Understanding how news gets managed exposes how social relationships get enacted in diverse ways, including how speakers (a) contingently display differential knowledge of the circumstances described, (b) describe the event by explicitly naming it or not (e.g., both the cancer itself and its diagnosis), and (c) construct the valence accorded to the "news", for example, through lexical (word) choice, intonational contours, and other prosodic markings (see Freese & Maynard, 1998; Schegloff, 1998). These demonstrations of social relationships are *reflexive* in the ways speakers work together to visibly accomplish their social identities, backgrounds, and fundamental understandings of "news" for each interactional participant.

News About Distant and Close Relationships

Moving beyond individuals' self-reported and written narratives to analysis of a large corpus of recorded and transcribed good and bad news deliveries, Maynard (1997) has substantiated a basic interactional pattern comprising News Delivery Sequences (NDS's). Though not rigidly enacted across diverse speakers, topics, settings, and predicaments, the following social actions routinely get achieved:

> **TIE:**   Topic Initial Elicitor (e.g., How's things?)
> **INI**   Itemized News Inquiry (e.g., Is something up?)
>   ↓
> 1 →   Announcement
> 2 →   Response
> 3 →   Elaboration
> 4 →   Assessment

Extending Button and Casey's (1985) work on how topics get initiated, an NDS may be pursued with a particular news inquiry (INI, e.g., "How is Dez anyway?"), or more generally (TIE, e.g., "What's new with you?"). The news may also be directly announced, as in Excerpt (2), as both L and M construct a distant relationship with "old Mrs. Cole":

2) H4Ba/Holt:X(C)1:1:1:2 (Maynard 2003, 128)

```
 1 L:1→      OH: uh:m (0.6) ≠Old Missiz Co:le is very ill d'you
 2           'member Philip Co:le, Carol's: (.) husba:n[d?
 3 M:2→                                      [↑Oh ↓ye:s?
 4           Ye-:s.
 5           (.)
 6 L:3→      She had a stroke in Cary last wee[k.
 7 M:4→                                        [↑Oh: ↓dea-:r.
 8 L:3→      And she seems t'be faili:ng
 9 (M):      °°(     )°°
10           (0.7)
11 M:        She's ↑ (quite'n) old lady wasn't she.
```

With L's reference to Phillip Cole (line 2), M is able to recognize a person known-in-common and respond with "↑Oh ↓ye:s?" in (2→). The eventual bad news, that Old Mrs. Cole had a "stroke" last week and "seems t'be faili:ng", is then elaborated by L in (3→). Following her "↑Oh: ↓dea-:r." (4→), a "standardized" assessment of the news (Maynard, 1997), M further reveals her limited relationship with the ill person by soliciting confirmation (line 11) that Mrs. Cole was indeed an "old lady".

Below, J and L display shared yet limited knowledge about a third party apparently diagnosed with "cancer":

3) (H26B/Holt:088:1:8:4—Maynard 1995, p .5)

```
 1 J:INI→    How is Gay Ma[rtin  ]
 2 L:1→                   [a-a-a-] Well she's (.) ^out'v^ hospit'l
 3 1→        v no [:w,]
 4 J:2→           [Is ] [she]
 5 L:3→               [ a]nd uh- you know it is: it is I thin:k v cancer
 6 J:4→      .tch v(w)e-:-:-o:-:ll
```

In response to J's specific inquiry about "Gay Ma[rtin" (INI→), L announces some "good news" in (1→) and J responds in a mildly surprised manner (2→). Next, and with some dysfluency and uncertainty, L elaborates with some "bad news" by stating "you know it is: it is I thin:k / cancer" (3→), which J assesses with some sadness (4→).

In Excerpt 3 (above), these speakers display some familiarity and concern with Gay Martin's condition by marking the news as worthy to inquire, report, and briefly comment upon. However as deliverer and recipient of the news, neither L nor J display that, or how, they may be affected by Gay Martin's having cancer. This stance is evident through both the standardized receipts and assessments provided by J (2→, 4→), and L's cautious report that she has "cancer". As noted in (3→), L's hesitation also displays uncertain knowledge, revealing further *distance* from the person and associated cancer problems. Thus, both speakers construct the news as events happening to someone else, *but not as consequential for themselves*: Neither L nor J claim ownership of the news as persons embroiled in the illness circumstances being reported on.

In contrast with Excerpt 1 (above) between dad and son, it should also be noted that talking about Old Mrs. Cole and Gay Martin were not the reasons for the calls. Rather, in Excerpt 2, L's "OH: uh:m" (1→) is a just-remembered and mid-conversation announcement. Similarly, in Excerpt 3 J's query about Gay Martin is not a primary reason for the call, but is an emergent topic as the call progresses. These moments thus stand in marked contrast with many of the NDS's in the Malignancy corpus (including those examined in this chapter), which do not reveal this by-the-way flavor. In the Malignancy corpus, the purpose of calling most often involves updating and discussing Mom's condition as the primary reason for initiating contact with a family member.

Sharing Knowledge and Concerns about Third Parties

In Excerpt 4 (below), with "Oh ^ dea:r" (line 7) L displays being unaware that Geoff is sick and queries about him (INI→):

4) (H17B/Holt:88:2:3:1 — Maynard 1997, 96–97)

```
 1 S:     Oh: Leslie sorry (.) beh to bother you? ∞h[h
 2 L:                                             [Oh: right
 3 S:     ^Could you a::sk Ski:p if- ∞hmhat- when you go: to
 4        this meeting tomorrow ∞hm could'e give Geoff:
 5        Haldan's a↓pologies through sickness?
 6        (.)
 7 L:INI→ ^Ye:s:. Yes. Oh [^dea:r what's the ^ ma]tter with Geeoff.
 8 S:                     [  Uh I  met)  ]
 9        (.)
10 S:1→   Well'e he's got this wretched um (0.3) he's got this
11  1→    wretche[d
12 L:1→          [d go[ut.h
13 S:1→              [gout.
14 L:2→   Oh: v ye[s. .hhhh
15 S:3→           [An' he-eh he: he's right flat on iz ba:ck.
16 L:4→   Ah: : : :. Poo:r Geoff
```

As S proceeds to announce something "wretched" in (1→), L reveals her prior knowledge by assisting S with a word search and simultaneously producing "gout". Although L had recalled being informed of Geoff's "gout", in (2→) she responds by treating as news its association with the "sickness" (see Maynard, 1997, p. 126). Following S's further elaboration on Geoff's condition (3→), L provides a sympathetic assessment with "Ah: : : :. Poo:r Geoff" (4→).

Contrasted with Excerpts 2 and 3 (above), L and S reveal shared knowledge about the third party, and their concerns about Geoff are more apparent: Geoff's sickness is emphasized with the "wretched" description offered by S (lines 10–11), followed by "he's right flat on iz ba:ck" (line 15). And the assessment in L's stretched and emphasized "Ah: : : :. Poo:r Geoff" (line 16) is offered with some intensity. In these ways, L and S construct themselves as informed and affected by the updated news about Geoff's "gout". But their delivery and response to the news is focused more on difficulties Geoff appears to be faced with in coping with *his* medical condition, rather than on how L and S are impacted by his sickness.

Consequential and Primary Figures in the News

Speakers can display concern for others' health problems, as overviewed in Excerpts 2-4 (above), yet at the same time exhibit distance and thus minimal personal impact from removed circumstances. These types of involvements can be contrasted with those where the deliverer and/or recipient of the news is a consequential and/or primary figure in the events being reported on. In Excerpt 5 (below), son calls long distance and requests a particular update (INI→), which gramma treats as a solicitation of information about "mother" (1→):

5) SDCL: Malignancy #35:2

1	Son:	INI→	.hh Is something u̱p?
2	Gramma:1→		Well your mother came home on Friday yesterday.
3	Son:	2→	O::h.
4	Gramma:3→		Uh- Friday.
5	Son:	4→	Wow. Well that's good.

Here gramma displays the ability to discern that son's ."hh Is something u̱p?" was in reference to updated news about "mother". This news was hers to deliver (1→), even though such information was about "your mother"—a familial reference explicitly naming son as a primary figure.[3] And with "came home" gramma invokes shared yet unstated knowledge (i.e., about the hospital), information that son's "O::h." (2→) receipts as a change of state in his understanding (Heritage, 1984a) but not a source for confusion or misunderstanding. Following gramma's repeat of "Friday" (3→), son upgrades with both marked surprise ("Wow.") and positive assessment (4→).

Speakers claiming access to events, such as gramma, may also produce *narratives* about their experiences when announcing and/or elaborating the news (see Maynard, 2003, Ch. 5). One instance appears below:

6) H08B (Maynard, 2003, 130)

1 L:1→	.hh Well I've ↑written to you in the letter
2	Ḵatharine's: ↓f̱ace is still hurting he̱:r?
3	(.)
4 M:2→	↑Oh ↓dea:r.=
5 L:3→	=S̲o uhm: she's going t'see our d̲octor when she comes
6	ho[me
7 M:	[( )
8	(0.3)
9 L:3→	.hh An' I'll g̲et her f̲ixed up with a d̲e:ntist too̱:.
10	(0.7)
11 M:4→	Oh w't a̱ ↓nuisance isn't ↓it. Is it̲ ↓ey̲:e tee̱:th?

By referencing an already written letter to her mother or "Mum" (M), L mentions a problem that Katharine (L's daughter) was having with her face. That such a problem was worth reporting demonstrates L's own involvement and thus relationship with Katharine.

Following M's receipt (2→), a standardized oh-prefaced assessment (see Heritage, 1998), L expands with a narrative (lines 5-6 & 9) in which she portrays herself as a *caregiver*: Katharine will see "our d˙ctor when she comes home", <u>and</u> she (L) will arrange a visit with a dentist as well.

Notice also that before inquiring about Katharine's teeth, M's "Oh w't <u>a</u> ↓nuisance isn't ↓it" (4→) addresses L's predicament and experiences. In these ways, L and M have collaborated in displaying concern about Katharine (the primary figure), but also in revealing L to be a more consequential figure in the news being updated and assessed.

SUMMARY: NEWS DELIVERY SEQUENCES AND "RELATIONAL" ISSUES

To summarize Excerpts 2-6 (above), a glimpse is provided of how it is possible that speakers involved in delivering and receiving news can exhibit distance and first-hand knowledge about newsworthy persons and circumstances. More distant relationships are evident as participants refrain from showing any (or minimal) consequentiality for them. The ability to know about, understand, and display concerns for others' health status is also limited. However, straightforward delivery and receipt of the news can occur among primary as well as less involved individuals tracking the news. In Excerpt 5 (above), when gramma informs son that mom came home (i.e., from the hospital), it is apparent that such a news update can also be abbreviated—even for family members who are more primary figures and therefore more likely to be impacted by the news. Although mom's return from the hospital was newsworthy, it was not treated (at least in relation to other news about mom) as deserving more attention or concern. The closer the relationship with the person figuring most prominently in the news, however, the more apparent are participants' methods for displaying concern and being personally affected by the circumstances reported on.

Other "relationship" issues become relevant when examining distance and closeness in the delivery and receipt of news. One barometer of intimacy, for example, is a greater likelihood that identification with a situation is revealed through actions tailored to unique individuals and events (e.g., through sympathy, compassion, excitement, willingness to help through caregiving). Deliverers and recipients of news exhibit the importance of their relationships to primary figures being talked about, and the very predicaments they are describing, as entitlements (Sacks, 1984b, 1992) to speak from personal experience about circumstantial details. Similarly, *relational history* becomes apparent as reportings are anchored within prior and shared experiences with primary figures in the news and with those who have established relationships with these newsworthy individuals. As with dad and son below, it also should not be overlooked that as primary yet absent persons (i.e., mom) are being discussed, it inevitably remains for the news participants themselves to manage their relationship with one another.

In the data above, by displaying differential knowledge about the events being reported and reactions to such news, speakers enact their social relationships with one another and the absent third parties (e.g., Gay Martin and mother). The following analysis, of how talk about cancer gets initiated during the first of a series of phone calls, compliments Maynard's (1997) extensive collection of *episodic* moments by investigating a *longitudinal* collection of family conversations addressing family cancer. A transcription of the opening moments of the first phone call, between dad and son, appears below:

7) **SDCL: Malignancy #1:1-2 ((1:24))**

((Ring))
```
 1    Dad:    Hello.
 2    Son:    Ola::.
 3            (0.5)
 4    Dad:    (.h) Como esta:? =
 5    Son:    = A:hh bien, bien? y tu::?
 6    Dad:    A::::hh (pt) yeah. $ he heh heh $ [ w h ] atever. =
 7    Son:                                     [(tsh)-]
 8            = Ran out already, h[ uh ] ?
 9    Dad:                        [Ra::n] out. We:ll, >late in the da:y<
10                     [ my::,  ]
11    Son:    [Ya gotta ] get past the como es↑ta: Pop come on.=
12    Dad:    = Ah°gch°. We(ll) (0.7) °.hh° l(h)a:te in the day.°hh°=
13    Son:    =Yeah I guess:, I'll forgive you this[ time.  ]
14    Dad:                                         [ °(.hh)° ]O:kay.
15    Son:    [°See to it-°]
16    Dad:    [ I'll be sh ]arper tommorow. =
17    Son:    = > See to it it doesn't happen again. <
18    Dad:    O:ka(h)y.
19    Son:    What's up.
20            (0.6)
21    Dad:    pt(hh) They ca:me ba:ck with the::: hh needle biopsy
22            results, or at least in part:.
23    Son:    °Mm hm:°
24    Dad:    .hh The tum:or:: that is the:: uh adrenal gla:nd
25            tumor tests positive.=It is: malignant.
26    Son:    O:kay? =
27    Dad:    = .hhh a::hh(m)=
28    Son:    = That's the one above her kidney?
29    Dad:    Yeah-
30            (0.3)
31    Son:    °pt° Oka:y, ah gee I didn't even re:alize there was a
32            tu:mor there. I knew sh[e had a ↑pr ]oblem. =
33    Dad:                           [ We:ll okay.]
34    Son:    = I thought it [w a s , ]
35    Dad:                   [ May-] (.) ma:ybe I'm not saying it
36            right. .hhh There is- I don't kno:w that there is a
37            tumor there. They nee:dle biopsied the adrenal gla::nd.=
38    Son:    = O:°[kay.°]
39    Dad:         [I gue]ss °that's what I should say° .hhh and tha:t
40            one came back testing positive.
41    Son:    Mm:k(h)a:y,
42    Dad:    pthh They di:d u:hh double needle biopsy of the(0.2)
43            lu:ng. .hh That one they do no:t have the results on.
44            (0.6)
45    Son:    °Je:[sus.°]
46    Dad:        [ pth ]h So: the doctor was in there tonight about
47            (.) sevenish:. .hhhh And he said ba:sically that >ya
48            know< ye:s she has a malignant tu:m- um she has a
49            mali:gnancy i:n: the: adrenal gland. = >He said< .hhhh
50            ((continues))
```

FORECASTING AND PREMONITORING BAD NEWS

As noted in Excerpt 1 (above), it is not until lines 24-25 that dad actually informs son "It is: malignant.". By first examining the outset of the phone call (lines 1-18) in some detail, beginning with son's initiation and dad's response to a Spanish greeting, it becomes clear how talk in a phone opening gives rise to opportunities for dad to *foreshadow*, and son to *realize*, the seriousness of matters associated with mom's diagnosis (lines 19→):

8) SDCL: Malignancy #1:1

```
      ((Ring))
1     Dad:    Hello.
2     Son:    Hola::.
3             (0.5)
4     Dad:    (.h) Como esta:? =
5     Son:    = A:hh bien, bien? y tu::?
6     Dad:    A::::hh (pt) yeah. $ he heh heh $ [ w h ] atever. =
```

In response to dad's "Hello.", son displays familiarity and recognition of dad's voice by offering a second "Hello" with "Hola::." (line 2). With "Hola::.", son not only offers a reciprocal greeting but invites dad to switch language codes and participate in a playful Spanish "language game" (Beach, 2000b; Wittgenstein, 1958). Following his (0.5) pause (line 3), dad next displays both recognition and acceptance of son's invitation with an appropriate "(.h) Como esta:? =" (i.e., "How are you?"). Since "How are you's" are typically initiated by the caller (see Hopper, 1992; Schegloff 1968, 1979, 1986), it is of some consequence that dad first queries son with "(.h)Como esta:? =."

As the news about mom is dad's to deliver, his acceptance of son's invitation to greet one another in Spanish extends a sequence referred to as *the Spanish lesson*. Several key actions are accomplished as this sequence unfolds. By expanding son's Spanish greeting, dad does not treat the news as sufficiently "urgent" to directly announce it then and there. Rather than immediately talking about mom's diagnosis, dad momentarily suspends consideration of any technical and medical details. And as recipient of the not-yet-delivered news, notice also that son's initiation of the Spanish greeting sequence has effectively transposed, and thereby postponed, outrightly asking dad "How are you?" Although "How are you's" are more frequently utilized by intimates rather than strangers in routine phone openings, as is the case with dad and son, son has (no doubt unintentionally) created an opportunity to first announce (line 5) "=A:hh bien, bien? y tu::?" (i.e., "Good good and you?"). Compared with "How are you" → "Fine. How are you" exchanges, son's altogether routine response functions to perpetuate an unproblematic orientation to the opening moments of this phone call. For son to respond otherwise to a language game he initiated may indicate possible trouble. In ordinary conversation, for example, when pauses follow "How are you's", a greeting or inquiry is not reciprocated and/or an utterance such as "pretty good I guess" is produced, speakers can be heard as premonitoring (see Jefferson, 1980a, 1980b) and projecting possible problems—actions revealing "special circumstances of some sorts" (i.e., divergences from routines). Not uncommonly, these and related types of sequential ambiguities indicate that "something is up", an orientation that son's actions actively avoid at this juncture in the call.

Son had not yet heard, nor requested hearing (see discussion of line 19, below), the updated and eventual bad cancer news from dad.[4] Prior to this call between dad and son, however, it should neither be overlooked nor discounted that both family members possessed some information and thus background knowledge about potential problems with mom's health. Specifically, son reported knowing that mom had previously been diagnosed with cancer at an early age (and thus was predisposed to a possible recurrence), was recently undergoing "tests", that "biopsy" results were due on or near the date he called dad, and that it was during this period of time that the family was involved in waiting for biopsy results. Such waiting is a common feature of cancer informings among families and friends who closely monitor a loved one's condition and diagnosis (see Kristjanson & Ashcroft, 1994). During "waiting", concerned individuals routinely provide and solicit new and/or updated information about whether "results" are available, and if so, just what they might be.

With these considerations in mind, it cannot be unequivocally stated that son's initiation and extension of the Spanish greeting sequence can itself be understood as purposeful *stalling* (Maynard, 1996)—designed to effectively delay and put dad's possible announcement (and thus son's hearing) on hold. It is not possible to advance such a claim of intentional action by son, or even that son may have been unaware—but influenced or motivated—by his possible anticipation of hearing bad news about mom from dad. Even close examination of son and dad's interactions on the telephone cannot verify that, or how, son's a priori knowledge about mom's impending biopsy results may have shaped his interactional conduct. What son knew, and how he subsequently oriented to talking with dad on the phone, is interesting and possibly consequential for better understanding the initial and unfolding moments of this phone call. But it remains speculative to claim empirically that son purposely initiated a delay in getting to anticipated, but not yet articulated, bad cancer news.

What can be stated, however, is that son and dad collaborate in producing opening actions on the phone that (for whatever reasons) delay consideration of possible and impending news about mom's cancer. Their displayed willingness to play together demonstrates at least a momentary orientation to "business as usual", actions essentially warding off potentially anxious and possible, expected trepidations associated with this family's inevitable "business at hand" (see Beach, 1996; Button & Casey, 1988-1989).

Returning to dad's (line 6), "A::::hh (pt) yeah. $ he heh heh $[wh]atever.=", he first searches for an appropriate response ("A::::hh") but quickly moves to pronounce, with recognition ("yeah."), one or both of two distinct possibilities: An apparent inability to continue in Spanish and/or an unwillingness to produce "Fine" in light of his knowledge about, and experiencing of, mom's circumstances. Because it is not clear that dad understood all or portions of son's prior "=A:hh bien, bien? y tu::?", his offering of a candidate extension of the greeting sequence in English (e.g., determining how to say "fine" in Spanish) may not have been possible. Even if dad did understand he faced the problem of (a) extending the ritual greeting, or (b) responding literally with "Fine", which he clearly did not do. What can be more directly discerned, however, is that through "$he heh heh $ [wh]atever." dad essentially *disqualifies* himself from the greeting with laughter marking his difficulty. He also finalizes his utterance in hearably *dismissive* fashion.

It is now clear that dad's prior "(.h)Como esta:? =" (line 4), produced as a native English speaker with restricted Spanish competency (as will soon become apparent), was more fully engaged in expanding a ritualistic greeting and language game with son than actually employing a "Topic Initial Elicitor/TIE" (Button, 1984; Button & Casey, 1985) designed to query son about how he was doing.

"Late in the day": Premonitoring Bad News

In lines 7 and 8 below, son initiates a series of playful admonishments by treating dad's "A::::hh (pt) yeah. $ he heh heh $ [w h] atever. =" as revealing limited Spanish abilities:

9) SDCL: Malignancy #1:1

```
 6  → Dad:   A::::hh (pt) yeah. $ he heh heh $ [ w h ]atever. =
 7    Son:                                      [(tsh)-]
 8             = Ran out already, h[ uh ] ?
 9  → Dad:                          [Ra::n] out. We:ll, >late in the da:y.<
10                                  [ My- ]
11    Son:    [Ya gotta ] get past the como es↑ta Pop come on.=
12  → Dad:    = Ah°gch°. We(ll) (0.7) °.hh° l(h)a:te in the day. °hh°=
13    Son:    =Yeah I guess:, I'll forgive you this [ time. ]
14    Dad:                                          [ °(.hh)° ]O:kay.
15    Son:    [ °See to it-° ]
16    Dad:    [I'll be sh ]arper tommorow. =
17    Son:    = > See to it it doesn't happen again. <
18    Dad:    O:ka(h)y.
```

Next, in line 9, dad's "[Ra::n] out. We:ll, >late in the da:y< [my::,]" first repeats and offers agreement by emphasizing son's prior description. Yet with a hint of *fatigue*, with "my::", dad moves quickly to excuse and possibly explain his actions. His elaboration is aborted, however, as son overlaps by further chiding dad's Spanish failure (line 11). Dad's next response, "= Ah°gch°. We(ll) (0.7) °.hh° l(h)a:te in the day." (line 12), is marked by an extended pause, followed by an even more noticeable display of tiredness: He *sighs* when uttering, for the second time (e.g., see Stivers, 2005), that it is late in the day—a more emphasized repeat displaying two key features: (a) That the course of action he is pursuing is *in progress*, and (b) that the stance he is taking makes available to son that dad bids to terminate play involving both the Spanish extension and the reprimanding son is initiating and pursuing.[5] Importantly, though dad does not at this moment report on mom's current and impending troubles, his line 12 can also be seen and heard as *premonitoring* and *forecasting* such troubles for the first time. The construction of his turn-at-talk thereby reveals the dual relevance of a tension between attending to the "trouble" and attending to the "business as usual" (Jefferson, 1980b, p. 153).

Nevertheless, in lines 13-18, son further delays exit from "play/business as usual". He first offers qualified "forgiveness" (line 13), in response to which dad offers a mock apology (lines 14 & 16). And intonationally, through a lower and hearably serious tone (e.g., see Beach, 2000b; Couper-Kuhlen & Selting, 1996; Freese & Maynard, 1998; Schegloff, 1998), son next sanctions dad's actions (line 17) and dad offers his assurance (line 18)—actions consequential for moving to the bad news (see Excerpt 10, below).

In the face of dad's displayed inability to speak Spanish, possible preoccupation with not being "Fine", and unwillingness to even playfully be admonished, son's continuations may come off as unnecessarily domineering. An alternative characterization, however, recognizes the "overbuilt" nature of his pursuit as anxious and compensatory: In response to dad's three contiguous responses exposing dismissal and progressive fatigue in the midst of attempted "play" (lines 6, 9, & 12), son is orienting not just to the *presence* of a trouble but the *imminence* of soon-to-be-reported bad news (see Jefferson, 1988). His actions, therefore, reflect situated attempts to enact stepwise progression toward actually hearing, not just anticipating, troubling news about mom (see Jefferson, 1984a).

Summary: Stepwise Progression Toward Bad News

To summarize, in the opening moments of the first phone call in the "Malignancy corpus" and prior to the first delivery and receipt of diagnostic news about mom, dad and son co-enact an extended phone opening revealing hesitancy to move directly to news of which dad was the *bearer* and son the *recipient* (see Jefferson 1984a, 1984b). Though clues were provided by dad that the as yet unarticulated news was bad, his premonitorings (see Jefferson, 1980a, 1980b) of forthcoming trouble did not lead him to announce the news without son's assistance. Yet through forecasting, dad did aid son in anticipating the *negative valence* of upcoming news. And just as the greeting sequence initiated and pursued by son may or may not be understood as stalling, he did not outrightly guess what the news might be, a common feature of conjecturing in the midst of bad news (see Schegloff, 1988). Although dad could have delivered the news at any given point, he does not; bearers of bad news often co-implicate recipients to pursue it (Maynard, 1992, 1997; Schegloff, 1988). Here, son was co-implicated by dad to ask about "it" (addressed in line 19 below). Thus, it is not dad (who possesses the news) who announces it, but son who calls to receive the news that will be shown to actually inquire about an update on mom.

This extended phone opening thus reveals delicately managed and progressive portents of bad news. As dad and son move toward dreaded issues surrounding mom's diagnosis, they collaborate (knowingly or not) in designing their talk cautiously and indirectly (Jefferson, 1980a, 1980b; Maynard, 1989; Peräkylä, 1995). Together, they delay moving to mom's biopsy results and, as an upshot of this *forestalling*,[6] son is positioned to discern information relevant to the valence of possible good or bad news. Though this interactional work occurs prior to dad's actual news announcement regarding mom's diagnosis, it should not be overlooked that (and how) dad and son appear to be coenacting shared ownership of an *ongoing* set of health conditions influencing dad and son as extended caregivers.

Stated more primordially, both son's "Hola::." and the actions it triggers, as well as dad's reluctance to announce the bad news directly, can be heard and seen as *elemental defense mechanisms* against bad news through which critical work is nevertheless achieved: Having not made an "undue fuss about the trouble", dad can now produce his initial reporting as a "troubles-resistant" teller by aligning his report with prior interactional resistance to announce the news directly (i.e., his dismissal and displays of fatigue). Son is now "prepared to track it [with] an affiliative, troubles-receptive hearing", being in a negotiable position to not only move the conversation toward the news *on his own terms* but (as addressed below) influence just "whose trouble it is and, thus, how it will be talked about" (Jefferson 1980b, p. 166). In these ways, a sensitive news environment was thus constructed in which forthcoming topics would continue to be delicately managed.

ANATOMY: SOLICITING AND DELIVERING THE INITIAL NEWS

At least initially, a "business as usual" orientation to the phone opening has been displayed as dad withholds and son collaborates in delaying movement to the news. It was also observed that son's line 17, "See to it it doesn't happen again.", sanctioned dad's Spanish inabilities through a hearably serious tone. Additional work is being achieved here, however, as son initiates a shift in *footing* and *stance* (see Clayman, 1992; Goffman, 1981; Wu, 2004): Son's utterance can also be heard as *terminal* as it moves toward closing down activities comprising the phone opening—an implicit but recognizable proposal "to start the conversation afresh" (Jefferson 1984b, p. 193), verified through both dad and son's next-positioned actions:

10) **SDCL: Malignancy #1:1-2**

17	Son:	= > See to it it doesn't happen again. <
18	Dad:	O̲:̲ka(h)y.
19INI→	Son:	What's u̲p̲.

```
20                     (0.6)
211a→    Dad:          pt(hh) They ca:me ba:ck with the::: hh needle biopsy
22                     results, or at least in part:.
23       Son:          °Mm hm:°
241b→    Dad:          .hh The tum:or:: that is the:: uh adrenal gla:nd
25                     tumor tests positive.=It is: malignant.
262a→    Son:          O:kay? =
27       Dad:          = .hhh a::hh(m)=
282b→    Son            = That's the one above her kidney?
29       Dad:          Yeah-
30                     (0.3)
312c→    Son:          °pt° Oka:y, ah gee I didn't even re:alize there was a
32                     tu:mor there. I knew sh[e had a ↑pr ]oblem. =
333→     Dad:                                 [ We::ll okay.]
342d→    Son            = I thought it [was, ]
353→     Dad                           [ May-] (.) ma:ybe I'm not saying it
36 ↓                   right. .hhh There is- I don't kno:w that there is a
37 ↓                   tumor there. They nee:dle biopsied the adrenal gla::nd.=
38 ↓     Son:          = O:°[kay.°]
39 ↓     Dad:              [I gue]ss °that's what I should say° .hhh and tha:t
40 ↓                   one came back testing positive.
41 ↓     Son:          Mm:k(h)a:y,
42 ↓     Dad:          pthh They di:d u:hh double needle biopsy of the(0.2)
43 ↓                   lu:ng. .hh That one they do no:t have the results on.
44 ↓                   (0.6)
45 4→    Son:          °Je:[sus°]
```

For the first time in the phone opening dad's free-standing "O:ka(h)y." (line 18) facilitates son's continuation by acknowledging, yet also refraining from elaborating on, possible implications of son's prior utterance. Once again, dad withholds from initiating transition to new topic/first informing (i.e., news about mom). Further, the prosodically serious and terminal construction of son's "See to it it doesn't happen again." is hearably projective of (i.e., carried over into, and embedded within) a forbidding "What's up." (line 19).

The emergent and hearably serious tone of "What's up.", following the preceeding and extended phone opening, reveals how son relies on his differential knowledge that indeed something was up with mom's condition—a state of affairs that, as consequential figures (Maynard, 1997, p. 94), both dad and son share considerable information about. It is this orientation that qualifies son's "What's up." as an Itemized News Inquiry (INI), a query focusing on not just any, but particular news that, as examined below, reveals an update about mom as the primary reason for the call, even though it had not as yet been articulated.

A Biomedical Announcement

Following a notable pause in line 20, dad treats son's "What's up." as a direct solicitation of news about mom and offers a *preannouncement* (see Terasaki, 1976) in (1a→):

11) SDCL: Malignancy #1:1

```
19       Son:          What's up.
20                     (0.6)
211a→    Dad:          pt(hh) They ca:me ba:ck with the::: hh needle biopsy
22                     results, or at least in part:.
```

```
23      Son:    °Mm hm:°
241b→   Dad:    .hh The tum:or:: that is the:: uh adrenal gla:nd
25              tumor tests positive.=It is: malignant.
```

By not directly announcing the news, dad's utterance continues to project a likely valence of bad rather than good news. And with "They ca:me ba:ck"—an indefinite, impersonal, and somewhat alienating reference (see Chapter 8)[7]—dad moves to deliver the news to son as a knowing recipient capable of recognizing both who "They" might be and just what "ca:me ba:ck" alludes to. In this way, dad's preannouncement sets the tone and scene for subsequent news, while also being "designed to handle a central contingency in the development of conversational news, which is recipient's prior knowledge of the occurrence to be reported" (Maynard 1997, p. 95). In response, son's restrained "°Mm hm:°" (line 23) acknowledges yet also facilitates a more complete report.

As dad continues in (1a→) he employs the vernacular of the medical sciences: By first mentioning "needle biopsy results", he enacts the responsibility and demeanor of bearing news by adopting technical terminology reflecting a distinct biomedical orientation. Next, dad qualifies with "or at least in part:" as an instruction that son hear the following announcement as incomplete, that is, subject to update and change as additional results become available.

With "The tum:or:: that is the:: uh adrenal gla:nd tumor" in (1b→), dad's deliberate and searching description attends to bodily/organic features (tumor = adrenal gland tumor). The insertion of "adrenal gland" specifies that (a) the tumor described is located within the "adrenal gland", though only one of several possible tumors undergoing biopsy, and (b) bodily location is critical to understanding the diagnosis rendered. As an extension of (1a→), laboratory results are cited as clinical findings giving rise to the possibility of a diagnosis, and a rationale is invoked whereby "tests positive" implies bad whereas negative findings connote good news.[8] And immediately, dad's "It is: malignant" is designed to minimize son's possible ambiguity by both clarifying and emphasizing the seriousness of the diagnosis. While dad further elaborates the language and description of traditional medicine, he once again qualifies by attempting to translate such information for son's hearing: "It" refers back to what is now shared "tumor" knowledge, and "malignant" is assumed to be understood by son as "cancerous" (and by so doing, *not* employing the term "cancer").

Several distinguishing features are apparent as dad relays to son his versions of being informed by medical professionals about mom's condition. As noted, dad obviously does not begin by announcing that mom has "cancer". He also refrains from describing both how mom is feeling and his own emotions about very troubling news. Rather, as dad relies upon technical and biomedical terminology, enacting the voice of medicine science and practice, he also momentarily suspends reporting any emotional reactions to mom's diagnosis. This is not to say that dad totally abandons his identity as husband and father. Rather, he enacts a line of action consistent with being a lay person attempting to summarize medical expertise he clearly does not possess, and as caught up in the process of reporting on medical procedures he obviously treats as necessary for producing a reasonable overview of mom's condition. His biomedical reporting, therefore, provides a resource for simply getting through a news reporting of this magnitude without *flooding out* (see Goffman, 1981; Chapter 10).

Dad's biomedical demeanor is designed in consideration of son's recipiency as well. Repeatedly, dad's actions are contingent and provisional alternatives for reporting, but not commenting on, potentially dire circumstances. By withholding any emotional reactions, yet also managing to instruct and clarify for son the incomplete yet serious nature of mom's medical problems, dad's (1a & 1b→) reveal "troubles resistant" attempts to not unduly influence nor contaminate either the "news" or son's hearing of, and reactions to, such information (see Jefferson, 1980b).

Stoic Response: Clarifying and Sharing the Trouble

The impacts of dad's emotional withholdings, achieved in part through close attention to technical details, are further evident as son responds with "O:kay?[+] That's the one above her <u>kid</u>ney?" (lines 26 & 28):

    12) SDCL: Malignancy #1:1-2
        241b→Dad: .hh The tum:or:: that is <u>the</u>:: uh adrenal gla:nd
        25   tumor <u>tests</u> <u>pos</u>itive. = It is: ma<u>lig</u>nant.
        262→ Son: O:kay? =
        27   Dad: = .hhh U::h(m)=
        282→ Son: = That's the one above her <u>kid</u>ney?
        29   Dad: Yeah.

This utterance is frequently commented upon, especially by those inspecting the opening moments of call #1 for the first time, as a curious and even somewhat strange reaction for a son having just heard that his mom was diagnosed with a malignant tumor. Numerous persons have stated the expectation that an immediate "Oh my God!" or "Oh no!" would be "normal" here. Yet analysis makes clear that the NDS in which son is involved is treated by him as hearably incomplete. As son responds (2→) to dad's announcement, his "O:kay?[+] That's the one above her <u>kid</u>ney?" *withholds* assessment by momentarily disattending dad's "It is: ma<u>lig</u>nant." (see Beach, 1993b, 1995a, 1995b). Having first heard dad's description that there was a tumor within the adrenal gland (line 24), son moves to seek clarification regarding the tumor's *location* in lieu of its diagnostic status and his affective or emotional response to it. Relying on his prior knowledge, and in reference to "one above her <u>kid</u>ney?", son's "location formulation" (Sacks, 1992; Schegloff, 1972) solicits understanding of *place* and its significance for the news just delivered by dad.[9]

  At this moment, son treats the news as complex and thus problematic in several distinct ways (see Local, 1996). By referencing "one" he displays recognition of having closely monitored dad's prior description (see Excerpt 11, lines 21-25), in which the biopsy results were characterized as both partial and focused on one of several tumors undergoing needle biopsy. Notice also that as son seeks clarification by soliciting unspecified information about location ("above"), he does so by relying on the "kidney" as a known point of reference. It is possible, perhaps even likely, that this reference is carried over from a prior description he has heard from medical professionals and/or family members. Finally, by attributing ownership of an organ, his use of the proterm "her" in "her kidney" invokes mom's body for the first time in this phone call series—references discussed more fully at the end of this chapter.

  In (2→) son's inquiry reveals himself as a fully competent family "member" capable of analyzing and sharing the trouble addressed. Though son is not the bearer of updated news, he shares knowledge and concerns about it. As son withholds assessment by inserting a locational query at this key moment in the delivery of news about mom, he is actually *being with* dad. He aligns with dad's inclinations to technically, not emotionally, work through news about mom's condition. He also accepts what is essentially treated as a prior (though indirect) solicitation by dad to continue stoic depictions of the bad news diagnosis. In these ways, son also displays a freedom and willingness to seek clarification in a manner that nonintimates or strangers are unlikely or unable to do.

  By aligning with dad and withholding emotive reactions to such news, repeatedly negotiable opportunities are made available for determining the nature of the trouble at hand (Jefferson, 1980a, 1980b). At this pivotal moment, son's clarification (2→) demonstrates that he is capable of being responsive to dad's stoic demeanor by withholding comments, emotions, and/or assessments about both mom's condition and any personal reactions to bad cancer news. He also further establishes himself as a knowledgeable family member who is capable of sharing the trouble by soliciting relevant details about the news in progress.

COMMUNAL ELABORATION AND REALIZATION
OF THE BAD NEWS

As son and dad mutually elaborate relevant details, the upshots of displaying a shared orientation to troubling news about mom are apparent:

13) SDCL: Malignancy#1:2

```
31 3→  Son:    °pt° Oka:y, ah gee I didn't even re:alize there was a
32 ↓            tu:mor there. I knew sh[e had a ↑pr ]oblem. =
33 ↓   Dad:                          [ We::ll okay.]
34 ↓   Son:    = I thought it [was, ]
35 ↓   Dad:                   [ May-] (.) ma:ybe I'm not saying it
36 ↓            right. .hhh There is- I don't kno:w that there is a
37 ↓            tumor there. They nee:dle biopsied the adrenal gla::nd.=
38 ↓   Son:    = O:°[kay.°]
39 ↓   Dad:        [I gue]ss °that's what I should say° .hhh and tha:t
40 ↓            one came back testing positive.
41 ↓   Son:    Mm:k(h)a:y,
42 ↓   Dad:        pthh They di:d u:hh double needle biopsy of the (0.2)
43 ↓            lu:ng. .hh That one they do no:t have the results on.
44 ↓            (0.6)
45 4→  Son:    °Je:[sus.°]
46     Dad:        [pth ]h So: the doctor was in there tonight about
47             (.) sevenish:. .hhhh And he said ba:sically that >ya
48             know< ye:s she has a malignant tu:m- um she has a
49             mali:gnancy i:n: the: adrenal gland. = >He said< .hhhh
50             ((continues))
```

As son continues (lines 31, 32, & 34), he moves from seeking clarification of the tumor (2→) to displaying his realization about the "tu:mor there". Although son neither argues nor disagrees with dad's prior news, he does persist by imploring and thereby further soliciting dad's assistance in making clear the discrepancies between what he *knew* and what he *realized*.[10] And even before son had completed his turn, it is worth noting that dad acknowledges the problem son has constructed, claims insufficient knowledge about what he has reported (see Beach & Metzger, 1997), and proceeds next to restate "They nee:dle biopsied the adrenal gla::nd.=" (lines 33-37).[11] In response to son's stated doubt and thus problem with tumor location, dad immediately backs off from his reporting by altering his description that a tumor existed within the adrenal gland. Of particular interest here is that dad's remedial action occurs despite its likely accuracy.[12] In this delicate way, dad displays sensitivity by giving priority to son's stated uncertainties rather than pursuing the correctness of a technical description. Dad addresses both the difficulty inherent to son's hearing of bad cancer news and (as noted above) acknowledges that he possesses neither the medical expertise nor ability to fully articulate and defend such a position.

Having been accommodated in this manner, son quietly receipts and apparently accepts dad's corrected version with "= O:°[kay.°]" (line 38). This utterance is produced in overlap as dad continues to qualify by restating "and tha:t one came back testing positive." (lines 39-40). In light of dad's updated reporting that a tumor didn't necessarily exist in the adrenal gland, "tha:t one" nevertheless, and curiously, makes indirect reference to *something* that tested positive. Yet such details are decidedly not taken up by son as his voice breaks in "Mm:k(h)a:y", (line 41), an aspirated and affective recognition marking the news as unequivocally bad (see also Chapter 4).

And finally in (4→), following dad's elaboration that results of the lung biopsy were incomplete (lines 42-43), son assesses the news thus far with "°Je:[sus°]" (see also Excerpts 2 & 3 in Chapter 8). This utterance is discernable as a quietly delivered and sorrowful assessment—something known and relevant to a son as increasing realization of bad news emerged (Goodwin & Goodwin, 2000). Best understood as a curious form of self-talk, offered less to dad than reflecting son's own subdued statement of disbelief, son enacts a subdued but revealing *response cry* (Goffman, 1981; see also Chapters 4 & 10) encapsulating recognition of the trouble such news might foretell.[13]

From son's actions, culminating in "°Je:[sus°]" (4→), it is clear that assimilating "It is: malignant." is an emergent, stepwise achievement. Such a rupture of daily existence is not entirely a matter of self-reflection and contemplation. Incrementally, son's actions reveal an emergent recognition and absorption of the seriousness and potential consequences of dad's report, not just for mom, but also for himself as a concerned son whose "life world" is undergoing "fundamental alteration" (Maynard, 1996, 2003).

Although he initially and actively sought clarification of dad's announcement, his cascading actions reveal an increasingly resigned and emotional assessment of mom's diagnosis. By inspecting such practical actions as son's four "Okays" (lines 26, 31, 38, & 41), increasing impact of the bad news is evident. As dad's news delivery unfolded, son's "Okays" became less proactive (i.e., designed to place dad's prior actions on hold and move to his next concern) and more reflective of the my-world inevitability that, whether there was a tumor in the adrenal gland or not, a needle biopsy produced a positive/malignant result. In the face of such news, it is seen how attention given to technical details can be supplanted with the tasks of hearing and emotionally coming to grips with a predicament each family member is variably yet deeply embedded within.

Following the initial delivery and receipt of news between dad and son, dad proceeds to report yet further details about what the doctor said regarding the adrenal gland (lines 46-49). Both the routine nature of dad's reporting, that is, the doctor making her rounds at "sevenish:", as well as dad's attempts to report "ba:sically" what the doctor had said, are instances of actions comprising *speaking like the doctor*. Subsequent chapters (e.g., 8, 9, & 13) more closely examine how it is not coincidental that talk about the doctor immediately follows the updating and reception of bad news. At or near critical junctures of interaction between family members, doctors get referenced as one set of resources for injecting some sense of stability into otherwise chaotic moments. Beyond the informational value of hearing how treatment regimens will be pursued by medical authorities, family members display being hopeful and optimistic about inherently uncertain and perhaps even dreaded future possibilities (Peräkylä, 1995; see also Chapters 12 & 13).

Moving Forward: A Delicate Future Unfolds

Rather than adhering to a rigid script for elaborating and assessing bad cancer news, dad and son have been shown to collaborate in producing fine-grained orientations to how such news gets delivered, received, and eventually assimilated. The moment-by-moment details comprising their mutual involvements are therefore impossible to determine in advance. And even though the valence of such news was forecast in their extended phone opening, it remained for dad and son to enact, on the cusp of interactional time, whatever premonitions and anticipations they may have experienced individually. Anchored in evolving and contingent practical actions, news delivery components thus "reflect dynamically concerted behavior of participants who offer and seek perceptibly relevant aspects of the news and concertedly provide for its suitable understanding and appreciation" (Maynard, 1997, p. 117).

Near the end of call #1, following an extended discussion of fixing "cars", attention is once again drawn to mom:

14) SDCL: Malignancy #1:20

    Son: We:ll ya think mom'll be up for a call in the <u>mo</u>rning.
    Dad: [O::h: I would- (.) Ye:ah I would] think so. =
    Son: [I thought I'd call her from work.]
    Dad: = Yeah [she wanted to be] =
    Son: [Okay.   ]
    Dad: →= Yeah su::re I <u>ca:</u>lled you, so I'm su:re <u>she</u>::'s gonna be
                  interested in your reaction. (.) So-
    Son: → °Mmkay. °
    Dad: → To at least be sure you're all right.
    Son: → Sure.
         (0.8)
    Son: →Well I'll give her a call tomorrow and (0.5) pt °an a:ll that°.
         I- I gave her a project today so .hhh

Here the focus turns to son speaking with mom tomorrow morning on the telephone. Notice that son does not first announce that he will make the call. Rather, he asks dad if "mom'll be up for a call", seeking dad's advice and assessment by relying on his more immediate knowledge of mom's condition. It is not just another routine call (from work) that son is addressing. Son's advice-seeking action displays sensitivity to mom's ability and willingness to not just speak with son, but inevitably to talk about her cancer diagnosis with him.

In response, dad confirms with "I would think so.", warranting his assessment by noting two relevant issues: That she "wanted to be" sure dad called son, thus, she's "gonna be interested in your reaction". What dad depicts appears to be a normal division of labor in families (and among close friends). On occasions when a loved one is sick, hurt, or otherwise in trouble a person "in the know" may be asked to make calls for them, with the explicit purpose of informing or updating significant others about the news—a right and obligation of intimacy. In this instance, mom now awaits son's "reaction", setting the stage for the following phone call the very next morning.

Son's initial reaction, a quiet °Mmkay.°, offers a reflective if not subdued orientation: What will it be like to speak with his mom about her recently diagnosed (and potentially serious) illness? What might such an encounter portend? How *does* one react to a loved one's health dilemma? Dad's response to son's restrained reaction, and to the inherent ambiguity of what son's "reaction" might consist of is incremental "To at least be sure you're all right". In this way, dad draws attention away from son's "reaction" and toward mom's concern with son's well-being. It is not known, of course, whether mom actually stated to dad that she wanted to make sure their son would be "all right". But her so doing is not inconceivable. Nor would it be out of character for a dad to assume that his wife would be concerned and to work to ensure his son's comfort for everyone's benefit.

Next, son's "Sure." acknowledges that it is indeed a parent's prerogative to care for his/her child's thoughts and feelings. And following an extended (0.8) pause, he reaffirms that he will call his mom tomorrow. Son ends with a quiet °an a:ll that°.", leaving unstated any speculation about what speaking with his mom might entail. The details that son had glossed, and could only anticipate, are revealed in the next chapter by focusing on call #2 (the very next morning).

NOTES

1. The *stoic* orientations exhibited here by dad and son, and as they gradually clarified, elaborated upon, and assessed bad cancer news, might be usefully contrasted with moments involving bad news in clinical settings. Heath (1992) and Maynard (1992) have both observed that although providers routinely provide immediate opportunities to talk about the just delivered news, patients avoid elaborating on the information conveyed—unless their illness conceptions differ from the medical experts' opinion. Even on occasions as these, where a disparate or even conflicting orientation to the news emerges during the consultation, the differential and asymmetrical status between patients and providers is maintained: Patients tend to affirm the objectified and scientific status invoked by physicians.

2. Regarding her data, Holt (1993) observes: "[M]y corpus consists of ten examples in which a teller announces the death of an acquaintance to someone who was not particularly close to the deceased. Also, none of those who have died were under sixty years of age. Thus it would be interesting to be able to compare instances in this collection with examples where the deceased was younger or was close to the recipient of the news in order to discover whether the sequential pattern identified herein is similar in those cases" (p. 211). The present study seeks to offer such a comparison, in that it is the wife/mother who is diagnosed with cancer.

3. Because son lived out of town, and gramma lived in the same community as mom, dad, and aunt, she was at times better informed of mom's condition and care.

4. This information was obtained by reading son's reflections and also, several forms of personal communication with him, including face-to-face conversations, phone calls, and e-mail exchanges.

5. It is perhaps not coincidental that the lexical terms "ran out" and "late in the day" are themselves tailored descriptions reflecting the very circumstances son and dad are caught up in and preoccupied with: mom's life/luck "running out", and her life being "late in the day". Further, as dad later employs "sharper tomorrow", might this also be tailored to soon-to-be-announced "needle biopsy" results (see Beach, 1993a, 1996; Jefferson, 1996; Sacks, 1992)? If so, such actions portray a preoccupation with the very predicament they will soon, and explicitly, address: mom's life possibly running out, uncertainty regarding the later stages of her life, and its ensuing but unknown character. Even son's "Ya gotta get past the como es<u>ta</u> pop" (line 11) may itself reflect problems in working through this local and co-created interactional environment: getting past the phone opening, and its attending "play" relevancies, and moving directly to discussion of mom's condition.

6. Regarding how interactants approach the delivery and receipt of news, Maynard (1996, p. 31) observes "Exactly how participants form and respond to them is needing further investigation for the reason that one person's or culture's *stall* might be another's *forecast*" (italics added).

7. I also treat "They <u>ca</u>:me ba:ck" as but one indicant of the often impersonal procedures inherent to reporting often critically important lab results: Those performing the tests remain anonymous to most medical staff and lay persons' alike, just as little is known or understood about where body fluids and tissues (i.e., "specimens" such as blood, urine, and tissues) are forwarded to nor the exact nature of the procedures being conducted. There is, then, an innate secrecy associated with removed and unseen, yet essential professionals' skills and actions. Further, "<u>ca</u>:me ba:ck" also invokes a decided sense of "powerlessness" for patients, as "results" are often anxiously awaited for yet emerge from mysterious labs on their own time tables, demand attention upon their arrival, and are not infrequently consequential for patients, family members, friends, and medical staff who "await" them to assess and prescribe subsequent courses of treatment (and thus impacts on "quality of life"). Although lab tests/results are routinely taken for granted as a normalized feature of medicine, such procedures are at times also treated as problematic by participants within the Malignancy corpus: Addressing the frustrations and fears associated with "waiting" and "uncertainties" are themselves recognizable as interactionally achieved matters, not sim-

ply individualistic nor mentalistic coping strategies. For reasons and predicaments such as these, patients and their significant others often feel "alienated" within the "medical industrial complex" (see Barbour, 1995; Cassell 1985; Illich, 1975).

8. The contrast between medical science and lay reasoning is once again evident as "positive tests" connote potentially "bad news" regarding cancer, whereas "negative tests" imply what is likely "good news". The adverse is apparent in lay persons' and patients' discourse: For example, "feeling good" is positive whereas "feeling bad" is negative.

9. Concerning how speakers display to one another "their membership in a same community", Schegloff (1972, pp. 91-92) observed nearly three decades ago: "Recognition involves, then, the ability to bring knowledge to bear on them, to categorize, see the relevant significance, to see 'in what capacity' the name is used. . . . And a show of knowledge about a place may prompt an inquiry. . . . It is by reference to the adequate recognizability of detail, including place names, that one is in this sense a member, and those who do not share such recognition are 'strangers.' . . . Where 'trouble' occurs, it can be seen either that the speaker's analysis was incorrect, or that the analysis was correct but the hearer is not a fully competent instance of the class of which he is (relevantly for the place term employed) a member. The occurrence of "trouble" can be most clearly recognized when the use of a place formulation produces a question or second question about the location of the initial place formulation".

10. Although not fully examined here, it is interesting that son's "I didn't even re:alize" (line 31) and "I knew . . . I thought it was" (lines 32 & 34) represent *reverse orderings* of typical "at first I thought 'X' and then I realized 'W'" devices. Originally analyzed in two lectures—by Harvey Sacks in the fall of 1967 (see Sacks, 1992) and by Gail Jefferson in a lecture at UCLA in 1978 (see Jefferson, 2004b)—and subsequently extended into patients' narratives in primary care visitations (Halkowski, 2006), these devices have been found to be employed by interactants to repair initial assumptions, provide mundane explanations for otherwise extraordinary events, and in essence to "normalize" how understandings evolve and are accounted for.

11. Several doctors and surgeons have informed me that a patient's adrenal gland might be "needle biopsied" for two primary reasons: (1) To assess the reason(s) for failure of function; (2) Following an "imaging" that had revealed a growth, a procedure to determine (through biopsy) whether a tumorous enlargement is benign or malignant. Needle biopsies are also performed to mitigate risks and costs of "open" biopsies involving general anesthesia and deep incisions.

12. Just as Maynard (2003, p. 36) has observed that "A recipient's state of knowledge regarding the event figures in heavily in whether it is accorded newsworthy status", it should go without saying that the status of teller's knowledge is clearly and equally consequential. Here, and elsewhere, dad *disclaims* his own knowledge as partial and thereby displays his lay understandings of biomedicine (see also Chapter 8).

13. Invocations of deities—at times abbreviated such as "Gees" (e.g., see S's "gee" in line 31) or "Gosh", but also in fuller form as with "Jesus", "Jesus Christ", "Holy Christ", "God", "Goddamn" and more—are routinely apparent in environments where speakers respond with not just surprise (see Wilkinson & Kitzinger, 2006), but where they lack control in times of apparent trouble. During these moments, speakers are most frequently *not* actively seeking "divine assistance" (e.g., comfort, intercession, and/or guidance) to remedy dire or potentially dire situations. Indeed, speakers producing invocations of deities do not display awareness of their actions and certainly need not profess religious or spiritual beliefs in the very deity invoked. Nevertheless, as revealed across a wider collection of these moments in this volume and more diverse recorded and transcribed materials, such invocations do occur in patterned ways, raising interesting implications for the investigation of relationships between language, interaction, and spiritual/religious orientations in everyday life (e.g., see Chapter 12.)

4

BETWEEN MOM AND SON

Talking About "The Verdict"

The morning following call #1 between dad and son, son called and mom answered the phone. This second call provided the initial opportunity for mom and son to speak directly with one another about her first-hand, postdiagnosis news. Although both had discussed (at some length) her diagnosis and treatment options with dad, it is in this call that mom elaborates her illness experience for son's hearing. In turn, son is now in a position to hear mom's rather than dad's versions of events and, as the call unfolds, is faced with responding to the experiences and bad news mom foretells. From the opening moments of this call, this conversation is marked by delicate and obviously difficult news about mom's diagnosis, treatment, and prognosis.

It would seem reasonable to assume that any conversation between a son and a mother involving talk about a serious illness at the outset of diagnosis will be fraught with a range of possible emotions: fear and anger, ambiguity and uncertainty, despair and hope, support and compassion. With the recordings and transcriptions, however, we needn't leave to our imagination just what might transpire under such ominous circumstances. In the ways talking through a cancer diagnosis is difficult, threatening, and tenuous (or not), it will be evident in the interactions themselves. In this chapter, specific actions to be examined include (a) how mom *forecasts* and son responds to her initial and ongoing characterizations of the news, (b) the construction and consequences of mom's blunt descriptions of the serious nature of her cancer, (c) moments where both mom and son display not knowing what to say about the worst-case scenario mom depicts (see also Chapter 10), and (d) the counterbalancing of hope and despair as interactional achievements, as their conversation cycles in and out of bad news (see also Chapters 12 & 13).

Phone call #1 (and other resources) are used and relied upon by both mom and son as they organize their interaction in call #2. Both possess and employ a stock of knowledge, generated primarily from their own experiences and from what they have heard others tell them about cancer. For mom, that includes doctors, medical staff, and her husband (dad)— for example, his informing her that he had spoken with son on the phone last evening. For son, that includes dad and, as we will see, what he and his wife discussed and thought about yesterday's family gathering (prior to his hearing about mom's diagnosis from dad during call #1). Informing and being informed about another's cancer, and being "in the know", are relative terms. In the opening moments examined in call #1, dad's informing son about mom's cancer is anchored in what the doctor(s) and mom have informed him about her medical circumstances. This can be contrasted throughout call #2, as mom authoritatively informs son and speaks as a person directly experiencing diagnosis and treatment of her own body.

The sustained relevance of what speakers know, and how they interact on the basis of their knowledge, will become increasingly clear as particular moments and longer episodes get examined from call #2. When describing how mutual understandings emerge as a result of speakers making available ongoing relevance for them, Heritage (1984b) proposes an *architecture of intersubjectivity*:

> Linked actions, in short, are the basic building-blocks of intersubjectivity. . . . By means of this organization, *a context of publicly displayed and continuously up-dated intersubjective understandings is systematically sustained.* It is through this "turn-by-turn" character that the participants display their understandings of the "state of the talk" for one another . . . because these understandings are publicly produced, they are available as a resource for social scientific analysis. (pp. 256, 259)

PREMONITORING AND FORECASTING TROUBLES AT THE OUTSET OF THE CALL

The following phone opening occurred between mom and son:

1) SDCL: Malignancy #2:1

1	Mom:	<u>He</u>llo.
2	Son:	Hi?
3	Mom:	Hi.
4	Son:	How ya <u>doin'</u>.
5 →	Mom:	↑O::h I'm doin' okay.=I gotta-
6		(0.6) I think I'm radio<u>acti:ve</u>.=↑<u>Ha::</u>.
7	Son:	He uh $Why's <u>that</u>.$

As son greets and mom reciprocates with "Hi.", their familiarity is revealed through reliance on voice rather than names for identification (see Hopper, 1992; Schegloff, 1968, 1986). What is not familiar are the details and circumstances surrounding mom's recently discovered illness and the kinds of troubling talk triggered by such a cancer diagnosis. This trouble gets displayed and organized in several distinct ways, even during opening moments of this call.

For example, son's "How ya <u>doin'</u>?" provides an opportunity for mom to depart from the canonical "How are you/Fine" inquiry/response adjacency pair typical of many phone call openings in which at least the appearance is managed that no or minimal troubles are present (see Jefferson, 1980a, 1980b; Sacks, 1992). With her hearably reflective "↑O::h I'm doin' okay.", mom's oh-prefaced response—marked by an upward shift in voice that is also extended—provides a standard yet revealing change in orientation to, and awareness of, her circumstances. It is both the initial placement of her "↑O::h", and its intonation contour, that reveal mom's attitude toward son's (otherwise benign) "How ya <u>doin'</u>?" as *inherently problematic*. Regarding oh-prefaced responses to questions, Heritage observed:

> Oh-prefacing of a response is a means by which the "change of state" proposal, carried by *oh*, can be deployed to indicate that a question has occasioned a **marked shift of attention**. Conveying a marked shift of this kind can imply that a question was unexpect-

ed, unlooked for, or "out of left field", and hence imply the existence of presuppositions which could have, or indeed, should have informed the question's design on this occasion. Oh-prefacing can thus be a practice through which a speaker indicates a problem about a question's relevance, appropriateness, or presuppositions. (1998, pp. 294-295)

Son's "How ya <u>doin'</u>?" occasioned mom to shift attention to her state of being and illness. She also treats son's question as though he *could* or *should* have known that she was not doing well. Mom knew that dad had delivered the news to son during last evening's phone call, and that son was informed that she had been diagnosed with cancer.[1] Her response to son's "How ya <u>doin'</u>?" thus gets produced as though his query was unexpected, inappropriate, and perhaps even taken quite literally. Whatever mom may have been thinking or feeling, there is an "inapposite" character to mom's response: "where the information is (or should be) 'already known' to the questioner, respondents commonly answer such inquiries with oh-prefaced responses" (Heritage, 1998, p. 297).

Despite stating "↑O::h I'm doin' okay.", mom nevertheless premonitors bad news about her illness circumstances by offering a "downgraded conventional" (Jefferson, 1980b, pp. 162-163) orientation to troubles. In all such cases, especially during phone call openings, there is fine-grained attention given to "business-as-usual" and possible troubles: "If there is a trouble (which there might not be) and if it is to be told (which might not occur), then it is being deferred while adumbrated in the interests of the business-as-usual of the conversation's opening, of which "pretty good" is an appropriate component" (Jefferson, 1980, p. 163). Both "pretty good" and "doin' okay" (e.g., as compared with "doin' ↑great!") make available a possible but not yet disclosed trouble, carefully straddling the "dual relevance" of ordinary business with other (more pressing) matters.

Giving Voice to a Wounded Body

With her next "=I gotta- (0.6) I think I'm radio<u>acti:ve</u>.=↑Ha::.", mom continues to forecast news regarding her recent diagnosis and treatment. This portion of her utterance delays offering further reportings on a treatment regimen she has already (less than one day following diagnosis) begun, as well as specific details about her cancer. She begins with "I gotta- (0.6)", which initiates a turn-extension that is abruptly cut off. The extended pause then provides an opportunity for mom to consider how to revise her immediately prior response with an alternative description, "I think I'm radio<u>acti:ve</u>.=↑Ha::.". Produced as a troubles-report followed by hearably "mocking" laughter, and in lieu of directly addressing a feeling or emotion, mom exhibits her "troubles-resistant" ability to somehow manage being overwhelmed by a very recent diagnosis (Beach, 1996; Heritage, 1998; Jefferson, 1980a, 1980b; Maynard, 2003)—which, as made clear below, is extremely serious. In making light of her situation by laughing it off, she also exhibits sufficient resilience to postpone describing further troubling, even dreaded and dire, circumstances (see Peräkylä, 1995).

Equally important, however, is that this is the first moment in the "malignancy" phone call corpus where, by referencing a shot she had in preparation for an upcoming bone scan (which she proceeds to elaborate upon as the conversation continues), mom speaks as a patient having just begun and thus subjected to radiation therapy. As described by Arthur Frank in *The Wounded Storyteller*, ill people are entitled to report experiences

through a wounded body. . . . The ill body is certainly not mute—it speaks eloquently in pains and symptoms—but it is inarticulate. We must speak for the body, and such speech is quickly frustrated: speech presents itself as being about the body rather than of it. The body is often alienated, literally "made strange", as it is told in stories that are instigated by a need to make it familiar". (1995, p. 2)

It is a new relationship to the world that mom offers for son's hearing, not from the outside looking in on diseased people, but a personalized perspective of being "radio<u>acti:ve</u>": a nonliteral depiction, voicing only one (yet a significant) portion of the experience of having begun a treatment designed for those diagnosed with cancer.

Even though she is at the very outset of what portends to be an extended cancer journey, mom invokes the authority to report an embodied residue of symptoms (Maynard & Frankel, 2006; Sacks, 1992): She hints at ("I think"), yet withholds elaboration of, the inherent indeterminancy and uncertainty associated with such treatments. As noted elsewhere about medical encounters, patients "make available the impacts of cancer they are currently experiencing. While seeking to minimize uncertainty and solicit assurance about their prognosis is a primary concern, patients also demonstrate being in the midst of varying degrees of emotional turmoil" (Beach, Easter, Good, & Pigeron, 2004, p. 895). Through mom's reporting to son a treatment she is undergoing and impacted by, such disorder can obviously be reported by patients when in the hospital, yet talking with family members on the phone.

In response, while son shares in mom's laughter with "He– uh $Why's <u>that</u>.$", he also provides both a confused and serious response to her self-description. It is clear that son is not yet fully informed about mom's treatment regimen, which she has begun so quickly following the cancer diagnosis. Thus, although son knows mom has been diagnosed with cancer, he displays not knowing that mom has already begun treatment. He is now in a position to hear and respond directly to mom's depictions and to initiate his own concerns about a family dilemma they are increasingly inundated with.

ENTITLEMENTS: CONTRASTING STORIES AND PERSPECTIVES BY MOM AND SON

Mom, dad, and son are each entitled to address the circumstances as their own, that is, as being in the very cancer journey reported on. The more that is known and understood about a specific "cancer journey" (Kristjanson & Ashcroft, 1994), the more "personal" the consequences. Family members delivering and receiving the news are thus differentially influenced by the course and progression of their unique, everyday experience. The following stories by mom and son further exemplify how each is experiencing unfolding events.

Mom: Controlled by Bone Scan Procedures and "the Verdict"

As we have just begun to see only mom—as a patient whose body has been diagnosed and is being treated for cancer—can speak to certain kinds of events surrounding her treatment and, eventually, to news she characterizes as "the verdict":

2) SDCL: Malignancy #2:1

```
1    Mom:   O:h I:'m doin' okay. = I gotta- (0.6)
2           I think I'm radioactive. ↑Ha::.
3    Son:   ts $Why's that.$
4    Mom:   Well you know when y'get that bo:ne scan so they
5    Son:   Oh did [ they    do  ] it already?
6    Mom:          [Gave me that.]
             Yeah they give you a shot. Then ya have ta- (.) .hhh drink
8           water or coffee (.) tea, >whatever the hell you want< (0.4) in
9           vo:lumes of it.
```

10	Son:	Mmm hmm.
11	Mom:	.hh A::nd I'll go down at about ten thir:ty.
12	Son:	Mm::k(h)ay.
13		(0.4)
14	Mom:	So (.) anyway.
15	Son:	Hm:m. =
16 →	Mom:	= Uh (But Pop do-) (.) I realized that I was told after (.) .hhh
17		you left here yesterday, that you had not al:ready heard the
18		verdict we had so. =

In continuing her story (line 4), mom acts as though son knew she had received a "bo:ne scan", an assumption son quickly disconfirms (line 5) . Her perspectives then shift from first → generic → first person references. When mom elaborates about the scan, the "shot" she received, and the liquid(s) she had to drink she refers to herself not in first person (e.g., "I/I'm") but generically (e.g., "y'get", "give you", "ya have ta", "hell you want"). (An exception is "Gave me that". on line 6). Then, on line 11, she states "A::nd I'll go down at about ten thir:ty".

One basic distinction between mom's first/generic person references hinges on her reporting of an experience and schedule (first person) and procedures initiated and performed by others (generic person). It is these latter activities that mom appears to distance herself from—as foreign procedures she does not control and must subjugate herself to. Even when reporting some control with ">whatever the hell you want< (0.4) in vo:lumes of it". (lines 8-9), mom displays disfavor for the inconvenience of being a patient whose plight is hellacious.

In response (lines 10, 12, & 15) son appears to have little to say. But these minimal contributions are meaningful, carefully monitoring and reflecting on the events mom portrays and withholding additional contributions in favor of attending carefully to a story that is mom's to reveal. His "Mm::k(h)ay" (line 12) is particularly revealing. By conjoining "Mm" and "okay"—and with the stretch and aspirated (h) articulation—son exhibits serious and marked consideration of mom's prior ".hh A::nd I'll go down at about ten thir:ty". In lines 13-14 mom next treats son as not having invited elaboration about her treatments nor schedule, but as being impacted by hearing news which may be distressing. Although "going down" for treatments will become an altogether routine feature of mom's schedule as time passes, this first and fleeting pronouncement was consequential for son's displayed realization of the seriousness of mom's illness.

Indeed, mom (lines 16-18) proceeds to offer her own realization that son was uninformed about "the verdict"—a continued foreshadowing of not yet disclosed details about her troubling diagnosis. Her choice of words is illuminating: Some external decision, judgment, ruling, or decree has occurred and is invocable; yet, binding and out of mom's control.[2] Typically associated with the outcome of jurors' deliberations following trial proceedings, a guilty verdict—even a "death sentence"—stands in stark contrast with what is portrayed later in this chapter to be, in all likelihood, a terminal cancer diagnosis. Ironically, terminal cancer patients may themselves be more or less innocent, and certainly unintending, victims of cellular degeneration promoting organ dysfunction and eventual failure. Yet, like sentencing following a trial verdict, mom and her family alike are on the cusp of receiving and reacting to bad news about a "large cell cancer".

Son: Accounting for "glib" Actions and Further Thoughts About the Family

The news mom has foreshadowed will be shown to be unequivocally "bad", yet also indeterminate. Just how long mom might live remains uncertain, and consequences for the fam-

ily are nebulous. In line 6 (below), son responds to mom's pronouncement about "the verdict" by informing her "that's" the purpose of his call:

3) SDCL: Malignancy #2:1-2

```
 1    Mom:    So (.) anyway.
 2    Son:    Hm:m. =
 3    Mom:    = Uh (But Pop do-) (.) I realized that I was told after (.) .hhh
 4            you left here yesterday, that you had not al:ready heard the
 5            verdict we had so. =
 6    Son:    = Yeah that's what >I was callin' to< talk about.
 7    Mom:    (( coughs ))
 8    Son:    Uhm::. (.) Yeah I think ma:ybe .hh $heh heh$ maybe Gina
 9            and I were a little bit glib an- an- an[d  all  of   that an-   ]
10    Mom:                                          [ No::  =  No  =  No = ] (.)
11            No that felt good.
12    Son:    Well good. .hh uh- 'Cause you know we were both- we
              kinda walked out and said ge:ez, .hh ya know. We both
              realize how serious this all is but it seemed like everyone
15            was being .hh (0.8) a:wfully down. .hhh =
16    Mom:    = Yeah. =
17    Son:    = And uh (0.8) pt we weren't enti:rely sure why and we both
18            thought well, .hh =
19    Mom:    = Well.=
20    Son:    =and maybe they're just ste:eling themselves for the worst,
21            and [>I guess we'd already heard<] it.
```

When mom coughs (line 7) rather than responds directly to son's informing, he initiates an
apologetic story (lines 8-9) about him and his wife (Gina) being "glib", acting as though
they may have taken too lightly (i.e., coming off as unconcerned about) the matters comprising yesterday's family gathering. Both his laughter ("$heh heh$") and awkward delivery ("an- an- an[d all of that an- "), which leaves unspecified what they did and how they
behaved, reveal some discomfort about their possibly inappropriate demeanor. Yet in overlap, mom's repeated "No's" exhibit a contrasting position: "that felt good" (line 10). And
to insure that son hears her position, following overlap resolution (see Jefferson &
Schegloff, 1975; Schegloff, 2000), she produces her fourth and free-standing "No". Taken
together, her repeated "No's" make clear that son's ongoing course of action is unnecessary
and should be halted (see Stivers, 2005).

It is with some relief that son states "Well good.", an emphasized repeat of mom's prior
"good". His utterance exhibits a reprieve from any harm they might have contributed, to
already tenuous circumstances, surrounding mom's biopsy news. As he continues to
account for their actions (lines 11-14), son offers mom a reasoned explanation for their
actions: how they walked out and with "ge:ez",[3] apparently, discussed that even though
they realized the seriousness of mom's illness, they considered everyone to be "a:wfully
down.". This is an assessment mom agrees with (line 15), en route to a soon-to-be-launched
fuller explanation. Thus, it follows (but is not made explicit) that their "glib" actions were
motivated by any number of possible and well-intended factors (e.g., nervous attempts to
humorously manage their own and others' tensions, one resource for coping with a difficult situation).

Whereas son reports that he and his wife remained uncertain as to why everyone was
so troubled (line 16 & 17), mom's topic initial "=Well." moves one step closer to addressing what son and his wife did not know. But son continues by reporting what they
"thought", namely, "and maybe they're just ste:eling themselves for the worst, and [>I

guess we'd already heard<] it.". Once again a word choice, as with mom's earlier "the ver-dict", is revealing: Son's "ste:eling" depicts a bracing or hardening for news qualifying as "the worst" (line 17) which, as shown below (Excerpt 4), is carried over and employed by mom four additional times as the bad news is finally made explicit and elaborated.

BUILDING AND RESPONDING TO EXTREME CASE FORMULATIONS ABOUT CANCER

The stances taken by son and mom regarding the news are markedly different. Son relies primarily on what others have told him, and what he has observed in the behavior of family members, to draw conclusions about unfolding events. For example, in lines 1 and 2 (below), son frames "they're" as anticipating and preparing for forthcoming but not-yet-finalized news:

4) SDCL: Malignancy #2:2-3

1	Son:	And maybe they're just ste:eling themselves for the worst,
2		and [>I guess we'd already heard<] it.
3	Mom:	[No it was the worst.] It was the worst. Yeah.
4		The a- (0.6) large cell cancer is- .hhh There's only one wor:se.
5		(1.0)
6	Son:	It's already being de:ad, perhaps.
7	Mom:	Huh.
8	Son:	$Heh heh heh$.
9	Mom:	There's an adenoma type that is uh- °worse°. But this is very
10		fast very rapid.
11	Son:	Mm hm.
12	Mom:	.hh Ah very difficult to tre:at. = There's a very sma:ll
13		percentage of people that that do: uh re:spond?
14		(0.8)
15	Mom:	A:nd we're talkin' uh (0.6) at that maybe °five years°.
16		(1.5)
17	Son:	H:mm::.
18		(0.6)
19	Mom:	So. (0.4) It's r(h)e::al °b(h)a:d°.
20		(0.8)
21	Mom:	((coughs))
22	Son:	pt .hh I guess.
23		(0.4)
24	Mom:	And uh: >I don't know what else to ↑tell you.<
25		(1.0)
26	Son:	.hh hhh Yeah. (0.2) um- ((hhhh)). Yeah, I don't know what to
27		say either.

He then states "we'd already heard it", apparently referring to what he and his wife had just heard family members talking about. But his reporting is not definitive, because the news from medical experts was delivered later that day—after son and his wife left mom and dad's home—making them reliant upon hearing news from other family members pos-sessing more direct information.

A related and notable difference is that son (with "And maybe" and "I guess" in lines 1-2), based on what he heard and observed about family members' actions, offers his claims as a speculation. He indirectly solicits from mom a current and informed update about her condition, one type of "fishing device" (Pomerantz, 1980) through which a speaker may disclose an experience "recognized as situated—that is, built out of particular, circumstantial details of an other's activity" (p. 188). In this way, son elicits information from mom he would otherwise not have access to.

In contrast to son having less direct access to information, with "No it <u>was</u> the worst." (line 3, below), mom begins to assert primary knowledge to speak authoritatively about her own cancer diagnosis. With a modified repeat (see Stivers, 2005) in next turn (line 3), mom repairs and transforms son's speculative understanding to a definitive position about the news. Offered within a beat of son's prior version of events mom does not anticipate son's extension ("I guess"). But with "No" she asserts an alternative position aligning with, yet upgrading, son's position. Both son's "heard *it*" and mom's "No *it*" rely on an indirect (i.e., indexical and deictic, see Hanks, 1992) method for referring to what may initially appear to be the same versions of "the worst". Yet a closer inspection reveals that while son's "it" refers to "worst" from the perspective of receiving bad news, mom's next "No it <u>was</u> the worst." confirms a depiction of an actual type or classification of cancer—a move that son's lack of knowledge constrained him from making.

Mom's utterance is not an exact reduplication (Couper-Kuhlen & Selting, 1996), however, as the emphasized "<u>was</u>" claims a primary right to characterize and advance the telling. With yet another repeat, to remedy the possibility of having not been heard (due to overlap in lines 2-3), mom continues with "The a- (0.6) large cell cancer is-." Typical of many moments where family members (as lay persons) refer to biomedical terminology (e.g., see Chapters 8 & 9), with a cut-off word and marked pause, mom displays some hesitancy and difficulty in moving to describe the nature of her cancer. Here, "large cell" denotes a classification or type of cancer, a lay description that is overly general and indefinite (especially by oncology and other medical experts' standards). Indeed, mom's "is-" aborts further and specific descriptions of this type of cancer in lieu of ".hhh <u>There</u>'s only one wor:se." (line 5), providing a sort of "metric" for assessing the extremity of what she is proposing (see Beach & Mandelbaum, 2005; Halkowski, 2000).

A Joking Response to Bad News?

Rather than move directly to articulating what this "one" is (line 2, below), mom leaves hanging the implication of what she is stating for son's next response:

5) SDCL: Malignancy #2:2

```
1        Mom: It was the worst. Yeah. The a- (0.6) large cell cancer is-
2    →        hhh There's only one wor:se.
3             (1.0)
4    → Son:   It's already being de:ad, perhaps.
5        Mom: Heh.
6        Son: $Heh heh heh$.
```

These moments have drawn repeated attention from students I have instructed who are involved in data/listening sessions of call #2 between son and mom. In fact, over the years, several students have taken the position—at times viscerally—that son's "It's already being de:ad? perhaps." (line 4) is an entirely inappropriate attempt to be humorous: How could son behave at mom's expense during such a sensitive discussion? It can be seen, for example, that with "Heh." mom next offers a hearably fake laugh, treating son's prior utterance as less than funny and possibly not appreciated, which son's "$Heh heh heh$." nervously recognizes. On these merits, students have claimed there is sufficient evidence, in the form of interactional consequences, to argue for the insensitivity of son's "already being de:ad?" formulation.

However, two alternative analytic positions shed a different light on students' position, namely, that son's response was behaving at mom's expense insensitively and/or inappropriately. Maynard (2003), for example, examines instances where recipients offer joking responses to bad news deliveries, as though the news was a "punchline to a joke" (p. 51). On such occasions, recipients may treat abruptly stated bad news in humorous ways, actions distancing the news from "truth" and thus delaying coming to grips with realistic interpretations of difficult events. Recipients may also laugh off and deny the existence of bad news, rupturing ordinary and normal features of everyday life. In response, deliverers of bad news may "counteract that interpretation" (p. 52), similar to how mom's fake laugh ("Heh.") makes available to son an unwillingness to take the situation lightly.

A related yet alternative analysis emerges when I ask students to consider the following: What was son responding to, and with what knowledge resources? Essentially, mom created a puzzle for son to solve, acting as though son might know what "one wor:se" is in reference to. But as a lay person, void of considerable technical understandings of cancer types and their extremity, is it not understandable that "one wor:se" is equivalent to "being de:ad? perhaps."? In this sense, son offers his response as one solution to mom's puzzle, advanced as a speculation rather than a pronouncement replete with confidence and certainty. And for these reasons, I encourage students (and perhaps now readers) to reconsider whether, in fact, son was *purposely* being insensitive or, and in marked contrast, simply trying to figure out mom's puzzle with available common sense: Many persons would agree that death is incrementally worse than even a serious cancer.

Understanding son's actions as responsive to a puzzle mom provided in the prior turn, one requiring a solution provided by son, reframes the position that he intentionally upset his mom—and any attributed blame grounded in his conduct being inappropriate. Such a position requires a mentalistic assessment of son's predisposition to respond, which these interactional materials do not provide. In contrast, a closer inspection reveals that son's response is interactionally contingent upon what mom left unspecified and how, following a (1.0) pause, son produced an understandable (lay) solution to an enigma mom proposed. Might son have said something different or handled this moment in another manner that did not (at least potentially) trigger a "fake laugh" from his recently diagnosed mom? Perhaps. But real-time involvements do not afford the convenience to change what has transpired. Speakers may seek to repair what has been stated, or otherwise seek to account or even apologize for their actions (e.g., see Robinson, 2004, 2006). But son does not pursue these alternatives here, the absence of which further supports an analytic position that his "It's already being de:ad? perhaps." was *not* offered to make his mom feel uncomfortable. Rather, son's utterance was an on-the-spot attempt to assess, understand, and respond to mom's prior description in a timely fashion.

Constructing the Extreme Case Diagnosis

As Excerpt 4 (above) unfolds, it is increasingly clear that mom continues to build a worst-case scenario of her diagnosis. On line 10, she states "There's an adenoma type that is uh-°worse°.", the fifth reference to "worst/worse" triggered by son's initial "ste:eling themselves for the worst." (line 1). This cumulative bad news environment is extended as, in lines 10-14, mom recruits "very" four times to characterize the "large cell cancer" she has been diagnosed with: "very fast very rapid...very difficult to tre:at...very sma:ll percentage of people that- that do: uh re:spond?". In describing how speakers routinely construct situations as *complainable*, Pomerantz (1986) observed how *extreme case formulations* (ECFs) are employed to justify and legitimate circumstances, in their strongest case, as "unfair, immoral, embarrassing, uncomfortable, or in some other way undesirable and/or intolerable. There is a shared assumption that the worse the problem, the more necessary it is to do something about it . . . . as demanding their actions" (p. 228). Through ECFs, mom's stance toward the extremity of her condition is laid bare, achieved in such a way that the investment she has in her failing health is increasingly obvious and compelling (e.g., see Edwards, 2000; Wu, 2004).

An additional and key feature of ECF's, of particular relevance to mom's actions, is how speakers compare their circumstances with others as a method for minimizing their responsibility for wrongdoing and possible blame. In lines 13-14, with "very sma:ll percentage of people that- that do: uh re:spond?", mom shifts from distinguishing features of the "large cell cancer" to how patients in general respond to treatment. By framing her plight as shared by others facing similar illness problems—people who even if they respond well to treatment, have "maybe °five years°" (line 16) to live—mom further evidences the extreme case she is advancing. Acquired from medical experts, she offers an objective, independent, and thus legitimate prognosis providing mom with little choice but to face undesired circumstances.

Though mom does not explicitly state that she may well be a new member of a particular category of ill persons—"terminally ill persons diagnosed with cancer"—her descriptions qualify her as a likely member of persons who face similar fates. Clearly, through mom's talk it is evident that events are on the horizon which cannot be fully controlled, are inevitably uncertain in outcome, and are enormously impactful for mom and family members alike.

Responding to Mom's Blunt Assessments

In lines 13-22 in Excerpt 4 (above), mom incrementally pursues a response from son (see Beach, 1996; Jones & Beach, 2005; Pomerantz, 1984b). When son does not respond to mom's prior reference to a small percentage of people that respond to treatment (lines 13-14), and following an (0.8) pause, mom increases the dramatic impact to "A:nd we're talkin' uh (0.6) at that maybe °five years°." (line 16). After another (1.5) pause, son's "H:mMom::.", and yet another (0.6), mom's voice breaks as she states "It's r(h)e::al °b(h)a:d°." (line 19). At this moment it is even further demonstrated that son is at a loss for words. Following a (0.8) pause, his "pt .hh I guess" is offered (see Chapter 10).

In her depiction and pursuit of response, mom utilizes a blunt approach to delivering bad news. Her orientation is succinct, direct, and draws focused orientation to informing son that her situation is serious and potentially terminal. When compared with forecasting and stalling bad news, Maynard (2003) examines how bluntness may actually inhibit recipients' realization of the bad news (e.g., see analysis of Excerpt 5, above), promoting responses such as joking, blaming the messenger, and maintaining ordinariness (pp. 51-54). The data below provide evidence that an additional (and fourth) type of response to blunt deliveries of bad news is possible—displaying not knowing how to respond, and just what to say, about the bad news:

6) **SDCL: Malignancy #2:2**

```
1  1→   Mom:   A:nd we're talkin' uh (0.6) at that maybe five years.
2               (1.5)
3       Son:   H:mm::.
4               (0.6)
5  2→   Mom:   So:, (0.4) it's °r(h)e::al b(h)a:d°. ((voice breaks))
6               (0.8)
7       Mom:   [[((coughs))
```

```
 8        Son:    [[pt .hh I guess.
 9                (0.4)
10 3→    Mom:    And uh: >I don't know what else to ↑tell you.<
11                (1.0)
12        Son:    .hh hhh Yeah. (0.2) um- ((hhhh)). Yeah, I don't know what to
13                say either.
```

These moments are marked by extended pauses, affective voice breaks, dysfluencies, and explicit statements that both mom and son have little else to say (see further discussion in Chapter 10). In response to (1→), son is reflective and withholding of further comment. In (2→), mom summarizes her prior news delivery with "So. (0.4) It's r(h)e::al °b(h)a:d°.", a formulation (see Beach & Dixson, 2001; Drew, 2003; Raymond, 2000, 2004) comprised of an aspirated and breaking voice indicative of nearly flooding out her emotions by crying (see Beach & LeBaron, 2002; Goffman, 1981; Hepburn, 2004). Again, her affectively delivered, bottom-line bad assessment is followed by an extended pause prior to son's "pt .hh I guess."—literally, an inability to assess the extremity of mom's condition due not only to lack of medical/technical knowledge, but the lived experience of being a cancer patient very recently undergoing diagnosis and treatment (e.g., bone scans). And in (3→), mom states that she has nothing more to tell son. Again, following an extended (1.0) pause—and with some difficulty—son's own choked voice is on the cusp of crying prior to "Yeah, I don't know what to say either.". With "I don't know" both speakers claim insufficient knowledge (see Beach & Metzger, 1997) to elaborate on bad news that appears to have run its course (but indeed has not, as discussed below).

Through these actions, mom and son appear to have completed an initial sequence terminating mom's blunt and bottom-line assessment of the severity of her condition. At least for the moment, neither mom nor son has more to say about unequivocally bad cancer news. They are, however, *sharing commiserative space*: Few words are necessary for expressing their feelings, and reactions, to facing her serious diagnosis together (see Chapter 10). Both mom and son exhibit voice breaks indicative of beginning to cry. In turn, by stating there is nothing else to tell or say about mom's condition, further discussion about the bad news is momentarily averted. Such closing actions appear almost compensatory, produced as aftershocks of having almost "flooded out". Rather than elaborate more details about mom's apparent terminal cancer diagnosis, these few words display that enough has already been stated and that a tolerance threshold (evident in their move toward topic closure) has been reached.

Although these closing actions may be recruited as a resource to briefly offset additional negative impacts of more fully addressing mom's condition, the grim nature of the problem obviously remains. On such occasions, having nothing more to "tell or say" offers only a transitory respite from anguish. As their cancer journey is just underway, considerable and ongoing work remains to talk through the technical details of biomedicine and to manage the distress inherent in continuing efforts designed to confront difficult truths and realities.

INTERACTIONAL DISPLAYS OF DESPAIR AND HOPE

Portions of mom and son's phone conversation are akin to a pendulum swinging between despair and hope (see also Chapters 12 & 13). Though mom had just stated "I don't know what else to ↑tell you." (line 25, Excerpt 4), her utterance prefaces additional talk by next disclosing what she does know and will do (see Beach & Metzger, 1997). The excerpt below begins as mom, with a marked uplifting (even "sing-songy") voice, shifts away from talking about her worst case scenario to visiting the "cancer man":

7) SDCL: Malignancy #2:2

```
 1   Mom:   No there's nothing to say. >You just-< .hh I'll I'll wait to talk
 2          to  Doctor (name) today. = He's the cancer man and =
 3   Son:   = Um hmm.
 4   Mom:   See what he has to say, and (0.4) just keep goin' forward. I
 5          mean- (.) I might be real lucky in five years. It might just be
 6          six months.
 7          (0.4)
 8   Son:   ↑Yeah.
 9   Mom:   °Who knows.°
10   Son:   Phew::.
11   Mom:   Yeah.
12   Son:   .hh hhh (.) Whadda you do: with this kind of thing. I mean-
13   Mom:   >Radiation chemotherapy.<
14          (1.2)
15   Son:   Oh bo:y?
16   Mom:   Yeah.
17          (0.5)
18   Mom:   My only hope- I mean (.) my only choice.
19   Son:   Yeah.
20   Mom:   It's either that or just lay here and let it kill me.
21          (1.0)
22   Mom:   And that's not the human condition.
23   Son:   No. (1.0) I guess [ not.]
24   Mom:                     [ No.] (.) So that's all I can tell you
25          (°sweetie°).
26          (0.8)
27   Son:   .hhh HHHUM.
28          (0.8)
29   Mom:   °Yeah I'm sorry.°
30   Son:   $Well::$ I should think yeah um- (0.2) Me too.
31   Mom:   °Yeah°.
```

The doctor is treated, in part, as a ray of hope in the midst of a threatening prognosis—a medical expert having the potential to disclose good news to counter the previously summarized bad news—one resource for managing optimism (discussed further in Chapter 12). Similar to earlier instances (see Excerpt 2, above), mom refers to herself in third person (">You just-<", line 1) when describing a visit (and possible procedures) conducted by another, the outcomes of which she cannot control—an integral part of "just keep goin' forward" (line 4). Yet the uncertainty surrounding such a medical encounter, marked by mom's voice once again becoming serious (line 5), also creates a scenario in which the doctor could deliver additional bad news, as summarized by "I might be real lucky in five years. It might be just six months." Like the co-presence of good and bad news (see Maynard, 2003), here it is seen that a glimpse of hope is overshadowed by the despair associated with facing "reality"—where good news is living five years.

At this juncture in her cancer journey mom projects a time frame that (and we can only speculate) was likely provided by her doctor(s), and is subsequently adapted here for son's hearing. In real time, the future always remains a tenuous and potentially "dreaded" landscape (e.g., see Peräkylä, 1993, 1995), the details of which emerge on the cusp of enactment and not before. It is, of course, a unique and removed perspective to be researchers and readers sharing knowledge that mom died in 13 months, by far closer to the six-month rather than five-year assessment. But who knows these exact outcomes prior to the time of their occurrence? Clearly, waiting yet being hopeful (e.g., to hear what a doctor has to say) is critically important as an illness journey unfolds (see Chapter 12). Living out these uncertain moments, as family members talking on the telephone, thus stands in stark contrast to the work involved in closely examining how mom and son, immersed in troubles, actually organized their conversations by talking through such delicate topics.

For example, as mom offers her "five years to six months" prognosis, it is left to son to respond to a topic that had just been closed, and about which there was (only moments ago) little more to tell or say. In this sense, son and mom are both involved in opening up a closing (Schegloff & Sacks, 1973). In lines 6-10, similar to Excerpt 6 (above), son again receipts mom's prognostic assessment with a pause (0.4) but follows with an acknowledging and aligned "Yeah.". Quietly and reflectively, mom's °Who knows.°" affirms son's recognition of the truthfulness of mom's assessment. This utterance also extends her prognosis by stating the uncertainty and lack of control which was previously only implied. Despite her first-hand knowledge of being a cancer patient and her authority to claim primary rights to speak about experiences only patients can report, mom's inclusive statement makes clear that she (and others) simply cannot know how the future might unfold. It is here that son offers an aspirated and emotional realization with "Phew::.", a response cry (Goffman, 1981; see also Chapter 10) treating mom's utterance "as something that has the power to elicit strong reaction visible in the cry" (Goodwin, 1996, p. 394; see also Good & Beach, 2005; Goodwin & Goodwin, 2000; Wilkinson & Kitzinger, 2006). Much of Goffman's (1981) analysis focused on privatized self-talk, "exclamatory interjections which are not full-fledged words" (p. 99) (e.g., "Oops!" if something was dropped when working in the kitchen, or "Ouch!" if touching a hot burner). For example, *Phew!* is described by Goffman as one type of "transition display" as individuals express discomfort from such activities as "leaving a hot place for a cool one." (p. 101). Yet certain descriptions offered by Goffman seem to capture how these nonlexicalized or quasi-syntactic (see Jefferson, 1981, 1993) utterances work in interactional environments as well:

> We see such "expressions" as a natural overflowing, a flooding up of previously contained feeling, a bursting of normal restraints, a case of being caught off guard. . . . Unable to shape the world the way we want to, we displace our manipulation of it to the verbal channel, displaying evidence of the alignment we take to events, the display taking the condensed, truncated form of a discretely articulated, nonlexicalized expression. Or, suddenly able to manage a tricky, threatening set of circumstances, we deflect into non-lexicalized sound a dramatization of our relief . . . (pp. 99-101)

The "relief" for son was not in managing these delicate circumstances, but in venting expression to being caught off guard about mom's prognosis. And with mom's "Yeah." she does not just agree but identifies with the emotion son's "Phew." exudes—a claiming of primary rights to know just what he is referring to. Taken together, lines 6-10 are another instance of moments where few words are enough, indeed all that is available, as mom and son share commiserative space while displaying the impacts of bad cancer news (see Chapter 10).

But is son's next query ".hh hhh (.) Whadda you do: with this kind of thing. I mean" (lines 11-12) tailored to mom's ability to personalize the impacts of a negative diagnosis and prognosis? It is not clear whether son designed his question to address (a) mom's emotional coping and/or (b) solicit her knowledge about treatment options. He did ask "Whadda ya do: with this kind of thing. I mean-", rather than "Whadda you do...", but what he "meant" was cut-off and remained unspoken. It is clear, however, that with ">Radiation chemotherapy.<" mom does not hesitate to invoke biomedical solutions to her cancer troubles. Any possibility of discussing how she feels and/or will personally manage her cancer remains unmentioned. She had just cited the importance of visiting her doctor as a resource for moving forward, and treatment options are one natural consequence of such a commitment.

For the third time in less than one minute of conversation, in line 13 a marked pause (1.4) occurs following a straightforward statement by mom. Son then produces "Oh bo::y. (line 14), a serious and reflective assessment which, with mild sarcasm, feigns the excitement that arises when looking forward to some joyful event (see Chapter 10). Having already heard that mom is undergoing bone scans, son further realizes—and makes available for mom's understanding—his recognition that forthcoming trials and tribulations are inevitable. And once again, mom's next "↑Yeah." achieves more than alignment: It avoids undermining son's displayed impact, while also asserting her right to speak as the patient whose body is ill and undergoing treatment (see Heritage & Raymond, 2005; Raymond & Heritage, 2006; Stivers, 2005).

This is further evident as mom continues with a revealing "my-world" assertion, "My only hope- I mean (.) my only choice." (see also Chapter 7, Endnote 7; Chapter 12). As a patient facing treatment for what is likely to be terminal cancer, hope and choice are treated as nearly indistinguishable by mom. Restricted choices needn't eliminate hope, however, and indeed may be the most rational alternative to hopeful (healing) outcomes. With "I mean" mom's self-correction and repair (Schegloff, 1992; Schegloff, Jefferson, & Sacks, 1977) also begins to make apparent that her choices have dire consequences: "It's either that or just lay here and let it kill me."(line 19). It is on this basis that mom justifies that it is *her* choice to avoid passivity in favor of proactive treatment. To do otherwise is "not the human condition." (line 20), a position emphasizing a primal urge toward survival that mom identifies with at such a critical juncture in her cancer journey.

The justification mom has provided is solely hers to offer. She does not seek son's advice. Next, son's "No. (1.0) I guess not."[4] agrees and, following reflection, exhibits some uncertainty but also does not assert an alternative to mom's commonsense position. It is in overlap that mom's "No." confirms son's alignment, prior to her endearing "So"-prefaced formulation—"So that's all I can tell you (°sweetie°)." (line 23)—that once again brings closure to this troubling topic. As before, mom's closing action is receipted by son with an extended (0.8) pause but also ".hhh HHHUM."—an emotional sigh, laying bare his difficulty with hearing and accepting, yet being unable to alter the truth and consequences of mom's position. His sigh expresses a feeling that is beyond words, a curiously exhibited mixture of being frustrated, overwhelmed, and anxious about successive waves of bad cancer news.

Two Revealing Apologies

The emotional turmoil encapsulated in son's ".hhh HHHUM." does not go unnoticed by mom. Following her own (0.8) pause, with "°Yeah I'm sorry.°" she quietly apologizes for having to share news that has caused her son to experience such consternation (see also Excerpts 4, 7, & 17 in Chapter 10). Robinson (2004) has recently examined how "sorry" is a primary method for constructing "social *claims* to have offended someone" (p. 295; italics in original). When apologies are the *primary* action being accomplished, as with mom's "°Yeah I'm sorry.°", they form the first part of an adjacency-pair sequence that solicits a range of preferred-dispreferred responses from recipient. Absolution from any harm being done, or even disagreement that an apology was necessary, are typical preferred responses. In contrast, dispreferred responses include recipients' delay and apologizers' pursuit of some type of preferred response.

In son's case, it is clear that being apologized to by an ill parent can trigger a tenuous reaction. What mom's apology does *not* receive is absolution nor disagreement that her "sorry" was necessary (given not just her recent diagnosis, but an inability to control cancer invading her body). Nor does son delay in a manner causing mom to pursue a withheld and preferred reply. Instead, son exhibits being surprised and somewhat confused. Marked by laughter, son's "$Well::$ I should think yeah um- (0.2) me too." (line 28) reveals how the verb "should think" is a gracious way to soften what he does think—which is not altogether clear as he appears, once again, to be caught off guard. And he continues with some difficulty by abruptly ending his talk, hesitating, and then offering a shorthand *reciprocation* of mom's apology with "me too." Thus, mom's apology does effectuate a confirming display of concern from son, but only following his momentary loss for words and direction—evidence of a perplexing orientation to not just hearing his mom apologize to him in the very midst of her calamity, but trying to discern just what to say and how to express it. With "me too" he only minimally claims the right to know what mom must be experiencing (see Chapter 10). Yet as her son, it is his right to feel sorry for his mom as well as himself, who is undergoing the turmoil of an exceedingly difficult set of topics and concerns in this phone call #2.

Although these touching moments may seem paradoxical—A cancer patient apologizing for telling the truth? A son not immediately absolving his diagnosed mom from any offense giving rise to her apology?—they represent basic and simple facts of everyday life. From mom's apology, it is clear that people abhor hurting the ones they love. Any parent disclosing bad news (health and otherwise) with a child can identify with this delicate moment, perhaps most especially moms and their sons, but caring for caregivers is a universal quality of everyday life: Ill persons routinely care for those who are (or will be) caring for them (e.g., see Frank, 1991; Morse & Johnson, 1991). And from son's response, it is evident that people do not always know what to say to loved ones, especially when unexpected actions (such as mom's apology) arise.

Normalizing and Revisiting Bad Cancer News

Following this pair of revealing apologies, son shifts from what he "should think" to a story where he explicitly addresses what he was thinking yesterday about mom's medication and depression (lines 1-9):

8) SDCL: Malignancy #2:4-5

1	Son:	I guess maybe it's good I didn't know yesterda:y. (1.5)
2		But uh- (0.2) here I was thinkin' (.) gee this medication's
3		sure makin' you depressed.
4		(0.2)
5	Mom:	°Yeah.°
6	Son:	I mean I understood that you would be depressed. But I just
7		thought (.) Wo:w. (0.6) .hh This is really- (.) really hittin' you
9		hard this medication. And I got all do:ne and then dad told
10		me. = And I thought (.) well (0.4) .hh the hell with th'
11		medication huh? tsh .hhh =
12	Mom:	= °Yeah.°=
13	Son:	= It's ahh-
14	Mom:	= Yeah. See it's already metastasized. It's already gone
15		↑°someplace else even.°
16	Son:	Mm hm.
17	Mom:	That's what makes it- >that's partially what makes it< so: (.)
18		ve:ry serious.
19	Son:	Mm hm.
20		(1.4)

```
21    Son:   .hhh hh
22           (1.2)
23    Son:   pt Sh:i:t. hh
24    Mom:   Yeah $I know.$
25    Son:   $Heh.$
26    Mom:   I kn:ow.
27    Son:   Well where's our magic wand mom.
28    Mom:   $It he$ (.) .hh °beats the hell out of me.°
29           (2.2)
30    Mom:   I guess the o:nly thing: (.) I: can do: is (.) after I'm done
31           ree:ling from  (this),=
32    Son:   Mmhm.
33    Mom:   =.hh is find a reason to keep fighting and (.) to keep being
34           hopeful. (0.5) >You know that- that's about all you can do.<
35           ↑That's all a person can do.
```

With "gee" (line 2) son begins to depict how mom's medication was causing depression—
yet another invocation derivative of the deity "Jesus" routinely employed in troubling situations that are difficult if not impossible to control and make people need comforting and
healing. So as to avoid blaming mom for her depression, son repairs ("I mean") his reporting (line 6) to make clear that such medication would understandably promote depression.
He then reports what was initially characterized by Sacks (1992) and later Jefferson (2004b)
as an "At first I thought…but then I realized." practice (lines 6-9)—a normalizing device
for explaining a pre-post shift of understandings occasioned by some particular event (see
also Halkowski, 2006; Heritage, 2002; Maynard, 2003). Here the event being referenced is
dad's informing son (in call #1) of mom's cancer diagnosis. This bad news is obviously a
more accurate and compelling explanation of just why mom would be so depressed. His
lay "theory" about medication as the sole agent for mom's depression has been proven
false. Indeed, with "tsh .hhh" son laughs off what he earlier thought as misinformed and
thus off the mark.

This story by son provides an opportunity for mom to further disclose knowledge
about her cancer, information that is hers to make available to son. From son's contrast of
medication versus bad cancer news, mom next cycles back to announcing additional bad
news with "Yeah. See it's already metastasized. It's already gone ↑°someplace else even.°"
(lines 13-14). As discussed previously, mom engages in a practice similar to dad when
announcing bad news to son (see Excerpts 1 & 10-11 in Chapter 3): A biomedical term
("metastasized") is defined for son in practical terms, that is, "it's gone someplace else
even." With "it's" another indirect reference to cancer is made, followed by a general reference to "someplace else"—in lieu of citing specific locations or organs in her body invaded by cancer—and "even" projects a more serious condition that she next articulates:
"That's what makes it >that's partially what makes it< so: (.) ve:ry serious." (line 16). As
serious as the spreading of her cancer might be, mom's repair interjects "partially" to
emphasize the inherent complexity and threatening nature of the illness she is facing.

As with mom's earlier depictions of the extremity of her condition (see Excerpts 4, 6-
7, above), the sequential aftershocks of her announcement include (a) marked silences and
a lamenting response cry ("pt Sh:i:t. hh") by son (lines 17-21), (b) mom's claiming primary
rights to assert and own her illness (lines 22-24), and (c) a hopeful attempt initiated by son
(e.g., see "magic wand", line 24), extended by mom as resources for coping with the bad
cancer news (lines 25-33)—actions designed to counterbalance and take an alternative perspective on the serious problems being addressed.[5]

Sharing Coffee and Being Together

As son queries mom about how she can "keep being hopeful" (lines 4-6) he acknowledges how tough it must be. With ("I mean–") he also works to insure that he doesn't come off "sounding like" . . . which never gets articulated, as mom announces "Here comes Papa::?" (line 8):

9) SDCL: Malignancy #2:5

1	Mom:	.hh is <u>find</u> a reason to keep fighting and (.) to keep being
2		hopeful. (0.5) >You know that- that's about all you can do.<
3		That's all a person can do.
4	Son:	How can you <u>do:</u> that. (0.2) That's [gotta] =
5	Mom:	[We::ll.]
6	Son:	= be tough. >I mean< I don't mean to sa:y that sounding like
7		a-
8	Mom:	Here comes your Pa<u>pa::</u>?
9	Son:	A:hhh.
10	Mom:	And he has brought me (.) the magic elixir called <u>cof</u>fee.
11	Son:	Ah (.) [well good you cou-]
12	Mom:	[Because]
13		I gotta pour all that stuff through me. = I might as well. =
14	Son:	= You guys can sip some coffee with me [>an' I<] =
15	Mom:	[Yeah.]
16	Son:	= I just poured myself a cup.
17	Mom:	>Wait a minute.< °What honey?°
18		(1.0) ((garbled talk in background with Father))
19	Mom:	Yeah okay. (.) Ju- uh (.) Bring my brown coffee cup too
20		'cause I've gotta drink sixty four ounces of <u>flu</u>id a:nd you
21		know how well I do that. (.) .hhh Yeah. =
22	Son:	= Tell <u>Pop</u> (.) good morning.
23	Mom:	Your son says good <u>morn</u>ing. ((away from phone))
24		(1.2)
25	Son:	.hhh I'm glad you're both <u>there</u>.
26	Mom:	Yeah. (.) We:ll he's (.) He's umm-
27		(2.0) ((sound of father talking in background))
28		Wait a minute. Hold on, <u>hold</u> on.
29		(4.0)
30	Dad:	>Good morning.<
31	Son:	Hi. (.) How ya doin'.
32	Dad:	O:kay. .hh <u>Hey</u> whadda'ya wanna do about your car. Is
33		there any chance you wanna try an jump <u>start</u> it?

Mom announces that her husband has brought her "the magic elixir called <u>cof</u>fee." (line 9), only moments following son's "magic wand" (Excerpt 8, line 24, above). These word choices are curious: "Magic" can be defined as wonder or miracle working, an "elixir" is a cure-all potion such as a wonder or miracle drug, and "wand" is an instrument for performing magical feats. Each description seems tailored to the precise circumstances mom and her family are faced with (see Beach, 1993, 1996; Jefferson, 1996; Sacks, 1992), namely, preoccupations with discovering remedies to what may otherwise be an untreatable cancer. Adapted here by mom in the midst of an otherwise daily routine—drinking coffee in the morning—it is seen just how interwoven a concern with healing and daily life can become.

At this moment, yet another contrasting orientation by son and mom emerges. Whereas son uses this opportunity to propose how sipping coffee together is a form of communal, family sharing (lines 10, 13, 15), mom again speaks as a patient undergoing treatment with "I gotta pour all that stuff through me" (line 12)—a preparation for her bone scan. Following talking with dad in the background, she continues with "I've gotta drink sixty four ounces of <u>flu</u>id a:nd you know how well I do that." (lines 19-20), invoking son's shared knowledge while also her resistance to the trouble by being able to humorously criticize herself.

After son extends dad a greeting with mom's assistance, son further pursues a communal course of action with ".hh I'm glad you're both <u>the</u>re." (line 24)—endearing actions, an attempt to be inclusive and express the importance of being together during this difficult period. As dad is speaking in the background, however, mom offers a limited response (line 25) before handing the phone over to dad. Thus, one consequence of mom and dad's discussion, while speaking with son on the phone, was to limit any opportunity mom had to offer affirmative responses to son's actions. Though son drew attention to sharing coffee together and, importantly, his being glad mom and dad were together, they remained unaddressed and did not significantly impact what was discussed next.

Instead, dad and son exchange greetings on the phone. In response to son's "How ya doin'.", dad's "Okay." minimally addresses prior query en route to asking son what he wants to do about possibly jump starting his car (lines 30-31). Readers may understandably wonder how it could be possible that dad would raise such a topic, and comparatively insignificant matters as fixing cars, in the midst of such a delicate and serious discussion about coping with cancer. At least a portion of the answer is relatively straightforward:

First, son's car was unfinished business from call #1. Indeed, son's car battery—which he assessed with "It's not inconceivable it just went to hell." (call #1, Excerpt 19, lines 22-23)—was the last extended topic prior to closing the call (i.e., by son's arranging call #2 with "We"ll ya think Mom'll be up for a call in the <u>morn</u>ing." in call #1, Excerpt 20, line18). Second, mom did not announce dad's presence until Excerpt 9, well into innately sensitive discussions examined throughout this chapter. Thus, any information dad could have gleaned as an eavesdropping third party was minimal. And finally, talking about cars is one of three prominent topics discussed by dad and son when *not* talking directly about mom's cancer throughout the malignancy corpus. Two other topics—dogs and food—are also recurrently discussed.[6]

TAKING STOCK OF CALLS #1-2

In the previous two chapters it has been shown how dad and son, and mom and son, talked through bad cancer news for the first time following diagnosis. By focusing on portions of two phone calls occurring one evening and the following morning, these case studies have begun to identify organized practices employed by family members as they manage the onset of a cancer journey. Before moving to the interactions examined in the following chapters—for example, as with how son calls the airlines to arrange travel plans (calls #4-9) examined in Chapter 5, and subsequently assumes the role of *news deliverer*, updating and passing ambiguous news about mom's condition onto other family members (as with calls #10–17, and beyond) examined in Chapter 6—the fundamental orientations dad, mom, and son have produced together, in calls #1 and #2, are briefly reviewed below.

Displaying unique and known-in-common understandings to *the news*, each speaker has contributed to the sustained relevance of a single event (mom's diagnosis) across repeat-

ed phone calls, but from alternative perspectives comprised of varying stocks of knowledge. Contrasting *epistemic territories*, and therefore hierarchical rights, have become evident as family members claim access and rights to own varying circumstances surrounding
mom's illness:

1. Dad exhibited primary rights to act as a conduit by reporting to son what doctors had informed him about mom's condition. This news was not announced
   directly, but subtly forecast by dad in the midst of the "Spanish lesson" son had
   initiated (e.g., "= Ah°gch°. <u>We</u>(ll) (0.7) °.hh° <u>la:</u>te in the day.°hh°= "). In the
   way dad did not disclose the bad news until son's "What's <u>up</u>.", he collaborated in stalling (in part) to facilitate son's readiness to hear and realize the news,
   and in constructing a stepwise progression toward mom's condition. And
   when the news was delivered, dad used technical, medical terminology as *stoic*
   resources for putting on hold any emotional reactions to the bad news they
   were facing as a family. His biomedical orientation solicited son to align by
   withholding emotions at the outset of receiving the news.
2. In contrast, mom asserted primary knowledge as a diagnosed patient who
   could speak authoritatively—with confidence and certainty—about *her* experiences and condition. Like dad, she *forecast* to son the troubling nature of her
   forthcoming news ("I think I'm radioactive."). Yet she also exhibited her resistance to the residue of ongoing symptoms from events such as bone scan procedures and, importantly, impacts of hearing difficult news from doctors. She
   emotionally depicts the quandary she is in as extreme—a worst case scenario
   that is "<u>r(h)e::al</u> °<u>b(h)a:d</u>°—and claims definitive positions about an uncertain
   and humbling prognosis (e.g., living from six months to five years). The interactional consequences of mom's continued bluntness include cycling in and out
   of bad news, and with few words, displaying not knowing what more to say.
   Mom and son thus repeatedly share commiserative space, delicate and transitional moments from bad news and new (and hopeful) orientations to the trouble at hand. With utterances such as "Yeah" and "I know", she also claims *epistemic superiority* over the realized impacts displayed by son as he assesses progressive news.
3. In calls #1 and #2, son is a recipient rather than bearer of bad news. He could
   not claim primary knowledge about what dad and mom had jointly experienced, namely, direct discussions with doctors about her symptoms and illness.
   Nor could son (or dad) speak directly to the experience of being a sick person
   and cancer patient. Son did know, however, that mom had not been feeling well
   (indeed, had been diagnosed previously with cancer), recently undergone a
   biopsy, and that the family was awaiting news about test results. The resulting
   stances he takes are therefore speculative rather than definitive. He can and
   does report what he thought and realized about mom's illness (e.g., location of
   mom's tumor above her kidney, what he and his wife were thinking about
   everyone being "<u>a:wfully</u> down", and what he thought about mom's medication making her depressed). Beyond these reportings, however, son is relegat-
   ed to assimilating and absorbing the bad cancer news that continues to come
   his way. His varied response cries (Jesus, phew, oh boy, shit) are situated displays of various orientations to the news, including being a recipient of troubling information he cannot control. Several moments—such as his initiation
   and pursuit of the Spanish lesson in call #1, his reporting about being "glib"
   and his reciprocal apology to mom's °Yeah I'm sorry.° in call #2—also reveal
   that son is managing tensions between appropriate/inappropriate conduct.

In these ways, it has been shown how a son reacts to talking with a dad and mom, in consecutive (evening/morning) calls, and the kinds of social activities involved in delivering, receiving, and assimilating bad cancer news.

The following two chapters draw attention to how son delivers news about his mother to various airline representatives, and to family members concerned about his travel plans and overall wellness. Others' responses to son's predicament, as a consequential figure in the news, are also examined.

NOTES

1. A variety of background assumptions are being relied upon in assuming that mom knew that son had heard about her cancer diagnosis. In call #1 son reported knowing for some time that mom had not been feeling well and had been undergoing tests including recent biopsies. And as examined at the conclusion of Chapter 3, dad reported that it was mom's request that he call son to inform him of the bad news. Son also announced that he would be calling mom tomorrow, and at the very end of the call, talking with dad as well. And finally, in call #2, son explicitly informed mom that he was calling to talk about what she depicted as "the verdict". It also seems likely, therefore, that dad had informed mom that he not only had spoken with son on the phone (call #1), but that son would be calling to speak with her the very next morning (call #2).
2. See also dad's use of the term "elected" in Excerpt 21/Endnote 6 in Chapter 8.
3. Son's "ge:ez" is invoked in a troubling set of circumstances that cannot be fully controlled, even though he and his wife had apparently tried to lighten the mood later characterized as everyone being "a:wfully down.".
4. Other "I guess" utterances produced by son are apparent in Excerpt 3 (line 21), and Excerpt 8 (lines 1 & 30), each analyzed in their own sequential environment.
5. A more extended analysis of these and related moments is provided in Chapters 10 & 12-13, where few words are enough and hope are established as patterns across single and collected instances of family interactions.
6. The relationship between topics such as cars, dogs, and food are only briefly addressed in this volume. A more detailed analysis about whether these topics are coincidentally raised and how they are connected to the cancer journey this family is undergoing remains to be conducted (but see the family interview in Chapter 15).

III

MANAGING LIFE IN TIMES OF UNCERTAINTY AND CRISIS

5

MAKING THE CASE FOR AIRLINE COMPASSION FARES

The Serial Organization of Problem Narratives

The focus shifts in two important ways in this chapter. First, as discussed in Chapter 2, 11 months have passed between calls #1-2 and #3. During that time, mom's health has diminished significantly. Her dying is now treated as imminent. Son has also moved away, requiring long-distance phone calls and, if necessary, immediate airline travel to visit mom and family. Second, as the recipient of dad and mom's descriptions in calls #1 and #2, and as time has passed, son has become an informed and impacted family member. He is uniquely positioned also to deliver news to others about his mother's illness.

Prior to Excerpt 1, call #3 (between son, mom, and dad) begins with mom informing son that "I don't want to be put on life support". She proceeds to announce being in considerable pain, and says she "can't go on":

1) SDCL: Malignancy #3:1-2

1	Mom:	U::m (2.4) the ↑pa:in is just- (1.4) unre:al.=
2	Son:	=Okay.=
3	Mom:	=There's no way=I can't go on.
4	Son:	Okay.
5		So: (1.1) >I said to Dad maybe I'm being te:rribly naive
6		but-< pt I want them to stop the pain.
7	Son:	[Ok:ay.]
8	Mom:	[°( ) °] Now i:f:=a:: (1.5) if they can do that, you
9		know I can sit there for five to ten da:ys an- .hh I
10		don't know.= I mean I: just don't know. I'm- I:'m (.)
11		not done it, so >I don't kno:w<.
12	Son:	O:ka[y.
13	Mom:	[I could sit the:re and they can- they'll ja:m me
14		with mor:phine and I'm,
15		(.) [((°dreamy voice°))]=
16	Son:	[And you can float for a while, °heh°?]
17	Mom:	=°Yeah°. .hhhh (°) the pain. Then I have
18		trouble ta(h)lking°. ((voice breaks))
19	Son:	Oka:y. hhh

As mom describes her pain and desires to have "them" stop it (line 6), and the uncertainties associated with such a treatment decision (lines 8-14), son continually acknowledges with "Okay" as he monitors and identifies with her elaboration (lines 2, 4, 7, 12, 19). In this excerpt, however, mom not only references problems with pain but experiences it as her utterance in lines 17-18 demonstrate.[1]

Excerpt 1 is obviously drawn from a complex set of circumstances involving an array of conversations not included in the recordings comprising the Malignancy corpus (e.g., between family members, medical professionals, friends and acquaintances). But from call #3 alone, it is not surprising that family members concluded it was quite possible that mom might die in the next few days.[2] With understandable urgency, therefore, it was mutually decided that son was to travel home as soon as possible (from the south-central to the west coast) to be with mom and family.[3]

Faced with the need to make last-minute and thus unexpected travel plans, son seeks to travel home to visit with his mother who is dying from cancer, and also to spend time with his family during this difficult period. His calls to the airlines reveal a need for discounted and timely airline reservations. Son works to legitimately make himself out to be a person in need, in the midst of a family crisis he did not ask for but is nevertheless embroiled within. In turn, the exhibited job of airline agents is to determine the legitimacy of the caller's need, what category of need caller falls within, and thus which services (if any) might be offered.

Interactions (from calls #3-10) consist of eight recorded and transcribed phone calls occurring within a 24-hour period (see "Timeline" in Chapter 2). Six of these calls were to major airlines within approximately one hour during that single day. Son's search for what he describes as "compassion fares" also involves a series of interactions with family members before (call #3) and after[4] (call #10) speaking with major airlines. For example, it is shown how son's initial call with mom and dad (call #3) forms the basis for subsequent problem narratives he contingently and progressively enacts for airline agents (calls #4-9). Following calls to airlines, son also offers a retrospective summary to an aunt whose advice about compassion fares was misinformed (#10).

A PREVIEW OF BASIC ISSUES AND QUESTIONS

These phone calls exemplify how routine interactions among family members and airline representatives are uniquely problematic and interwoven throughout everyday life. As summarized in Figure 5.1, when familial and institutional calls are examined together as situated in a natural chronology of everyday encounters—in the present case, a series of calls drawn from a single day—it becomes possible to examine how different interactional problems require distinct interactional solutions.

Attention is drawn to the serial organization and cumulative impact of calls over time, a primary advantage of working with longitudinal data. Specific interactional devices are examined as son (a) delicately initiates phone openings with airline agents, (b) makes initial requests for information about *compassion fares*, (c) constructs narratives offering a persuasive case for urgent and affordable assistance (i.e., soliciting special understandings regarding the legitimacy of his troubling circumstances as a person in need of help), and (d) modifies and streamlines his actions as he adapts to interactional contingencies.

Across multiple calls, it is revealed how son displays learning-in-action about the airline system. It is also possible to examine how pre- and post-interactions with family members influence, and are influenced by, the airline calls.[5] And numerous ironies common to everyday life are identified: What kinds of unavoidable disjunctures occur between airline representatives and lay persons? How does son talk with different strangers about person-

In a discussion with his dying mother, son is initially faced
with making a choice and committing to travel home.

↓

Later, during the same call, he must next inform his dad about reasons
underlying his decision to travel home, as well as seek dad's financial assistance.

↓

Once familial travel decisions are made, discussed, and financed,
son next pursues his travel reservations by calling airlines, whose offerings
and restrictions influence his abilities to travel quickly and cheaply.

↓

Having completed calls to the airlines, son is now in a position to inform
his aunt (a flight attendant) about how his experiences from these calls differed
from her earlier travel advice regarding "compassion fares".

Figure 5.1. *Summary of Key Events in the Serial Organization of Calls #3-10.*

al and family matters? And as time unfolds and mom's condition fluctuates, how do predictions about imminent death become susceptible to modification and change (see also Chapter 6)?

Three basic research questions are addressed in this chapter:

- What practices are recruited by the son as he delicately requests information, and through portrayal of his troubling circumstances, attempts to legitimate (i.e., make his case for) being a candidate for discounted fares?

From the opening moments of son's calls with the airlines, actions are designed to deformalize, personalize, and treat as delicate subsequent disclosures about his family crisis. In each call son repeatedly relies on the same basic set of resources for narrating his problem and thus making his case (e.g., being a graduate student with little money). However, specific and contingent actions are shown to emerge *on the cusp* of interactional moments (e.g., agents' questions) that could not be intuited nor fully planned out by son in advance.[6] Son's a priori approaches to calling airlines, including his stock of knowledge at hand, become improvised social involvements revealing the emergent and progressive character of son's actions. How does son, as an upshot of accumulated experiences with family members and prior agents, adapt and thereby alter his orientations to contiguous and subsequent airline calls to the airlines? The *serial and sustained ordering* of airline calls is thus a focal concern of this analysis: Any given set of interactional circumstances can be laid bare as progressively built, developmental orientations to tasks extending beyond a single encounter (i.e., getting the best rate offered by airlines).

A related and secondary focus addresses the following:

- How do agents respond to son's requests for "compassion fares"?

In all but one call, airline agents inform son that despite his stated problem narratives, he does not qualify for "compassion fares" because they are not offered by their airline.

Finally, conversations with relatives, prior to and following calls to the airlines, shape son's actions:

- How do familial conversations influence subsequent interactional conduct when talking with institutional representatives? How do institutional encounters get reconstructed to family members following calls?

Son's prior conversations with mom and dad function as essential background understandings and motives informing action, that is, as resources for shaping subsequent airline involvements. The final call #10 to be examined in this chapter, between the son and his aunt, includes son's retrospective accounting to his aunt about her advice regarding "compassion fares"—a description contrasting with his accrued experiences from talking with airline representatives.

Taken together, these calls aid in framing how son's subsequent calls to the airlines were influenced by interactions occurring before his calls, and retrospectively, in an attempt to explain his a priori versus post-hoc experiences. Collaborative strategies for affording and soliciting discounted fares also become apparent. To continue preserving a sense of the natural evolution of these chronological activities, analysis will proceed by examining calls in the order in which they occurred.

SITUATING "COMPASSION CALLS"
AS SERVICE ENCOUNTERS

Airline representatives receive thousands of calls yearly from individuals who, facing a crisis due to critical illness or death of a family member, are in need of arranging last-minute travel plans to be with distant relatives. Searches for discounted and open-ended tickets are set into motion by family members, activities that may involve initiating numerous telephone calls with major airlines.[7] Airlines offer "compassion" fares to facilitate bedside vigils for grieving family members, as well as "bereavement" fares to attend funerals for those who have already died.[8]

Calls to the airlines may be usefully contrasted with other types of emergency (911) assistance, and an array of other service encounters.[9] Previous research has examined what might be characterized as "customer service telephone calls," encounters in which "people [call] an institution of some sort for some sorts of assistance" (Sacks, 1992, p. 377). For example, analysis has focused on suicide prevention hotlines (Sacks, 1992), calls for 9-1-1 emergency assistance (e.g., K. Tracy, 1997; K. Tracy & S. Tracy, 1998; S. Tracy, 2002; Wakin & Zimmerman, 1999; Whalen, 1990; Whalen & Zimmerman, 1987; Whalen, Zimmerman, & Whalen, 1988; Zimmerman, 1992), a poison control hotline (Frankel, 1989), a mental health peer-run "warm line" (Pudlinski, 1998), a consumer help line (Torode, 1995), a software help line (Baker, Emmison, & Firth, 2001) and a travel agency (Mazeland, Huisman, & Schasfoort, 1995). From these studies, two features might be noted at the outset as having particular relevance to the airline calls examined in this chapter.

First, it appears universal that call takers, as institutional and thus bureaucratic representatives (see Heritage & Drew, 1992), transform the caller's inquiry into a routine call comprising the call-taker's standardized "day's work." (Whalen, 1990). A pre-existing institutional arrangement awaits callers. Staff who are otherwise detached (but not necessarily uncaring) individuals regularly perform tasks involving callers' problems with which they may be quite unfamiliar (e.g., traveling home to be with a dying mother). Thus, lay persons' lives often require them to enter into relationship with call takers whose daily work involves transacting a considerable volume of arrangements (urgent and nonurgent alike).

It is normal, then, for discrepancies to be apparent between callers' presented needs and call takers' service-oriented actions. Whether attention is given by call takers to categorizing the seriousness of the reported trouble in ways delaying service (Frankel, 1989; Sacks, 1992; Whalen & Zimmerman, 1990; Whalen, Zimmerman, & Whalen, 1988), addressing inherently adversarial help line calls (Torode, 1995), or even negotiating satisfactory descriptions of vacations sought by customers (Mazeland, Huisman, & Schasfoort, 1995), call takers enact "gatekeeping" functions (see Baker, Emmison, & Firth, 2001; Maynard & Schaeffer, 1997, 2002a, Endnote 10). Because representatives' actions are inevitably constrained by institutional offerings (i.e., categories of product, service, or information), a call taker "tries to create an overlap between possibilities of the agency and the preferences of the customer by interpreting the categorization in the vicinity of the customer in such a way that contains categories to satisfy both" (Mazeland et al., 1995, p. 281). And fundamentally, however unique callers' problems might be, they remain "just another problem" in a series for call takers whose work involves processing large numbers of service calls.

Second, urgency alters participants' orientations to the time-sensitive nature of information exchanged, and in all cases is interactionally negotiated. Calls to a 911 emergency or poison control center operator, addressing potential or actual life-threatening issues (i.e., heart attack or a child who ate rat poison), stand in marked contrast to less urgent discussions about utilizing software or planning vacations. Airline calls #4-9 are midpositioned between these more/less urgent extremes. A basic continuum depicting service calls according to urgency appears in Figure 5.2.

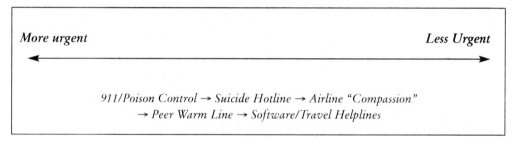

Figure 5.2. *Continuum of Customer Service Telephone Calls According to Urgency.*

A call to a poison control hot line could vary from immediately to less urgent (e.g., what to give a child who just ingested poison vs. information about risks associated with using home pesticides). So too might a customer's call to the airlines be even more urgent than what son presents for agents' consideration in the calls examined herein (i.e., a need to travel in the next few hours rather than few days).

PROLOGUE: GROUNDS FOR FAMILY CRISIS

The first of eight calls examined in this chapter provides sobering and poignant glimpses into why this family is undergoing crisis. As seen in Excerpt 1 (above), mom informs son that she does not want to be placed on life support, her " ↑pa:in is just- (1.4) unre:al.=" line 1), and that she is incoherent at times as a result of the morphine she has been taking to minimize her pain. In lines 9-11, she also explicitly addresses the inherent uncertainty of not knowing how long her dying might take: "I don't know.=I mean I: just don't know. I'm- I:'m (.) not done it, so >I don't kno:w<.".[10] Excerpt 2 begins with her articulation of the dilemma she is facing:

2) SDCL: Malignancy 3:3-4

```
1     Mom:    = A:h, (.) But I don't know if- if I say no life support? (0.2)
2             a:nd I get in ther:e and it's >r(h)eal r(h)eal ↑quick.<
3     Son:    Mm hmm.
4             (1.1)
5     Mom:    Which of course >I have no way of knowing?<
6     Son:    Yeah.
7             (1.2)
8     Mom:    Then maybe you can't get here. = And maybe you don't
9             <wa::nt,> to get here. .hh [(                                    )]
10    Son:                                [ > Yeah I want to get there. < ]
11    Mom:    Yeah? Yeah. .hh >I said to dad you know- or da:d said to
12            me.< Says you want- you wanna be here for this, or the
13            service. (0.5) 'Cause now we're ta:lkin' mo:ney.
14    Son:    Um hmm. hhh
15    Mom:    .hh Which we know you have little o:f?=
16    Son:    =Ye:ah.
17            (0.6)
18    Mom:    You're° not wealthy. =So we gotta- (0.4) ↑A:nd we're
19            talkin' your, (.) job °and your school an al[l that. ]°
```

As a background and preview to a more extended analysis of son's airline calls, only three fundamental activities occurring throughout Excerpt 2 are briefly overviewed. First, in lines 8-9, mom states "maybe you can't get here", which is qualified to "maybe you don't <wa::nt,> to get here.". Immediately, however, son next makes clear that he can and wants to be with mom by responding "Yeah I want to get there." (line 10). Second, additional and very practical problems arise even though son has just displayed his willingness to travel home: "Cause now we're ta:lkin' mo:ney...↑A:nd we're talkin' your, (.) job °and your school an al[l that.]°". Obviously, a genuine urgency occasioned by critical illness does not alleviate limited financial resources or job/school responsibilities. Apparently, in lines 11-13, this is why mom reports a discussion with dad—a curiously repaired reference, leaving hanging whether mom or dad initiated the idea—about son's choosing to travel home now or for her memorial service (see also Endnote 4). Although such constraints can be addressed, they require organized efforts and workable solutions as responses to mom's health status. These are unstable and often ambiguous developments subject to daily fluctuation (see Chapter 6).

Updating and Planning Travel with Dad

During the same phone call, shortly following Excerpt 2 (above), mom requests that son inform dad about his decision:

3) SDCL: Malignancy 3:4-5

```
1     Son:    Well what I told mom is- is as far as I'm concerned if the
2             question is do I want to be there for- for this or the memorial
3             service...I kinda feel like now would be a good (0.4) time to
4             ah- (.) to be there with Mom, when she's still got (.) any- any
5             time left ah and to be there together (.) you know (.)wi- with
6             everybody now I think it would make more sense. (.) ah And
7             (.) you know yes? I can't come for an: indefinite period an: I
```

```
8           certainly can't come back an forth a couple of times 'cause I
9           know as sure as hell I can't afford it. ((continues))
```

Son reports to dad a summary of his prior discussion with mom. He states an unequivocal preference to travel "<u>now</u>", stating in lines 4-5 what had not previously been articulated: "when she's still got (.) any- any time left ah and to be there together". Problems associated with repeated visits and money also reappear: "'cause I know as sure as hell I <u>can't</u> afford it" (lines 8-9).

Once dad is informed of son's intentions to travel immediately, attention is given over to what is known about "compassion fares" as a result of son having talked with aunt Carol, a flight attendant:

4) SDCL: Malignancy 3:6

```
1    Dad:  Allright let me talk to Carol and find out what I do about
2          plane tickets. = [ Um.]
3    Son:  = [Yeah] you can ca::ll- there's a couple of different airlines.
4     →    They have something called <compa:ssion
5          fares>, which means that they waive all restrictions and
6          basically give you (.) um the best de:al .hhh that's possible
7          without all of the restrictions...And I guess Continental, US
8          Air, and American all do them...An:d I guess you can buy
9          you know like (.) relatively <open-ended> hhh (.) tickets and
10         all of that kind of business. But I got this information from
11         auntie Carol, .hhh so she'll know this. So >give her a holler<
12         um- (0.3) and (.) if you need me to do anything from this:
13         end, you know if you want me to just go down to the airport
14         and- and buy a ticket here ah an: just come home fi:ne. (.)
15         You know call me. .hhh (.) an I- I may have to get you- you
16         to wire me some money or something.
```

It is important to notice how son initially defines "compassion fares" as "they waive <u>all</u> restrictions and basically give you (.) um the best <u>de:al</u>" (lines 4-7). This preconception is repeatedly qualified by son, however, as he twice states "I guess" in lines 7-8. Finally, and once again, practical issues involving money are raised as the son lays out possible scenarios for enacting travel.

To summarize, it has been shown that son's interactional involvements with mom and dad gave rise to calling the airlines. An urgency was thus created for travel, which son subsequently initiated and pursued. Several practical considerations (e.g., job, scheduling, and money) also emerged as relevant issues to be addressed and resolved. The relevance of seeking information about "compassion fares" was specifically raised and discussed (with dad and aunt). In short, this background provides an essential framework for understanding how, during son's subsequent calls to airlines, he relied upon earlier family conversations as resources for organizing requests for information.

ANALYSIS OF AIRLINE CALLS

Within approximately one hour, son initiated six calls to major airlines. Two calls are not analyzed: a hang-up by son following four minutes of listening to a Continental Airlines recording,[11] and a 16-second (wrong number) encounter with a PAN AM representative while attempting to contact US Air. Prior to examining son's "problem narratives," three fundamental features of call openings are examined:

- Pre-Beginnings
- Institutional Identifications and Greetings
- "Hi" + "question for you" Format

Pre-Beginnings

> Work on calls for emergency (911) assistance has made clear that the process of project-
> ing the character of the call is initiated through a "pre-beginning" . . . the opening seg-
> ment of emergency calls rests on a prior action presumed to have a particular relevancy:
> dialing an emergency number projects a need for help *prior* to the alignment ordinarily
> achieved by the identification/acknowledgment portion of opening sequence [just as]
> call-takers answering a 911 call (or other emergency number) are primed to hear it a
> request for help *before* the first word is spoken. The pre-beginning thus establishes the
> alignment of identities which provides a particular footing for the call . . . the relevance
> of which continues in force until an alternative alignment is proposed through some
> action of the participants. (Zimmerman, 1992, pp. 403-404)

Son initiated calls-in-a-series which included American, US Air, Continental, and
Southwest. Understanding son's pre-alignment with airlines, as resources for travel help,
reveals how each successive call shapes subsequent involvements (see below). Further, during son's first attempt to speak with Continental, he was placed on hold and for four minutes waited to speak with a representative before terminating the call. Waiting, then, is a
normal and inevitable course of activity when soliciting airline assistance. Urgencies receive
no preferential treatment prior to contact with an agent and, as evident below, only then as
the agent becomes responsive to the case being made that attention being given to a problem (i.e., by the caller) actually merits such categorization by the call taker (Sacks, 1992).

Institutional Identifications and Greetings

Opening moments of the four calls appear below:

5) SDCL: Malignancy 4 (Airlines Call #1)

1	AA:	American Airlines. Greg Ga:ines?
2		(0.2)
3	Son:	pt Hi. I got a question for you.=

6) SDCL: Malignancy 7 (Airlines Call #4)

1	US:	US Air: reservations. This is <u>Mon</u>ica?
2	Son:	Hi::. Uhm (.) question for you.

7) SDCL: Malignancy 8 (Airlines Call #5)

1	CN:	Continental Airlines. <u>Linda</u>?
2	Son:	pt .hh <u>Hi:</u>. Um (.) got a <u>qu</u>estion for you.

8) SDCL: Malignancy 9 (Airlines Call #6)

1	SW:	Good evening? Thank you for calling Southwest Airlines?
2		This is <u>Jes</u>sica. How may I help you?
3	Son:	Hi? Do you have such a thing as what they call a <compa::ssion fare.>

Obvious similarities of the first three calls are compared, and a contrastive analysis with the final call to Southwest Airlines is offered.

Most telephone calls are triggered through summons/answer sequences, typically "rings" occasioning call takers to pick up the phone. These actions must somehow occur for parties to gain focused access to interaction (Hopper, 1992; Schegloff, 1986), giving rise to identification/recognition as parties next display for one another their "situated identities." Consider the following two openings in 911 emergency calls (from Zimmerman, 1992), in which institutional affiliations are followed by caller's reportings of circumstances requiring help:

9)   [MCE:21:1:1] (CT=Call Taker, C=Caller)
    1   CT: Mid-City=emergency:
    2   (.)
    3   C: Yes."I'd like tuh report ur disturbance in an alleyway:,
    4   behind our building?

10) [WC:EMS:1:JW]
    1   CT: Nine one one what is yur emerg- ((cut off by transmit static))
    2   (.)
    3   C: GO:D MY WIFE JUST SHOT HERSELF (.3) TWENTY TWO
    4   SIXTY EIGHT (GRANT) AVENUE HURRY U::::P

In each instance, CT's open by stating their institutional affiliation and in (10) move to query caller about the emergency. In these ways, they establish their status as bureaucratic representatives ("Mid-city emergency", "Nine one one"), but do so anonymously because no further self-identification (i.e., names) or information is provided (see Whalen & Zimmerman, 1987). Next, C moves to report problems requiring assistance and, as with Excerpt 10, explicitly (and urgently) requests help.

Similar to 911 calls, airline calls also begin not with the "Hello" commonly occurring in ordinary phone calls, or even with a name (as with certain business/organizational interactions), but by official reference to the particular airline they represent:

11) Three Airline Openings: Affiliations + Self-Identifications
    AA: American Airlines. Greg Ga:ines?
                        ↓
    US: US Air: reservations. This is Monica?
                        ↓
    CN: Continental Airlines. Linda?

With US Air, the agent further specifies that "reservations" have been accessed. Unlike 911 calls, however, airline call takers self-identify with first and last name (AA)—which as Sacks (1992) observed, allows next speaker the opportunity to choose whether to move to retain this formality or move toward a more informal tone—or just by stating first name (US, CN).

In contrast, consider son's call to Southwest Airlines:

12) A More Personalized Airline Greeting
    1   SW: Good evening? Thank you for calling Southwest Airlines?
    2   This is Jessica. How may I help you?

This opening is elaborated and more personalized in two ways: (a) Before identifying that SW has been reached, caller is bid "Good evening" and thanked for calling; (b) Following self-identification with first name ("Jessica"), the opening is brought to close with an explicit offering of "How may I help you?"

In contrast, earlier examined calls all begin with an institutional greeting followed by the representative's name. None of them offer an initial greeting or thanks for calling, and none of them ask how they may help son. The SW greeting is thus designed to be friendlier than any of the other companies. It is also interesting, and perhaps only coincidental, to note that in the end SW was the company who was able to provide son with the lowest fare. The interactional consequences of this more tailored opening,[12] contrasted with the first three calls, are examined below.

Repeated "Hi" + "question for you" Formats

Opening moments of the first three calls appear (once again) below. Notice that son does not immediately announce his problem. Rather, he first provides an anonymous yet repeated "Hi" response to agents' greetings (affiliation and offering of names), followed by "question for you":

13) SDCL: Malignancy 4 (Airlines Call #1)

        1   AA: American Airlines. Greg Ga:ines?
        2   (0.2)
        3   Son:→pt Hi. I got a question for you.=

14) SDCL: Malignancy 7 (Airlines Call #4)

        1   US: US Air: reservations. This is Monica?
        2   Son:→Hi::. Uhm (.) question for you.

15) SDCL: Malignancy 8 (Airlines Call #5)

        1   CN: Continental Airlines. Linda?
        2   Son:→pt .hh Hi:. Um (.) got a question for you.

It was Sacks (1992) who initially observed that when people call various institutions requiring help for a problem, the first way to "catch the special status of this sort of call happens right at the beginning of the call" (p. 377). Schegloff's (1986) later inquiries more fully revealed how telephone openings are rich environments for examining "the vicissitudes of telephone interactions between both known and unknown parties" (p. 174). For example, whereas institutional representatives somehow announce their identities and provide a name, callers typically do not. Both Schegloff (1986) and Hopper and Drummond (1992) have observed how the absence of greetings is routine among unacquainted strangers: Callers often delete the greeting and initial inquiry, as well as withhold self-identification, en route to moving directly to the business of the call.

Contrasts between ordinary and service provider calls have revealed two key features: (a) Increased specialization, and thus the pursuit of identification over recognition responses to telephone summons; (b) a general reduction in opening sequences, including an absence of "greetings" or "how are you" responses, which is consequential for earlier movement to first topic and thus "reason for the call" (Schegloff, 1979; Whalen & Zimmerman, 1987; Whalen, Zimmerman, & Whalen, 1988). In these ways,

> The reduction of the opening sequence . . . exhibits participants' orientations to and appreciation of the contingencies of seeking and providing assistance, through an anonymous encounter in which the sequential achievement of prompt response to urgent need displays and reproduces the institutional features of the interaction. (Whalen, Zimmerman, & Whalen, 1988, p. 178)

Such practices and canonical forms are subject to variation. Specifically, "If one speaker greets another by saying 'Hi' at the start of a telephone conversation, this ordinarily invokes the relevance of the category 'previously acquainted . . .' (Hopper & Drummond, 1992, p. 193). Of what relevance, then, are son's repeated "Hi" usages (above) at the outset of interactions with unknown airline representatives? Each of S's "Hi's" are instances of routine divergences displaying how "special, problematic, urgent, or strategic" (p. 197) matters get enacted, circumstances which

> simulates an opening for acquainted parties; then caller exploits this virtual pretense of acquaintance to ask a special favor. That is caller acts like an acquaintance as part of a **persuasive line of activity**. . . . Callers augment the reduced forms . . . in order to pursue transparent goals . . . in certain telephone openings callers do use greetings to enact transparently-motivated social gestures. (pp. 192-193; **bold** in original)

Son's "Hi's" are devices for simulating, and in this way beginning to establish familiarity with major airline representatives. These actions are designed by son to deformalize and thus personalize his calls, set up his subsequent requests for information that resemble *solicitations for favors* (see Maynard & Schaeffer, 2002), and thus create an environment conducive to requesting information about discounted fares.[13] Because son's repeated "Hi's" are themselves preliminary to his following "question for you's", however, "Hi's" per se are accomplice to paired actions leading up to "problem narratives." A variety of turn formats have been shown to involve preliminaries to what a speaker may be proposing to do, orientations designed to influence recipients' possible involvements in such actions (see Beach & Dunning, 1982; Sacks, 1992; Schegloff, 1968; Terasaki, 1976). To better understand the working features of "Hi + question for you," it is useful to first contrast them with actions initially identified by Schegloff (1980) when examining how callers participate during radio talk shows. For example, when asking "Can I ask you a question?" callers orient to their calls as "conversations in a series" by announcing the "type of call one means to be initiating" (p. 106). Aside from functioning as basic practices for gaining recipient's attention, such utterances are also centrally understood as marking "preliminariness" en route to prefiguring next and potentially *delicate* pursuits (e.g., requests, favors, apologies). With son's "Hi + question for you" formats he is, in similar fashion, enacting "preliminariness" to personal/delicate matters that, and importantly so, are being disclosed to a stranger on the telephone. That son is pre-announcing his question and not delivering it directly reflects his continual recognition of the importance attributed to agents' hearing his next-positioned actions not simply as informational requests, but as petitions for "personal" help. By extending his "Hi" greeting son's actions are designed to insure not just any hearing or response by the representatives and by enacting a more personal, less formal tone, son works to set the stage for agents to hear subsequent disclosures about his mother, and lack of money, in ways granting legitimation for his case and possible empathy for his family crisis. Again, as discussed more fully below, these preliminaries contribute to how son's actions qualify as not only "requesting" but, as he builds his case, a form of "favor asking" in pursuit of a specialized and sensitized identification with his troubling circumstances (see Maynard & Schaeffer, 2002a).

RESPONDING TO A TAILORED OPENING

Similar to the prior three calls, son responds to SW's elaborated opening with "<u>Hi</u>?", but here with emphasis and upward intonation:

16) **SDCL: Malignancy 9 (Airlines Call #6)**

    1   SW: Good evening? Thank you for calling Southwest Airlines?

    2   This is <u>J</u>essica. How may I help you?

    3   Son: →Hi? Do you have such a thing as what they call a

    4   <<u>compa</u>::ssion fare.>

Unlike prior calls, however, son does not follow his greeting with a pre-announcement about a forthcoming question. Essentially, SW's prior offering of "How may I help you?" pre-empted the son needing to make such an announcement. The upshot is how son designs his query by directly asking "Do you have such a thing as what they call a <<u>compa</u>::ssion fare.>". Is it possible that "such a thing as what they call" is an upshot of having spoken with prior airlines who offered only bereavement and <u>not</u> compassion fares? Perhaps. But son is at least objectifying, and thereby treating "<<u>compa</u>::ssion fare.>" as a "social fact" and established category. He thus treats his reference as not his invention, but a normal type of request for reduced fares routinely initiated and responded to by other cultural members.

To summarize, analysis thus far has examined pre-beginnings, the openings of serial airline calls, comprised of institutional greetings/identification and son's responsive greeting ("Hi"), and son's repeated "pre-announcement" in the form of "question for you". Attention has also been given to son's response to SW's tailored opening. We are now in a position to address how son formulates his additional "requests" for "compassion fares" and, in so doing, narrates his predicament for agents' hearing in ways legitimating his family crisis. Preliminary attention is also given to agents' responses to son's problem narratives.

PROBLEM NARRATIVES
AND INFORMATION EXCHANGE

Excerpt 16 (below) includes son's extended narrative and AA's initial responses. In this and three subsequent calls, son's problem presentation includes five basic features listed in Figure 5.3. From the prior overview of son's prior conversations with mom and dad (and son and dad's reported conversations with aunt), it is clear that these features are not coincidental but carried over from these interactions. Essentially, (1→5) are son's formulated upshots of the basic gist of these conversations, paraphrased and adapted into a "script" or "template" for presenting his case to airline representatives (see Beach & Dixson, 2001; Heritage & Watson, 1979, 1980). Although these descriptions are variously configured in construction and ordering in the excerpts below (e.g., see 2/3→, below), the same numbers with arrows are employed throughout. And in all but the Southwest call, some versions of these narrative components are articulated before making a specific request (5→).

Interactionally, then, son's pre-discussed topics eventuate as scripted/templated portrayals of his predicament. These resources are designed to enhance the likelihood that he will not only qualify, but receive discounted rates associated with compassion status. It must again be emphasized, however, that although recurrent features appear across each of son's four contiguous calls (1→5), each call is contingently enacted as speakers respond to and shape emerging interactional circumstances—actions that cannot be fully planned for nor anticipated in advance.

> Reference to being a graduate student (1→),
>
> ↓
>
> who doesn't have much money (2→),
>
> ↓
>
> yet needs to travel home in a hurry because his mother is dying (3→),
>
> ↓
>
> has prior knowledge that "compassion fares" exist (4→),
>
> ↓
>
> giving rise to a specific request about "compassion fares" (5→).

Figure 5.3. *Five Basic Features of Son's Problem Narratives.*

Analysis begins with a longer excerpt from son's call to American Airlines:

17) SDCL: Malignancy 4 (Airlines Call #1)

1	AA:	American Airlines. Greg Ga:ines?
2		(0.2)
3	Son:	pt Hi. I got a question for you.=
4	AA:	=Yes?
5	Son: 1 →	I'm (.) a **graduate student** here at the University of [name]
6		and uh-
7	AA:	[°Yes, uh huh.°]
8	Son:	[I jus- jus'] got a phone call: pt (.) ah and apparently my
9	2→	**mother's going to die:** pt (.) and **I need to get back** to
10	4→	[city]. (.) **I am told there is such a thing as a compassion**
11	2/3→	**fare for poor fo:lks like me who need to go somewhere in**
12	5→	**a hurry. (.) ↑ Do you have such a thing?** hhh
13		(0.3)
14	AA:	↑ Well let's check out. Uh Do you wanna leave uh like leave as
15		soon as possible?
16	Son:EN	Yeah uh well tomorro:w I've got- I'm a teacher I've got
17	↓	some <u>stuff</u> I have to do first thing in the morning.
18	↓	And .hh conceivably (.)tomorrow afternoon. I'm- I'm
19	↓	waiting for one more phone call before I'm:: sure,
20	↓	but I want to figure out what I have to do (.) ah to
21	↓	pull this off. So-
22	AA:	Okay. Let me check just one second please.

In the following ways, son adapts his a priori concerns to the contingencies of this particular call with AA:

Son's reference to "here" in (1→)—the only such reference in the calls examined—invokes a shared demography with an AA agent assumed to be headquartered in Dallas, Texas. Referencing a shared place is one device for producing affiliation and thus assistance by a representative who is at least employed by a Texas airline, perhaps even a Texas resident, and for these reasons better positioned to accommodate son's request.

Son also initiates an attempt to make his case for urgency by referencing "I jus- jus'] got a phone call: pt (.) ah and apparently **my mother's going to die**:"(lines 8-9). The construction of his utterance could not have been fully formed in advance. Rather, it was built on-the-spot to invoke both recency of a call and inherent ambiguity ("apparently"). These are central issues testifying to the nature of the crisis at hand and son's role as a consequential family member awaiting updated news (see also Chapter 6). In response, although son has just informed AA that his mother is dying, AA's response to this personal information is not compassionate but service-oriented. Immediate attention is given to establishing flight information, as the agent neither grants nor declines son's informational request and does not acknowledge that such a fare exists. Rather, she asks a follow-up question.

It is in response to AA's query "Do you wanna leave uh like leave as soon as possible?" (lines 14-15), an apparent and natural upshot of son's just prior depiction of his urgent situation, that he provides an elaborated narrative (**EN**). This extension contains information that, had it not been occasioned by agents' prior query, would likely not have emerged. Once available, however, son (as question recipient) offers further details about his work as a teacher, schedule, and reliance on additional phone calls from family. Taken together, this information clarifies how and why son does not yet know for sure just when he needs to depart. It offers resolution to a potential disjuncture, emerging on the cusp of interaction. Son's expressed urgency to travel, yet inability to articulate when "as soon as possible" might be, was thus not pre-formed.

Only in this first call to AA does son make separate references to being a "graduate student" with implications for not having much money. Here, although son identifies himself as a "graduate student" (1→) at the outset, "**poor fo:lks like me who need to go somewhere in a hurry**" (2/3→) is delayed. His being both "poor" and "in a hurry" is conjoined immediately prior to making an indirect request (5→) (Brown & Levinson, 1987; Schegloff, 1988; Streeck, 1980): He queries about whether the airline offers the service ("such a thing?"), rather than making a direct request for the service itself. By so doing, son cautiously requests information in a manner providing the agent an *out*, allowing for the possibility that the airline might not offer such fares. He also defines and operationalizes his lay notions about what compassion fares might be, including why he might qualify for a reduced rate (see Chapter 6).

Essentially, son's build up to making his indirect and cautious request (5→) is constructed to delay agents' yes-no answering of his question. It may appear that son is asking a favor by imploring the agent to respond to his dilemma, which "implicates different answering options . . . a sense of being *solicited for a favor* rather than simply being *asked to comply* with a request . . . [which] can more strongly compel a positive response" (Maynard & Schaeffer, 2002b; italics in original).[14]

Yet a closer examination of son's appeal reveals that the fundamental significance of a "favor"—in the generic sense, an act of kindness, goodwill, and/or special treatment—does not sufficiently capture several key features of son's actions. In his narrative, son nominates the category "compassion fare" (lines 10-11), and then proceeds to provide criteria for why he qualifies as facing a family emergency (e.g., mother's going to die). Even though this is the only relevant criterion from the airline's perspective, son also orients to his financial status as relevant ("poor fo:lks like me"). In these ways son attempts to make his case for receiving discounted fares, but he does not seek special treatment, such as requesting that the airline go against policy to grant him reduced rates.

Thus, although son's actions may be described as an active pursuit of empathic consideration for the fix he is in, which may (and does) qualify him for receiving a timely and cheaper ticket, such actions are not tantamount to favor asking per se.

Becoming Routinized: A More Deliberate Orientation

As subsequent calls to airlines are initiated, occasions emerge (as with Excerpt 18, below) where son is informed that because compassion fares aren't offered, his stated criteria do not meet the requirements. In these moments, son does not actively pursue reconsideration in light of his special circumstances (though he may briefly comment on them). Rather, he displays understanding of bureaucratic categories and policies and moves to closing the call.

The second call to US Air, which eventuates in a shortened encounter because "We don't really have a compassionate fa:re", appears in full below. Prior to agents' announcement, however, son proceeds to narrate his troubling circumstances:

1) **SDCL: Malignancy 7 (Airlines Call #4)**

```
 1    US:     ((Recording)) Thank you for calling US Air reservations?
 2            (.) All of our agents are busy? (.) However please stay on the
 3            line, as your call will be handled-
 4    US:     US Air: reservations. This is Monica?
 5    Son: 4→Hi::. Uhm (.) question for you. pt .hh I understand that
 6            there is something ca:lled a <compa:ssion fa:re>. .hhh I just
 7            3→ found out that I need to: (.) get home, my mother's about
 8            1/2→ to di:e? .hhh U::m pt and I'm a graduate student and
 9            have no:t got much money>. .hh [ U:m ]=
10    US:                                    [Umm:]
11    Son: 5→=[Do you-
12    US:     [>We don't really have a compassionate fa:re. We have
13            what we call a bereavement fare. < =
14    Son:    =Oka[:y. hhh
15    US:     [And unfortunately <tha:t is when> someone has
16            a:lready passed awa::y.=
17    Son:    =All right.=
18    US:     =We do u:m we do offer, that fa:re when people are going to
19            a fu:neral:.=
20    Son:    =Ok(h)a:y. ↑Well fu:neral won't happen 'til after I get there,-
21            I('ve) suppo:se. .hhhhh ↑O:kay. Well thank you anyway. hh=
22    US:     =>I'm: sorry I couldn't help [you.<
23    Son:                                [That's all right. Bye.
      ((End of Phone Call))
```

One preliminary observation is that this call to US is produced more slowly and deliberately (see "Uhm/Um") than son's prior call to AA. As a second presented problem narrative, son begins to enact an "assembly line" demeanor: He exhibits becoming acclimatized to involvement with the airline system. Several marked differences from talking with AA (Excerpt 17, above) are evident as son produces adjustments arising from his earlier call:

- Unlike the first call to AA, son's "question for you" is more streamlined as his agent and verb ("I have a") are deleted. This utterance is followed by a lips-mack and inbreath ("pt .hh"), which provides only a brief slot for the US agent to respond following "question for you". (In the previous Excerpt 17, agent's "Yes?" response is latched onto the end of "question for you", with no intervening space.) Next, son moves directly to "I understand that there is something ca:lled a <compa:ssion fa:re>." (4→).

- Rather than beginning with his justifications for needing the fare, as with AA, he straightforwardly announces his purpose for his call.
- Son retains a sense of recency with "I just found out that I need to: (.) get home". He withholds mentioning ["city"] in favor of "get home", a different locational reference than with AA in Dallas (and him in another city).
- He alters "apparently my mother's going to die" to an upgraded, less ambiguous, and emphasized "my <u>mother's</u> about to <u>di:e</u>?". These latter actions imply a greater certainty of the imminence of mother's death.

Son also makes his request for compassion fares more urgent by conjoining "**I'm a graduate student and have <u>no:t</u> <u>got</u> <u>much</u> <u>money</u>>."(2→)**:

- With his first call to AA, it was left for the agent to connect his being a "graduate student" with a "poor folk". With US, son makes this connection explicit.
- He emphasizes "<u>no:t</u> <u>got</u> <u>much</u> <u>money</u>", perhaps as an upshot of his first call where son was unsuccessful in obtaining a good price.

Yet just as son begins to formulate his specific request with "Do you-" (5→), he is informed by US that "we really don't have a compassionate fare" but a "be<u>reavement</u> <u>fare</u>.". In this way, son's request is pre-empted even before it is articulated. Agent's response is shaped as an informing that implicates rejection, rather than a rejection of son's request for other reasons. The agent does not refuse to help son, but displays not being institutionally empowered to offer information about the fare requested. This initial and official response by US attends to institutional offerings while essentially disattending son's solicitations for consideration of his personal disclosures about a family crisis.

Notice that agent's pre-emptive response is receipted by son with a slightly stretched and downward intoned "<u>Oka[:y</u>."(line 14), displaying both some lingering doubt about just what a "bereavement" fare might be and whether he qualifies for it, and some incongruity between son's presented case and the pre-emptive, "official" reply. Son's response, however, is not addressed by the US agent because, in overlap, the agent was en route to defining the fare with "And un<u>fortunately</u> <tha:t is when> someone has a:lready passed awa::y.=" (lines 15-16). With "un<u>fortunately</u>" she displays some sensitivity to son's dilemma (i.e., mom's dying but not dead), because the fare she is describing is not helpful to son.

Son's reaction, an immediate and emphatic "<u>All</u> <u>right</u>.", accepts his "non-qualification" status with finality. Son does not respond as though the narrative he presented was treated by the US agent as not compelling. Nor does son attempt to quibble with having had a request refused or declined, thus pursuing agent's reconsideration. Instead, the agent continues by further describing that the fare they offer is only for "a fu:neral:", which son displays acceptance of yet some frustration with his next "Ok(h)a:y [+] ↑Well fu:neral won't happen 'til after I get there,- I('ve) suppo:se." (lines 20-21).

Several features of son's elaboration are of particular interest. For example, son's response succinctly states the double bind this leaves him with, namely, that he will likely qualify for the fare offered only after he gets home and his mother dies. Also, this statement is not just a pursuit of response (see Pomerantz, 1984b), but a venting of son's frustration. In this instance, despite the inability of the airlines to assist, son makes his predicament available for agents by stating "just the facts": not to provoke or out of hostility, but to go on record by indirectly complaining about the lack of fit between son's dilemma and US's bereavement offering. His actions also make available an opportunity for agent to provide some sympathetic understanding, and US's "=><u>I'm</u>: sorry I couldn't help [you" (line 22) does apologize for the inability to assist while also withholding a more personal offering of sympathy or concern. (A small collection of these types of moments are examined more fully later in this chapter.) Notice, however, that son also displays a recognition of the constraints this agent, as a bureaucratic representative, is operating under. He thanks the agent and, in response to agent's qualified apology, replies "That's <u>all</u> right. Bye." as the call is terminated.

To summarize, in this second call to US son enacts a more deliberate orientation, initially apparent as "compassion fare" is raised as a first item of business. Son also retains recency and urgency, removes ambiguity about mother's condition, and conjoins his graduate/money status. Taken together, son's actions document his having learned from the first AA call in ways allowing for subsequent modifications in narrative presentation. He exhibits a *streamlined* character not apparent in his initial encounter with AA. His enacted and more business-like demeanor, however, does not eliminate but works toward optimization of his personal appeals designed to solicit discounted fares. Nevertheless, because son is informed that he does not qualify, he becomes subjected to constraints imposed by the US agent as a bureaucratic representative. Son is accepting of agent's inability to assist and thus does not exhibit having had a reasonable request declined for no good reason. But he is frustrated (and understandably so) and makes his dilemma available for agent's hearing in light of her reply. Yet he does so without blaming her for it. In response, son receives an apology for agent's incapacity to assist, rather than personalized sympathy for what son must be undergoing.

Fundamentally, even though son's problem narrative is itself becoming more routinized, he cannot escape being subjected to institutional criteria for qualifying appropriate customers. This is an inevitability that son's own closing remarks seem resigned to acknowledge.

The Irony of Shortened and Elaborate Problem Narratives

The third airline call-in-a-series, a two-part call to Continental Airlines (CN), appears in full below:

19) SDCL: Malignancy 8 (Airlines Call #5)

((Son places his second phone call to CN reservations. His first call resulted in hanging up in response to four minutes of a recorded message. This recording reports that "all of our agents are temporarily busy. Please remain on the line and your call will be answered in the order in which it was received. If you already have a reservation please have your date of travel and flight number available. Thank you."))

Son waits 2:50 from the outset of the recording (see Endnotes 8 & 9), and then agent (CN) comes onto the phone and eventually a Customer Service Manager (SM).

1	CN:	Continental Airlines. <u>Linda</u>?
2	Son:	pt .hh Hi:. Um (.) got a <u>question</u> for you.
3		[pt]
4	CN:	[Ok]a:y.=
5	Son:	4→= Do you <u>do</u>: such a thing as a compa:ssion <u>fa:re</u>.=I just
6		3→found out my <u>mother's</u> going to di:e,
7		1/2→and I need to get back to San <u>Diego</u>:=<u>and</u> I'm a
8		<u>student</u> and I got <u>very</u> <u>little</u> <u>money</u>.
9	CN:	Oka:y. Um <u>how</u> soon did you want to travel.=
10	Son:	=We:ll like to<u>morro:w</u>.
11	CN:	°Tomorrow°. Okay, just a [moment.
12	S:	[Maybe tomorrow after<u>noon</u>.

```
13      CN:     Okay one moment?
14                      .
15                      ((Recording comes on for 00:14; same agent comes back on
16                      line))
17                      .
18      CN:     Okay sir. Thanks for holding [(I'll put a supervisor) on the=
19      Son:                                  [Sure.
20      CN:     =line to help you.=
21      Son:    =Okay.
22      SM:     Hello sir. My name is Peter, I'm the customer (.) service
23              manager. How can I [help you.
24      Son:                       [Hi: well I- I'm tryin to find out
25          3→something. I just (.) r:eceived this wonderful phone call,
26              that it looks like my mother's gonna die. .hhh Uh and I
27              need to:, find o:ut. They're gonna let me know for sure in
28              the morning, but I think I need to get back to [city] from
29      1/2→[city].   .hhh U:h (.) and I am a graduate student, and do not
30          4→have a lot of money. I was told there was such a thing as
31              compa:ssion fa:res, and that you're one of airlines that
32              offers them.=Is that true? .hhhh=
33      SM:     =No: we do:n't.=
34      Son:    =↑O::[k(h)ay.
35      SM:          [(Actually) what we do: have is a fare only (.) to attend
36              funerals.=
37      Son:    =O:h oka:y. My misunderstanding then. .hhh All right, well
38              thanks very much anyway.=
39      SM:     =Thanks fo[r calling.]
40      Son:              [ O k a y. ] Bye bye.
```

Son's opening to his problem narrative is designed as an upshot of having been informed, in his call to US airlines, that they don't offer a "compassion fare". He shifts from "I understand that there is something ca:lled a <compa:ssion fa:re>." (US), which cites his prior knowledge, to a more direct and even blunt "Do you do: such a=thing as a compa:ssion fa:re." (line 5). This adjustment downplays his understandings in favor of more pragmatic concerns: Does CN do (i.e., offer) these fares or not? Without waiting for response, son follows his straightforward query with a more quickly produced, concise, and efficient listing of his narrative. His deliberate presentation to US was replete with filled pauses ("Uhm/Um's") and delivered at a slower pace. This presentation to CN again retains his appeal to recency and unequivocal urgency (3→). But it involves no filled pauses, eliminates "graduate student" for an abbreviated "student", and provides a shortened "have no:t got much money>." (US) to "I got very little money" (CN,1/2→)—a grammatically incorrect, yet basic description that nevertheless encapsulates his dilemma.

It is apparent, therefore, that to this point son's third call is comparatively simplified and streamlined. His optimizations are natural inclinations for interactions in a series: Each subsequent presentation promotes a more basic, well organized, and adept portrayal of the basic issues.

In response, however, the agent does not answer son's initial query about "compassion fares." Rather, and similar to AA's query ("Do you wanna leave uh like leave as soon as possible?"), she asks how soon he wants to travel. Following his response of tomorrow/tomorrow afternoon, CN places him on hold with "Okay one moment?". Once again son is listening to a recording[15] yet, unbeknownst to him, is soon to be informed that the agent has turned his call over to a supervisor "to help you." It cannot be determined whether, for example, this agent was new on the job and/or simply did not know about such fares and thus required assistance. What is clear, however, is that following the "customer service manager's" institutional greeting and offering of "help", son is now faced with presenting his case for the second time in a single call (his fourth problem narrative thus far).

What emerges is a noticeably longer and more complete problem narrative. Produced specifically for SM's hearing as a representative in a position of authority, son constructs his quandary for a recipient he did not choose yet who is capable of granting special assistance/discounted fares he is pursuing. After stating he is "tryin to <u>find</u> <u>out</u> <u>something</u>", notice that son also begins this narrative ironically: "**I just (.) r:<u>ec</u>eived this <u>wonderful</u> phone call, that it looks like my <u>mother's</u> gonna die.**" (lines 25-26). It is possible that this irony, the only instance produced by son across all airline calls, is triggered by son's just prior listening to a recording describing alluring vacation opportunities. This stands, of course, in stark contrast to his reasons for calling the airline to address a family crisis (see Endnote 8). Interactionally, however, this ironic opening is recruited by son in three related ways.

First, the opening is produced in a manner similar to how speakers invoke idiomatic expressions (Beach, 1996; Drew & Holt, 1988, Chapter 7), namely, in environments where producers treat others as potentially withholding sympathy and/or affiliation to a complaint and/or problem. Son's opening of his second problem narrative is designed to garner SM's support in the very face of the irony he is proposing. Clearly, there is nothing "wonderful" about receiving an unsolicited call sated with bad news, and son employs his ironic expression in a self-effacing manner.

Second, son's opening reflects an enactment of Goffman's (1961) conceptualizations of "role enactments":

> . . . by introducing an unserious style, the individual can project the claim that nothing happening at the moment to him or through him should be taken as a direct reflection of him, but rather of the person-in-situation that he is mimicking. . . . Sullenness, muttering, irony, joking, and sarcasm may all allow one to show that something of oneself lies outside the constraints of the moment and outside the role within whose jurisdiction the moment occurs. (pp. 105, 115)

It has been emphasized how son is caught up displaying being a person in need of help. He also exhibits for SM's recognition that although he is aware of the dilemma he is embroiled within, he is not totally consumed by it, at least to the extent that he cannot (at least momentarily) be unserious or ironic.

Third, in producing such an ironic utterance, son employs an alternative device for deformalizing this call. In a troubles resistant manner, he puts on hold more explicit displays of his emotional concerns and by so doing distances himself from the predicament within which he is embroiled. Sometimes when a troubles-teller is referring to a topic that might "reoccasion tears," he or she may replace an emotional description "with a description biased toward less than serious treatment. . . . He is exhibiting that, although there is this trouble, it is not getting the better of him; he is managing" (Jefferson, 1984b, pp. 351, 353). Yet by exhibiting the prerogative to treat his dilemma lightly, son also invites SM to be even more receptive to the troubles he is experiencing.

At the completion of son's narrative (lines 30-32) is "**I was told there was such a thing as compa:ssion fa:res, and that you're one of <u>airlines</u> that offers them.=Is that <u>true?</u>**". This utterance stands in marked contrast to his earlier query designed for CN, "**Do you <u>do:</u> such a = thing as a compa:ssion fa:re.**" (line 5). Similar to calls with AA and US, son relies again on "I was told" but here ends with "Is that <u>true?</u>". By citing other sources, son creates for himself an out should he come off as misinformed (see Bergman, 1992). And, indeed, such is the case. Immediately SM responds with an emphatic and blunt "<u>No:</u> we <u>do:n't</u>." (line 33). Following son's somewhat incongruous "O::[k(h)ay" (see Beach, 2002c), which (like the US call) may have but did not occasion an already launched explanation by SM about "funerals," son marks SM's informing as news, acknowledges his misunderstanding, and thanks him anyway. Unlike the call to US, however, son neither verbalizes his dilemma nor solicits SM's sympathy for what are obviously troubling circumstances. His passing on doing so may itself be an upshot of having already attempted and failed to solicit personalized support from the US agent. In absence of this recognition, SM does not offer an apology (like US), but a reciprocated "Thanks for calling." as the call moves to closing.

To summarize, there is an irony about son's repeated efforts—shortened and efficient, as with CN, and more elaborate when speaking with SM—in that despite his adaptations from prior calls and ongoing claims for urgency, these efforts have essentially been to no avail. When airlines don't offer compassion fares, there is apparently little business to transact and calls quickly move to closing. In essence, airline calls examined thus far reveal how son's journey through airline industry offerings requires, at the very least, an articulation of his personal circumstances—yet without assurance of receiving cost-effective and timely compensation. And as noted, agents have withheld expressing sympathy and compassion for his dilemma.

Streamlining the Problem Narrative

A portion of the fourth and final call, to Southwest Airlines (SW), appears below:

20) **SDCL: Malignancy 9 (Airline Call #6)**

1	SW:	<u>G</u>ood evening? Thank you for calling Southwest Airlines?
2		This is <u>J</u>essica. How may I <u>help</u> you?
3	Son:	4→**<u>Hi</u>? Do you have such a thing as what they call a**
4		3→**<<u>compa::ssion fare.</u>> (.) Um- I just found out it looks like**
5		**my mother's gonna <u>di:e</u>? and I need to get back to [city]**
6		1/2→**from [city, state] and I'm a graduate student and do <u>not</u>**
7		**have a lot of money.**
8	SW:	Let me check and see: umm (.) <u>exactly</u> what the fares: would
9		be:. I know we <u>do</u> not have anything like tha:t.
10	Son:	Okay?
11	SW:	Our fares are usually much less than u:h American, Delta,
12		(.) people like tha:t.
13	Son:	All right.
14	SW:	Ah the normal fare sir is one thirty three one way?
15	Son:	Okay.
16	SW:	Are you under twenty <u>two</u>.
17	Son:	<u>No:</u>, I'm twenty seven.=
18	SW:	= >All right sir.< You might want to try um (2.5) u- um
19		America <u>West</u>.
20	Son:	Okay.
21	SW:	They may have ah- is it a p<u>a</u>ssion fare or bereavance fare.
22		Something like tha:[t. =
23	Son:	=[Yeah ah- there's a couple places that
24		°will° do this when (.) if I want to go for a funeral? But I'd
25		just as soon get there before she dies and [that's] =

26   SW: [R:ight.]
27   Son: = a matter of <u>days</u> at this point. And um hhh

((Agent and son continue to talk about fares, other airlines, and scheduling.))

In this fifth problem narrative, son retains his initial and direct inquiry addressing the root issue underlying his calls: "compassion fares." This narrative is the most complete and succinct of the five. Exact information is provided for the SW agent, but little more, and produced not just in an assembly line but a list-construction manner (see Jefferson, 1990). Pauses and dysfluencies are essentially absent as son constructs his narrative. This presentation can be attributed to son's becoming acclimatized to encounters with airline agents. As such, the information that son offers about specific matters (e.g., his mother's dying and lack of money) have become increasingly refined and shaped. *They are presented less as affective displays of urgent need and more as required list components for meeting institutional requirements.*

Son's actions are now efficiently built in an order tailored to SW's needs: request for information, urgency, locations, and cost. This recipient-designed ordering can be understood as a natural evolution of presentational skills, designed with airline requirements in mind yet adapted to the precise contingencies of his SW encounter.

Next, SW responds to son's narrative by informing him that she will check the fares and then stating that she knows SW does not have a compassion fare. Son stays on the line at this juncture to hear what fares would amount to, even though SW does not have compassion fares per se, and is soon told that SW fares "are usually much less" than other airlines. This is quickly confirmed: The normal one-way fare is $133, what amounts to a $60 roundtrip savings over AA's quoted compassion rates.

Despite these savings, the agent next suggests that son try a competitor, "America West." Because the agent treats as primary not the selling of a SW ticket to this customer, but the best possible price for a man faced with a family crisis, priority is given to son's needs. Notice also that her references to "passion fare or bereavance fare" (line 21) are not accurate. She exhibits being uninformed of alternative fares, concluding with "Something like tha:[t.", which son next treats as a teaching moment rooted in his residual experiences. Without correcting her inaccuracies, he simply informs her of the difference between "funeral" fares and the option of "get[ting] there before she <u>dies</u>" (lines 24-27), an obvious preference for him that is acknowledged by agent. The call then continues with an extended discussion of travel details.

EPILOGUE: COMPASSION FARES REVISITED

Prior analysis has made clear how son's conversations, prior to calling the airlines and particularly with his dad and aunt, strongly influenced his preoccupation with and search for compassion fares when speaking with airline representatives. The final call in a series is examined below: a conversation with his aunt, a flight attendant who initially informed son and his dad that "compassion fares" were available and provided the lowest discounted rates. This excerpt begins as son somewhat delicately draws his aunt's attention, "for professional curiosity sake" (lines 1-2), to his assessment that she was basically misinformed about the advice she was offering:

21) **SDCL: Malignancy 10:4**

1   Son: Ye:ah, (.) .hh <u>interestingly</u> jus- just because um (.) for
2   pro<u>fess</u>ional curiosity sake I thought <u>you'd</u> be interested to

```
3              know this. (.) Ahh um most of these places that do (.) what
4              you're calling compassion fares >oh there they are .hhh
5              don't do it until the person is already dead.< (.) They do it
6              for funerals. (.)The only one that did it (.) for these kind of
7              circumstances that I found was American.
8    Aunt:    Yeah. =
9    Son:     = .hhh But Southwest because of (.) being Southwest actually
10             was cheaper. (.) .hhh I can buy ah on the spot one-way ticket
11             from Southwest .hhh a- and then just buy another on the
12             spot one way ticket when I'm done and come back (.) and
13             still have it come up (.) to be .hhh A::h .hhh let's see
14             ((mumbling)) .hh seventy dollars cheaper than American
15             Airlines (.) compassion fares (.) so-
16   Aunt:    Well that is why I gave you the infor[mation.]
17   Son:                                          [ .hhh   ] Yeah I- I called
18             about six places .hhh and hh th- the details would be uhh I
19             would leave here two twenty my time go through [city]
20             end up there five thirty your time.
21   Aunt:    Uh hmm Okay. (.) Alright. Uhm by- I would- (.) the way
22             <normally> things work with Dr. Wylie is she makes rounds
23             in the morning.
24   Son:     Um hmm. Yeah that's what dad said.=
```

What can be gleaned from this excerpt has little to do with aunt's reception of son's update. She fails to acknowledge any culpability for her actions (line 16), which were no doubt well intended despite being inaccurate. Rather, what is provided by son, and thus available for analysis, is a capsulized and retrospective summary of his just completed airline experiences. In less than one minute, son sketches the "gist" of his efforts: compassion versus bereavement fares (lines 4-7), Southwest's offering of cheaper and convenient tickets (lines 9-15), and his eventual flight schedule (lines 17-20).

Son begins by describing a key distinction he has learned between "compassion" and "bereavement" fares—the latter being for "funerals," and thus not applicable to son's need to promptly travel home to be with mom and family. It is somewhat curious that son would, essentially, be educating a flight attendant on such fare distinctions. Yet, as it was earlier noted how SW's agent mispronounced "passion fare or bereavance fare," there is no guarantee that those working for the airlines are fully knowledgeable about the full range of services offered. In this sense, a lay person (son) can emerge as more of an expert than some airline employees.

The knowledge undergirding son's expertise is also apparent in lines 9-15, in which SW is overviewed as both cheaper and more convenient than AA, the only "compassion fare" offered by any of the airlines he called. Following aunt's disavowal (line 16), son next summarizes by stating "Yeah I- I called about six places" before offering his flight details including late afternoon arrival (lines 17-20). Finally, aunt next updates son (lines 21-23) about when mom's doctor "makes rounds in the morning", which son acknowledges and informs her "that's what dad said".

Cumulative Impacts of Calls-Over-Time

Being in a crisis, and even bereaved, is rarely a matter of personal choice. Difficult circumstances emerge throughout the course of daily affairs, events that may be anticipated but at times arrive unexpectedly. These exigencies set into motion a series of practical activities that would (if choice were an option) be otherwise avoided altogether. Yet when individuals are faced with the need to make last-minute and thus unforeseen travel plans to visit dying family members, it becomes necessary to arrange affordable and timely airline reservations. The interactions examined in this chapter provide a glimpse of one families' attempts to manage such activities, across a series of family phone calls (involving son, mom, dad, and aunt) as well as encounters with several airline agents.

Analysis has revealed how son worked in unison with mom and dad to make key travel decisions, how he subsequently makes his case to airline agents, and reconstructions (to aunt) of these airline experiences. Particular attention has been given to the serial organization and cumulative impact of calls over time. By examining specific features of how the son initiated and elaborated calls with airline agents delicately—from "Hi → question for you → [problem narrative]"—attention has been given to not just request making and yes-no compliance, but two additional and key features: attempts to make the case for being qualified for discounted rates (i.e., meeting institutional criteria for a "fare category") and eliciting understandings from agents who might therefore accommodate son with timely and discounted fares.

Beginning with son's initial calls to mom and dad, the ontogenesis of his personal decision and commitment to travel were laid bare. Also pressing were inherent uncertainties surrounding death and dying, and thus an urgent need to be with his mom and family. Clearly, as noted previously, no analysis of these interactionally sensitive moments can adequately capture such complex and unsettling circumstances faced by family members. The obvious and personal turmoil experienced by each family member can never be fully encapsulated. But is has been possible to trace how son enacted (and agents responded) to a form of urgency comprising son's airline calls.

The initial and most apparent influence on these airline calls was son's being informed by his aunt and dad that "compassion fares" existed and should be pursued. From these family encounters, as introduced in Figure 3 (above), we have identified the interactional foundation and base components of son's subsequent "problem narratives": **being a graduate student → with little money→ who just found out his mother is dying →who is aware of "compassion fares" and → needs to find out if each airline offers such discounted fares**. It is indeed rare to have access to materials revealing the interactional roots of what eventually amounts to a "presentation format." And whenever any script/template gets repeatedly enacted by speakers, especially to different and first-time recipients, such actions will reveal how speakers' a priori conceptions about interaction inevitably get tailored to real time and thus contingently organized interactional moments. Such is the case regardless of the participants involved and tasks/problems addressed.

This is especially the case when a son requires assistance organizing travel in the midst of a family health crisis. With access to such materials, an enhanced understanding and appreciation of an array of interactional moments is acquired—events and activities that are typically not available when researching single case or episodic interactions in everyday life (see Chapter 2). Specific attention can be given to how relevancies comprising a single interactional encounter between family members (i.e., a phone call between son, mom, and dad) utilized as resources for constructing narratives for subsequent airline calls. Over time, son's narrative adaptations across subsequent interactional involvements could also be tracked. Although only portions of eight contiguous calls have been examined in this chapter, a case has thus been made for the value of longitudinal observations.

It is curious that son persisted with presenting his narrative, especially following repeated failures to receive adequate compassion fares. Yet his actions exemplify how each time he speaks with a different airline the agents exhibit being first-time recipients, unaware that son is reenacting versions of prior appeals. Even though son's problem narratives were increasingly adapted to the kind of recipients airline agents showed themselves to be, son's basic orientations remained the same because his recipients were uninformed as to whether they were called in a series. Son, then, was in a position to adapt his presentations without agents' knowledge that he was increasingly working to optimize his likelihood of receiving timely and discounted fares.

Progressive Routinization: Streamlining Calls to Agents

Son's adaptations to airline agents' agendas is increasingly self-evident as these calls emerge. The more son interacted with airline agents, the more he adapted his problem narratives through brevity, less hesitancy, and forcefulness indicative of more practical modes of delivery. Over time, his informational requests were more tightly constructed as urgent needs for travel were laid bare. From the first to last airline call, a gradual diminishing of son's wordiness is apparent. These changes may be a basic upshot of repetition and practice. But it should not be overlooked that son was also influenced by not receiving discounted fares that are indeed compassionate, and being informed (at times) that he cannot qualify for fares airlines don't offer. These residual experiences are evident as son's presentations increasingly resemble assembly-line productions replete with items/lists. This is not surprising because stories themselves, let alone narratives about here-and-now personal crises, become increasingly streamlined and to the point through repeated retellings (see Beach, 2000a; Norrick, 1997; Sacks, 1992).

Interactionally, as each agent initiated contingent actions during greetings, replies, narratives, and even closings, son was in a position to respond accordingly. But it is curious that with each progressive call to airlines, son built his narrative presentations not necessarily with specific recipients in mind—indeed, each agent was a stranger—but for more generalized and routinized airline protocols he was increasingly learning about.

Related ironies have only been hinted at: As son repeatedly discloses personal dilemmas occasioned by his mother's dying from cancer, his own presentations take on some of the same characteristics as those enacted by otherwise institutional representatives. A central part of son's efforts are direct reflections of his necessary immersion into the world inhabited by major airlines. Eventually, the son is even capable of teaching some airline employees (e.g., SW agent and aunt/flight attendant) about fare structures he only recently learned about.

Pursuing Withheld "Compassion"

It must be re-emphasized that with two exceptions (the calls to US Air in Excerpt 17, and Continental in Excerpt 18), only the opening moments of airline calls have been examined thus far. Following greetings, focus has been given to how son initially and explicitly requests information about *compassion fares*. To a limited extent it has also addressed how son describes his dilemma to airline representatives in ways that make the case for being a person in need of help and requiring special assistance, and solicits special understanding (e.g., legitimacy or sympathy) regarding his personal circumstances.

Further attention could be given to specific practices employed by son as he pursues what is treated as prior and withheld empathy, sympathy, or compassion by airline representatives. For example, consider the following example from near the end of his call to AA:

22) **SDCL: Malignancy 4:3-4 (Airlines Call #1)**

1   AA: Okay. The flight number tomorrow is ah flight one twenty
2   three. =
3   Son: = One twenty three.

4	AA:	Yeah an' that departs [city] at four forty six. = Now it
5		connects in [city], to flight sixty seven.
6	Son:	Okay. And °sixty seven° (.) All right.
7		(0.8)
8	Son:	→Well? ↑I wish I was traveling under nicer circumstances. Um=
9	AA:	→=Well we do too sir.
10	Son:	→$Huh.$ Well thanks very much for your help and I will
11		probably call you back first thing in the morning then.
12	AA:	All right.
13	Son:	Thank you. (.) Bye bye.
14	AA:	↓Thanks for calling American.

As a bid for closing this call, and indeed as one form of a "sequence closing assessment" (see Jefferson, 1980a, 1980b, 1981, 1993), son here states the obvious: "Well? ↑I wish I was traveling under nicer circumstances." (line 8). This and/or some related utterance could very well have been offered by a recipient having heard and sympathized with son's travel predicament. In ordinary conversations, such actions might be understood as offerings of "condolence", provided as a means of comforting and supporting a person in trouble. But because no such offering is offered by the AA agent, son enacts one type of "fishing device" (Pomerantz, 1978, 1980) to elicit a reply that son treats as having been noticeably absent. And in response, "Well we do too sir." (line 9), the agent aligns with son's assessment, otherwise retains his institutional identity ("we"), and thereby withholds offering any personal commiseration. With "$Huh.$" (line 10) son receipts this minimalized offering with laughter, once again showing himself to be somewhat resistant to events triggered by mom's dying.

Throughout the airline calls it can be seen how son repeatedly attempts to strike a balance between maintaining the composure and interactional distance that is expected during normal business interactions and presenting himself as a sympathetic figure who is in trouble and deserves compassion. This is often a precarious line to straddle:

> Where it is certainly the case that although a troubles-teller can be overly upset by and receptive to his or her own troubles, the teller can as well be overly troubles-resistant, can be seen to be taking a trouble too well or too lightly, which can be assessed as a matter of irresponsibility or incompetence. (Jefferson, 1984a, p. 355)

Such is certainly not the case with son's "$Huh.$" above. But this moment does exemplify how it is interactionally problematic to manage troubles, let alone solicit from an unacquainted troubles-recipient (agent) empathy surpassing what airline representatives typically offer. It cannot be overlooked that for agents, son's call is just another in a series of what amounts to dozens of calls per day, perhaps hundreds over the routine course of a week's employment.

It becomes clear, then, that "While in a troubles telling the focal object is the 'teller and his experiences', in the service encounter the focal object is the 'problem and its properties'" (Jefferson & Lee, 1981/1992, p. 535). The troubles facing the parties are differentially distributed: for son, facing a solitary and pressing family crisis requiring timely and affordable travel; for airline agents, determining whether services are offered and can be provided—a business as usual approach to handling numerous calls. Left hanging are more than fleeting and institutionally constrained attempts to pay focused attention to callers' personal circumstances—experienced but temporarily disadvantaged troubles whose full disclosure and resolutions extend well beyond what a single reservation agent might possibly provide. In short, son must manage the social fact that offering personalized service for airline customers is not tantamount to counseling services nor, even minimally, *being compassionate*. Indeed, activities comprising the "pursuit and withholding of commiseration" are commonplace in everyday affairs (e.g., see Beach, 1996; Mandelbaum, 1991) and by no means limited to encounters between institutional representatives and lay persons.

Yet the SW agent appears to be somewhat of an exception to this rule. She improvised and provided a more personalized institutional greeting, made son's needs a priority over making a sale, and in the end represented a major airline that offered less restricted and cheaper fares than other airlines called by son. A more detailed analysis of the remainder of the SW call (not provided here) would reveal her to be somewhat more sympathetic than other agents examined in our corpus. It is the son's encounter with SW, then, that forces reflection on what, pragmatically speaking, is really meaningful about compassion fares. It is paradoxical that even when compassion fares per se are not offered, as with SW, services rendered can far exceed programs built for the explicit purpose of helping customers embroiled in the trials and tribulations surrounding death and dying of family members.

And continued problems emerge. The *sustained relevance* of cancer-related dilemmas are evident in the following Chapter 6: Son is involved with a series of calls with his recently divorced wife, and dad, about his pending yet tenuous travel arrangements to visit mom and family.

NOTES

1. Considerably more can be said about troubling interactional environments involving discussions of pain and medication. This excerpt is drawn from collections of related moments where diverse activities get accomplished: how an ill person specifies and others respond to preferences for treatment (e.g., no life support and pain management); how activities such as "uncertainty" and "pain" might be understood as social constructions (e.g., see Capps & Ochs, 1995); and how references to medical professionals are achieved, in this case involving "them" as authorities whose technical skills and knowledge allow for the possibility of "stopping" pain (see Chapters 8 & 9).

2. Exact details about medical professionals' opinions of mom's impending death are not known. However, beginning with phone call #3, son is encouraged to be ready to travel home to see and speak with mom before her death. Later in call #3, mom and son speak in some detail about whether he would rather visit now or at mom's memorial service, a reality dad confirms when he gets on the phone to discuss arrangement of travel plans.

3. Specifically, as discussed in Excerpt 2, son states that he would rather visit mom now than attend her "memorial service". His decision is strongly influenced by normal matters such as budget and scheduling. It is paradoxical that factors such as money and time influence how family members spend time together, even under dire circumstances. Even in the midst of life's most challenging events, however, the realities of budgets, work, and related commitments must be managed.

4. In call #10, following son's calls to airlines, he has an extended discussion with his aunt (mom's sister) about mom's condition: how the doctors are treating her considerable pain with morphine, advice regarding travel (aunt is a flight attendant), and how the family (including both of them) was coping with uncertainties and troubles regarding the looming inevitability of mom's death.

5. Subsequent moments throughout these calls are analyzed later in this chapter, when son describes his dilemma to airline representatives in ways that continue to (a) make the case for being a person in need of help and requiring special assistance, and (b) solicit special understanding (e.g., legitimacy or sympathy) regarding his personal circumstances. Airline agents' responses to son's compassion-seeking activities are also analyzed.

6. Analysis might usefully be compared to Maynard's (1997, 2003) work on News Delivery Sequences (NDS's) overviewed in Chapter 3. Although news informings display universal and even canonical features, such features are neither dependent on the events themselves nor rigidly enacted. Rather, news deliveries and their receipts are part of a generic NDS, through which participants assemble matters or events in the world as news for them of a particular kind.

Produced contingently in real-time NDS's, as well as son's narratives, get coenacted within and across turns at talk through the mutual articulation of in-course interactional adjustments.

7. In addition to phone calls directly to the airlines, travel agents may be consulted during family crises. So too may an array of websites, providing updated information on discounted and efficient travel (e.g., a search with key terms "bereavement fares" will produce a long listing of such options). Given that the phone calls examined herein were collected in 1988-89, internet access was not an option. Yet it is an interesting and common feature of these websites that recognition is made of travelers' troubling circumstances. One website noted that "Dealing with travel plans in the face of the death or illness of a loved one is incredibly difficult" (http://www.independent-traveler.com/). And in an article entitled "Getting Home Soon: Finding the Best Bereavement Fares," ABCNews.com observes that "When you're faced with the critical illness or death of a family member in a distant city, negotiating a good air fare is the farthest thing from your mind. . . . Sad as the subject may be to contemplate, a little advance thinking can save you a great deal of worry and money should the need arise."

8. The *offering* of discounted fares, designed by airlines to accommodate urgent situations involving family illness or death, needn't be synonymous with receiving the lowest and most convenient fares. If possible, customers are encouraged to shop around for cheaper discount tickets, because prices and travel restrictions vary widely across major airlines. Even though airlines often waive advance and full-fare prices to assist travelers, less expensive fares can still be found (see Jeffrey, 2000). Nevertheless, many family members simply do not have the time to shop fares in times of crisis and thus rely on calls to the airlines to solicit information about reduced rates. Unfortunately, in their haste, many people fail to request information on bereavement or compassion fares, let alone seek cheaper rates from other airlines. Ironically, reduced rates may be offered by the same airline due to sales promotions in particular markets. For these and related reasons, "the majors are not going to give you a deal you might deem compassionate" (Parsons, 2002, p. 1).

9. For example, recent work on the interactional organization of survey interviews (see Maynard et al., 2002; Maynard & Schaeffer, 1997, 2002a, 2002b) reveals how interviewers proactively work to insure respondents' participation, and how it is *call recipients* who are in the position to grant or decline requests to respond to telephone surveys: "It is "citizens" or household members, rather than members of some institution or organization, who are keeping the gate" (Maynard & Schaeffer, 2002, p. 201). In marked contrast, airline agents are gatekeepers in the calls we examine. As recipients of son's calls, agents represent institutions that regulate service offerings (i.e., fares, prices, and scheduling). It is the son who works to persuasively make requests in pursuit of their being granted rather than declined, who initiates such actions as "personalizing the opening of the call", and even behaves in ways akin to "soliciting a favor." Our data, then, allow for interesting comparisons with telephone surveys, especially grounded understandings of the "front end" of calls and how requests are made, responded to, and dealt with throughout assorted encounters.

10. The inherent uncertainties associated with death and dying represent unrivaled mysteries defining the human condition. The vast spiritual, religious, clinical, and palliative care literature addressing how people make sense of, cope with, and communicate about death and dying cannot be adequately summarized here (but see Kubler-Ross, 1969b). Nor can we, as analysts, do justice to the sensitivities of such revealing family moments. For example, inserted into mom's emphatic "I don't knows" is her "I:'m (.) not done it,". This is an obvious statement, of course, but raises a fascinating and complex set of issues addressed (in part) in a patient-narrated video entitled *I've Never Died Before* (1999, Kaiser Permanente, Department of Preventive Medicine/San Diego).

11. There is distinct irony in son's listening to soothing classical music mixed with intermittent recorded messages—invitations to "Make it a memorable Christmas" by traveling to St. Thomas, or nonstop service and easier routes to Honduras, Scandinavia, or other world destinations—escapisms standing in marked contrast to the family business son needs to attend to. These recorded messages are hearably receipted by son with loud "sighs", preceding his hanging up the phone and calling the next airline on his list (US Air).

12. Maynard and Schaeffer (2002b) describe a single instance where a survey interviewer engages in tailoring the script: "Tailoring is facilitated at the front end of the interview because interviewers

are not required to adhere strictly to a standard introduction" (p. 220). Rather than stating "Hello, I'm Bob Roth calling from Indiana University," the interviewer stated, "Hi my name's Bob Roth, I'm calling from Indiana University." The observation is made that the latter format is an instance of "personalizing" a call. In contrast it is not known, however, whether the SW agent had an actual written script to follow (as did the survey interviewer). What can be noted is that it departs from the three prior agents' introductions and greetings, and son next (in all cases) designs his response in consideration of these specific features.

13. These "Hi's" may be usefully contrasted with a caller's "Yes", which briefly confirms receipt of call taker's opening identification immediately prior to requesting assistance:

[CDV31B-A/080: D=Dispatcher, C=Caller)] (Whalen & Zimmerman, 1987, p. 176)

> D: Nine one one emer:gency.
>   (0.6)
> C: Yes, I need a towing tru:ck (continues)

14. When examining how survey interviewers improvise telephone "scripts", Maynard and Schaeffer (2002b) note the following:

> The crafting of his opening talk, and its departure from the more conventional script, can be working interactionally in at least two ways. First, "May I please . . ." occasions the relevance of a straightforward yes-no answer as a reply to the request for an interview, while "we'd like a chance . . ." implicates different answering options, in particular the granting or withholding of an opportunity. (p. 227)

With the son's case-making to airline agents, pursued answers have less to do with "granting or withholding of an opportunity" in favor of being treated as a legitimate candidate for receiving discounted fares.

15. Once again, as noted in Note #6 (above), this 14-second recording encouraged son to consider traveling to distant and exotic travel locations for vacations, which, as noted, stand in marked contrast to demands arising from his urgent family business.

6

STABILITY AND AMBIGUITY

Living in Flux
With Mom's Cancer

Problems with travel and scheduling do not end once son has completed his calls with airline representatives. In this chapter, excerpts are analyzed from four phone calls involving family members: three with Gina (his recently divorced wife) in calls #11, 17-18, and a surprising news update from dad in call #12. Each call involves discussions of how son's travel plans are intertwined with mom's changing health status. In three phone calls over a two day period, son delivers and updates news to Gina about the stability of mom's condition. His updates arose from prior informings. When updating Gina about travel plans and mom's condition, son relies upon reconstructions from both family members' and health professionals' reportings.

Several distinct features and problems enacted through these cumulative News Delivery Sequences (NDSs, see Chapter 3) are identified. Behaving as if mom would soon be dying, news announcements and elaborations are shaped by inherent and practical ambiguities associated with mom's prognosis (e.g., stabilizing of her condition, when doctors will visit her, and what they know). Son and dad repeatedly display frustration and fatigue from being primary family members preoccupied with how to simultaneously manage mom's health, work, travel, and scheduling plans, and a host of related matters in their daily lives. For Gina, responding to and assessing son's news updates will also be shown to be problematic. Displaying concerns for mom and son, yet also distancing from reported troubles, require different interactional solutions. The achieved character of social relationships (e.g., closeness and distance) is once again evident as speakers demonstrate being differently affected by the news.

These interactions make clear that understanding the social organization of family cancer journeys requires close examination of single moments, but also the sustained and managed relevance of topics and concerns across multiple interactions. During extended periods of illness, family members have little choice but somehow to adapt to the evolving nature of diverse relationships. So too must family members continually alter their practical decision making and plans, and collaborate in producing their own ongoing lay diagnoses about an illness they neither fully understand nor control.

FAMILY UPDATES: MONITORING AND TRACKING AMBIGUITIES ABOUT MOM'S STABILITY

In Excerpt 1 (1→) son's announcement to Gina, that he may not be coming home, occurs as first topic following their phone greeting (lines 1-11). Analysis begins with the delivery of son's news (lines 12-13) and will return to the phone opening in a later discussion:

1) **SDCL: Malignancy #11:1**

```
 1    Son:     He̲llo ↑Doug here.
 2    Gina:    I ↑lov:e yo:u:.
 3    Son:       ↑Hi::.
 4    Gina:    I wanted to te̲ll you tha:t.=
 5    Son:     =Well tha:n[ks.
 6    Gina:              [°(You're the one.°)
 7             (0.2)
 8    Son:     .hhh Thanks. hhh
 9    Gina:    °(He's)° the little one, I love him.
10    Son:     hhh Thanks.=
11    Gina:    °I haven't left him.°
12    Son:1→   .hhhh hhhh Well there's a po::ssiblility I might
13             not be ↑coming now.
14    Gina:2→  °Why?°
15    Son:3→pt Oh- hh .hh [Because- ]
16    Gina:2→              [ °(   )° ] pull t[hrough)]?°
17    Son:3→                              [ well? ] =
18             =↑Not pulling throu::gh but at least s:ta:bilized=an:d
19             of course I̲ can only be gone so: lo:ng.= So .hhh if it
20             looks like she's gonna (.) ha̲ng in for another (0.2)
21             couple of wee:ks, then I'll wanna wait a couple of
22             weeks but,=
23    Gina:4→  = Oh my $G(h)o[::d.$
24    Son:                   [Ye:ah ri̲:ght, .hh uhm, hh So >that's
25             in fact< that's what I thought this pho:ne call was,=
26             I'm- I'm wa̲iting, (.) to hear from,=
27    Gina:    =(  ) Did they call you last ni:ght?
28    Son:     Yeah.
29             (1.2)
30    Son:     Yeah we- e- u::m- pt a:nd she's gotta .hhhh a do̲ctor
31             who's gonna see her this mo̲rning, but (.) you know (.) the
32             ti:me difference an    every̲thing. .hhh uhm pt Th- they won't
33             (.) kno::w anything for a little whi:le yet. So it's kinda puts
34             me in an awkward spot ↑here. 'Cuz ge:ez I̲ >ya know< pt .hh
35             I got everything arra̲nged to go::, and .hh >ya know< got
36             somebody to pick up the ma:il, and got somebody to take
37             my classes and all that. And if I end up sta̲:ying I'll (0.2) f-
38             feel a little we̲ir:d. But- .hhh uhm =
```

Prefaced with a sigh (1→), son displays a sense of frustration and fatigue associated with making (and altering) travel decisions. He is not yet reporting directly on mom's circumstances (see 3→), but does reveal himself as a family member caught up within and impacted by mom's uncertain illness trajectory. By not referencing mom throughout this excerpt,

Gina is treated by son as having some prior knowledge about mom's health and as a person affected by son's ongoing predicament. She is also involved in his travel plans, which explains his updating efforts.

In (2→) Gina queries "°Why?°", yet next (line 16) proffers a guess as a knowing recipient: The reason for son possibly altering his plans may be that mom might "pull through". This description stands in contrast to her dying, in which case son would not be postponing his visit. This is not an apt description, however, as son's immediate correction to "s:ta:bilized" in (3→) indicates. Although mom's stability is comparatively good news, especially given the unstated alternative (i.e., dying), it creates other ambiguities of waiting, which son must now deal with (lines 18-21). A delicate balance is revealed between how long mom has to live, how long son can be gone (e.g., from work), and thus problems with discerning exactly when to travel home.

In reporting these looming decisions to Gina, son depicts himself as double-binded by a quandary of interwoven professional and personal commitments. Because there is no way of knowing for sure just how long his mom might live, the fluctuating circumstances he is faced with cannot be remedied by locking in plans and schedules. It is clear that mom's stabilization does not necessarily simplify son's daily affairs. Nor does it significantly improve his abilities to cope with her illness (e.g., the pain and suffering mom may be experiencing). Rather, mom's stabilization complicates son's own situation, as portrayed in the narrative account of the dilemma he is in: He can only be gone for so long, and if mom is going to "hang in" for a while he needs to wait "but..." (line 21) — and what remains unsaid is the contrast to her not hanging in — that is, dying.

In the face of these ambiguities, however, there are also distinct certainties: Mom is seriously ill, and son is committed to travel and be with her (and family). However, the fact remains that travel plans require careful monitoring of a situation in flux: Schedules and even expectations are often volatile in everyday life, and son's dilemma offers only one poignant example.

Responding with "Oh my $G(h)o[::d.$"

In (4→) Gina offers "Oh my $G(h)o[::d.$" as a display of surprise to son's just-stated news, one routine device for assessing some prior action as worthy of such a reaction (e.g., see Maynard, 2003; Wilkinson & Kitzinger, 2006; Excerpt 3, below). It is significant that her "Oh my $G(h)o[::d.$" occurs precisely in response to son's reference to "a couple weeks". In this way, son creates a metric for assessing how long mom might have to live: He provides Gina with a more specific resource for understanding just how serious mom's condition actually is. With "Oh" she registers awareness of new information and knowledge, a noticeable shift in her "change of state" about mom's health and what family members are facing (see Heritage, 1984a, 1998, 2002). Constructed as a "my-world" realization of the circumstances son has described, Gina also exhibits being negatively affected by the news about mom. It cannot be overlooked that as prior daughter-in-law, Gina has a relational history with mom and son's family.

Central to an understanding of these paired and key moments (i.e., between son's 3→ and Gina's 4→) is not overlooking that, and how, Gina prosodically constructs "$G(h)o[::d.$" through laughter, aspiration, and vocalic stretch. As an expletive rather than a substantive evaluation, Gina's "Oh my $G(h)o[::d.$" does not formulate the specific target of what she is assessing, even though it does occur (as noted) precisely in response to son's "a couple of weeks" (lines 21-22). But by inserting a laugh token in the middle of her invocation of "$G(h)o[::d.$" — once again, in troubling circumstances she does not control — Gina does display a delicate orientation to son's reporting. For example, Jefferson (1984a, 1984b) has shown that laughter produced by tellers of troubles indicates their resistance to the predicaments reported. However in this moment, as troubles-*recipient*, Gina's laughter is designed to lighten the expletive assessment and thereby display that it is ultimately son's trouble, not primarily her own, that is being addressed. Although Gina demonstrates that she is affected by troubling news surrounding mom's illness and mom's condition, she simultaneously distances herself from those very troubles. Yet she also shows appreciation for son's dilemma, that is, the distressing and consequential impacts of such news for son. As noted, his daily affairs (e.g., plans, schedules, expectations) are correspondingly in flux. In this way Gina is momentarily being with son, showing recognition of the inevitable tensions he is facing: maintaining flexibility, yet understandably seeking closure, in the midst of making decisions that can instantly change because of mom's changing health status.

In noticeably delicate moments in medical interviews, for example, patients' laughter may indicate their own embarrassment about a trouble they have reported (see Beach & Dixson, 2001; Haakana, 2001). In moments like these, patients are not inviting shared laughter, evidenced in part by providers refraining from laughing. Similarly, in Excerpt 1 (above), son does not laugh in response to Gina's "$G(h)o[::d.$". In overlap, with "Ye:ah ri:ght" (line 24), he ratifies the stance Gina has constructed with respect to the news, thereby accepting her assessment and the distancing mechanism embedded within it. Son's response, which precedes his reporting that he was waiting for a phone call to receive a current update of mom's condition, effectively reconfirms and emphasizes the intensity of his owned experience as a central figure in the news he has delivered (see Heritage & Raymond, 2005; Raymond & Heritage, 2006; Chapters 7 & 10). Son is able not only to show agreement (line 24) but own the quandary he is attempting to deal with by claiming epistemic priority over unfolding events. In stating that he thought this was another phone call that he was waiting for, he elucidates the urgency of the situation *he* is faced with and *his* preoccupation with it (lines 23-25).[1] His dilemma is further exemplified when son reports that because "they won't know anything for a little while yet" he's in an "awkward spot here", and because everything is arranged to travel home, "if I end up staying I'll feel a little weird" (lines 32-37).

Consequently, the present call with Gina is placed in temporal perspective by son: not as unimportant, but as comparatively less in touch with *current news* about mom's condition, the very issues prior talk with Gina had been about. As son shifts attention to a (potentially) incoming call, further evidence is revealed that the situation is a serious one, a predicament in which son is a prominent figure as news develops and gets disseminated, and that additional and relevant news is forthcoming. And it is these matters about which Gina next queries with "=( ) Did they call you last ni:ght? " (line 27), as she further collaborates on talk about ensuing troubles, information that only son can report on when he states that there is a "doctor who's gonna see her this morning." (lines 30-31).

Managing Ongoing Uncertainties and Frustrations

Yet another paradox is faced by the son and his family: After all the efforts to arrange travel plans, so apparent in calls between son, mom and dad (call #3), son and airline representatives (calls #4-9), son and aunt Carol (call #10), and son and Gina (call #11 and Excerpt 1, above), son does not travel home to be with his dying mother and family until weeks later. Within 24 hours following calls with his aunt and divorced wife, he received another call from dad:

2) **SDCL: Malignancy #12:1**

```
1    Son: INI→A::lri::ght? What's the scoop. hhh =
2    Dad: 1→=↑We: :ll (.) stay there.
```

```
 3    Son:  2→Stay here. hh
 4    Dad:  3→Stay there. =
 5    Son:  4→= .hh Oh:::y hh .hh o-↑okay. hh =
 6    Dad:PAE=  Ye::ah I know. This >been a damn up an down an up
 7      ↓   an down.< I °ya know° ya- ya don't know whether to be
 8      ↓   p:le:ased or not ple$ased [hah hh$]
 9    Son:  ↓                        [$huh hh$] .hhhh=
10    Dad:  ↓[Hu::m.]
11    Son:  ↓[ .hhhh ]
12      ↓   (1.0)
13    Dad:  ↓Hhhh hhh <I d:o:n't kno::w ye:t.> (1.1) Ya know, the trip was
14      ↓   gonna come about. It's just that ya know (.) i::f ya wanna
15      ↓   come this week, this is not gonna be an e:nd week kinda
16      ↓   thing. . hhh So:::o, (.) your mother's answer was na::h stay
17      ↓   there ya know. She's- she is ↑much better this morning,
18      ↓   ((continues by talking about what the doctor said))

           ((10 lines deleted))

29    Dad:  >Ya know< as I said her ans[ wer ya s ]tay there. =
30    Son:                              [.HHHHH ]
31    Dad:  = For the time being [ ( mean ) time. ]
32    Son: →                     [Tu huh huh .hh]hh Ya guys gotta stop
33          doin' this to me.
34    Dad:  Uhh.
35    Son: →Ha:::::ah $.hh hhh [ huh hhh .hh hhh hhh .hh hh hh hh ] =
```

Here it is clear that, and how, uncertainty is realized and evident in practical actions.[2] As dad updates and announces to son that he should "stay there", reactions amount to a mixture of frustration and relief. In lines 6-8 (during his PAE or Post Assessment Elaboration) dad himself states "This >been a damn up an down an up an down.< I °ya know° ya- ya don't know whether to be p:le:ased or not ple$ased [hah hh$]"—a disclaimer marked with laughter, which son shares through his own aspirated response (lines 9 & 11).

In retrospect, it can be determined that mom does not die for an additional six weeks (see Timeline in Chapter 2). This is the case even though doctors, who advised mom and dad to contact son and urge his travel, anticipated a high probability of mom's imminent death. Yet doctors can be and frequently are wrong. Just as hindsight is a 20-20 resource not applicable to future events, so too is it an understatement to note that death is difficult to predict (see Excerpt 8 in Chapter 9). But if and when experts believe death is imminent, and even the patient (mom) concurs (as evident in call #3 as mom states her preferences about life support), what else is a family to do but arrange their lives as if mom were dying sooner rather than later? These are only some of the exigencies giving rise to calling and updating family members about a loved one's illness—increasingly familiar, yet inherently unpredictable, illness circumstances.

Ongoing Volatility of Mom's Condition

The next day Gina calls son, in response to a message from him she had "finally" gotten on her phone recorder (see also Excerpt 11, Chapter 7). She reports that the message wasn't clear ("chopped"), and that she had called to find out what had happened. Several moments later and within the first minute of this phone conversation, Gina's "What's up" solicits news about mom's condition, which son next delivers:

3) SDCL: Malignancy #18:2

```
 1   Gina:INI→ What's up?
 2   Son:1-3→  We:ll (.) the:y've sta:bilized 'er again.=A:nd ba:sically
 3             what they said i:s .hhh keep you're le:sson pla:ns
 4             current:, a:n don't unpa:ck your ba:g comple:tely.=But-
 5             (.) I don't need ta sho:w up: quite ↑(ch)yet.=So:=
 6   Gina:4→   = < O:h my G(h)o::d. >
 7             (0.3)
 8   Gina:4→   You poor thi::ng. hhh
 9             (0.4)
10   Son:      pt So tha:t's:=↑really all I can tell ya.
11   Gina:     (°W(h)ow-°) How long (they) think she's gonna hold o::ut?
12             She still in the hospital?=
13   Son:      =Ye:ah, yeah. She's still in the hospital. They don't
14             kno::w. 'Could be a couple a weeks?
```

This segment, a mixture of good news about mom's stabilization yet ongoing bad news about son's travel predicament, can essentially be parsed as a four-part NDS. Because son latches (=) his continuation (line 2), Gina's response to his announcement is missing but not noticeably absent. Next, son moves to elaborate his news (lines 2-5), which is then assessed twice by Gina (4→).

By initiating his reporting with "the:y've stabilized er aga:in.=" (1→), son treats as unnecessary the need to specify that "they've" (treated collectively and anonymously) is in reference to medical staff caring for his mom. Such indexical and medical references occur frequently in this corpus (e.g., see lines 2, 3, 11, & 12 above; Excerpt 4, below; Chapter 8). And as a focal issue in the news update, "stabilized" is repeated from the prior phone call (see Excerpt 1, line 18, above). With "again" son adds emphasis to the in-flux character of mom's condition, a qualification implying the omnipresent threat of her instability.

Having provided the gist of his news for Gina, son next reports basic features of "what they said" (line 3). Although "they" is unexplicated, it is likely referring not to medical personnel but to an earlier discussion with dad in call #12 (see Chapter 7, Excerpt 11). Produced as hearably grim yet wise advice that was given to him, son depicts not necessarily what "they" actually said, but a version directly reflective of a situation son had previously articulated: He will need to coordinate his teaching responsibilities while remaining ready, at a moment's notice, to travel home. The conjoined phrases, "keep you're le:sson pla:ns current:, a:n don't unpa:ck your ba:g", are figurative expressions (e.g., Beach 1993a, 1996; Drew & Holt, 1988, 1998; Holt & Drew, 2005; see Chapter 7). In ordinary conversations, it has been shown that speakers routinely employ formulaic constructions when attributing figurative meanings to situations they are attempting to summarize and/or complain about, while also pursuing affiliation and alignment from recipients. Both phrases also represent a state of readiness as responsive to the urgency this family is facing (see Chapter 7).

As son collapses an update about mom with a description of his travel situation, he makes his troubles available for Gina's response. He then provides the practical upshot of this news (lines 4-5) by stating "I don't need ta sho:w up: quite ↑(ch)yet.". With "sho:w up:" the details and importance of his actual reasons for traveling home are glossed. However, "quite ↑(ch)yet" succinctly retains the impending nature of the situation he is imparting: an ongoing and unresolved circumstance in which son's travel plans are contingent upon updates about mom's health status.

In (2→), yet another "< O:h my G(h)o::d. >" uttered by Gina shows her involvement in and being affected by son's precarious situation, treated by son as a knowing recipient capable of hearing an update carried over from a prior call (Excerpt 1, above). Once again (see the previous Excerpt 1, line 23), Gina invokes an emphasized, aspirated, and stretched "G(h)o::d." as a second-party recipient for whom troubling news is consequential. And marked by the small aspiration "(h)" in "G(h)o::d.", she further displays that although the news affects her, she is nevertheless not undergoing the turmoil that son reports (i.e., as the primary consequential figure). In this moment, her assessment is directed more to son's own involvement in the situation and the effects it appears to be having on him, rather than impacts on her life. Followed by silence (line 7), son's lack of response is treated by Gina as further evidence of the chaos *he* must be experiencing. In response, with "You poor thi::ng.", she shifts attention more directly to sympathy for son's well-being, concern offered by Gina as a person less involved and impacted by mom's cancer diagnosis and treatment.

Marked by another delay (line 9), by stating "pt So tha:t's:=↑really all I can tell ya." son continues what his earlier "So:" (line 5) appears to have been initiating. His word repeat, and the utterance it is embedded within, essentially proposes closure to further talk on this topic. Any further elaboration would be available only from son's narration about his experiences (see Schegloff, 1998), which he has introduced as a primary figure dealing with the news. He thus treats as unnecessary the need to explicitly and further acknowledge the dilemma he is squarely in the midst of. By remaining silent, son is enacting being in a difficult situation about which little more can be said at the moment, an option available to a primary and consequential figure embroiled in managing ongoing bad news.

But there is more here, actions further revealing the nature of son's relationship with Gina. In line 10, son's ""pt So tha:t's:=↑really all I can tell ya."" shifts focus away from himself and his experiences of the situation, and (as noted) toward the news and the finality of its reportage. By not further elaborating on the situation and how it is affecting him, and by not displaying "letting go" (Jefferson, 1988, p. 428), he fails to comment on Gina's "You poor thi::ng." Line 8). Jefferson (1988) has described how news recipients frequently exhibit affiliation following a troubles-telling, or what Maynard (1997, 2003) terms an "elaboration", and that is clearly what Gina has offered. Yet her affiliative display was not treated by son as an opportunity to produce "emotionally heightened talk, 'letting go', and/or turning to or confiding in the troubles/recipient" (p. 428). In marked contrast, son noticeably refrains from such talk by avoiding disclosures about his dilemma and finalizing his news delivery. Through his actions, an opportunity for further intimacy (including additional commiseration) is bypassed. Instead, son continues by offering a story about mom's "cigarettes" (see Excerpt 3, Chapter 11).

Negotiating Ongoing Relationships in Times of Trouble

What other plausible explanations might be provided for son's actions? One possibility is that his failure to respond directly to Gina's stated concern is reflective of the ongoing status of their divorced relationship. Consider the phone opening below between son and Gina (from Excerpt 3, above):

4) SDCL: Malignancy #11:1

1	Son:	Hello ↑Doug here.
2	Gina:	I ↑lov:e yo:u:.
3	Son:	↑Hi::.
4	Gina:	I wanted to tell you tha:t.=
5	Son:	=Well tha:n[ks.
6	Gina:	[°(You're the one.°)
7		(0.2)

```
8    Son:      .hhh Thanks. hhh
9    Gina:     °You're the (  ) one, I [know that.]
10   Son:                           [ .hhh ] Thanks.=
11   Gina:     (°  loved him.° )
12   Son:1→    .hhhh hhhh Well there's a po::ssiblility I might
13             not be ↑coming now.
```

Here, too, son passes on repeated opportunities to pursue actions related to Gina's endearing comments. He first withholds reciprocation of Gina's "I love you" (line 3). As this phone opening unfolds, Gina does not implore but hearably pursues more than what son continues to offer (see lines 4, 6, & 9): He thanks her, but noticeably does not respond in kind with endearing compliments.

Nevertheless, Gina initiates a stepwise shift and further queries son about mom's condition (lines 11-12). Her wondering about "How long (they) think she's gonna "hold o::ut?" closely resembles her "pull through" in an earlier call (see Excerpt 1, line 5, above). But it is clear in son's response (lines 13-14) that although mom's being in the hospital is easily confirmed, "They don't kno::w." references medical professionals' uncertainties about when, where, and how mom might live or die.

A GLIMPSE OF HOPE ABOUT MOM'S DELICATE HEALTH STATUS

Later that same day, Gina called son to speak about a number of matters, including an update about mom. Immediately prior to the excerpt below, son had informed Gina that he had told his parents that she was moving. When Gina inquired, son informed her about their reaction. Next, Gina moves to query son about his parents and, more specifically, "Talked to your mom?"(line 1):

5) SDCL: Malignancy #18:11

```
1    Gina:INI→Your parents? Talked to your mo:m?
2    Son:       No:.= >I talked to my fa:ther<.=
3    Gina:      =°Hm:.°.
4               (2.0)
5    Son: 1→    [ No  mom- mom's ] mom's in the hospital.
6    Gina:      [(°     your fa:ther?°) ]
7               >Well that's when you said that I thought-< =
8    Son: 1→    Although the:y ↑think she might come ho::me?
9               (0.2) Uhm, pt I mean (.) se- since- sh- once- once
                they stabilize her, they don't need her in the
                hospital again. .hhh Uhm I guess what it is now is
                it's in all of her lo:ng bo:nes, an they're- they're-
                afraid that .hh her bo:nes are gonna just start
14              breaking.=hh .hh Uhm=
15   Gina:2→    =°Uh huh?°
16              (0.5)
17   Son: 3→    So they're gonna- (0.4) what they think they're gonna
                do is- >is do her out patient, you know let her< spend
                the nights at ho:me, .hh an' then take her into the
                hospital during the days for radiation (.) .hh uh on
                her legs. hh That's the next thing. (1.0) But I haven't
```

23   Gina:4→   pt .hhh Well anyway an' I thought about jus' saying
24   that I'm staying with a friend of Ma:rk's.

After stating that he talked not with his mom but father, thus specifying his father as the source of any updated information, Gina's "Hm:" (line 3) reflectively acknowledges yet awaits for news that only son may deliver. Following an extended pause (line 4), son announces that mom's in the hospital. Left unstated are reasons why her hospitalization precluded son from talking with her. And to insure that Gina adequately hears his inform- ing, son repeats mom's name until the overlap with G's talk is resolved and thus "in the clear" (Jefferson, 1973; Schegloff, 2000).

Something about son's informing triggered a "thought-" by Gina (line 7), which is cut off and left unspecified as son announces his news (in lines 8-14). With some difficulty and uncertainty, son next provides background information about her hospitalization. His ori- entation is reflective of the very treatment protocol and troubling diagnosis offered by the medical professionals he is attempting to depict. He begins with "the:y ↑think she might come ho::me?", an intonationally marked and audibly upbeat attempt to offer possible but not unequivocal good news about mom's condition. Moments such as these reveal practices that manage hope and optimism about difficult health circumstances (see Chapters 12 & 13). But notice that his next "I mean" precedes a series of dysfluencies and false starts (line 9), an initiated repair that her coming home is contingent on "once they stabilize her". Of particular interest here is the delicacy involved in first reporting what medical profession- als "↑think", then moving to qualify that what has just been stated is (more or less) inac- curate—perhaps even an embellishment overstating son's own optimism. Although her sta- bility will lead to a release from the hospital and is treated in part as an eventuality by son, such an outcome is not guaranteed. This is revealed in son's next utterance (lines 11-14), prefaced by his "I guess", where he reports that "they're" afraid of mom's bones breaking.

Balancing Medical Experts' Reports, Uncertainty, and Hope

This announcement by son is a striking example of inherent difficulties that emerge when updating news about another's health condition. There is an obvious and delicate balance between attempting to report accurately about ongoing treatment by medical professionals, yet maintaining a stance whereby hoped-for good news (i.e., mom coming home, stabiliza- tion) is not altogether abandoned. This problem is exacerbated when uncertainties about mom's condition are omnipresent, revealed in part when examining the indexical references employed by son when referring to medical personnel ("they/they're" in lines 8, 10, 12, 17; chaps. 8 and 9). Uncertainty is a key element as son describes both the work medical per- sonnel are attempting to accomplish (i.e., stabilize her, get her out of the hospital to outpa- tient status), and their thoughts and fears (e.g., see "afraid" in line 13; Beach et al., 2004).

By quietly responding with "=°Uh huh?°" in (2→), Gina displays that she has been attending to son's announcement, yet withholds any surprise or concern. Next, notice that son pauses (line 16) before elaborating his news. At this moment it is not possible to dis- cern whether son treats Gina as having produced a minimal response exhibiting lack of interest, a restrained orientation to having heard the serious uncertainties and consequences which he has constructed, or is simply awaiting further commentary by Gina. What can be observed in (3→), however, is that son's next offers a "So"-prefaced move to elaborate the upshot of his prior news delivery (see Beach & Dixson, 2001; Drew, 2003; Heritage & Watson, 1979, 1980; Raymond, 2004). He once again addresses matters involving "what they think they're gonna do" (lines 17-18). Strikingly similar to (1→, lines 8-10), son repairs his reporting from what "they're gonna" do to "what they think they're gonna do". By so doing, son takes care to accurately report news for Gina's hearing, yet retains the treatment uncertainties inherent to cancer therapy.

In extending his prior description about the hospital (line 11), it is also interesting that son defines for Gina what "out patient" means (lines 18-20). Additionally, prefaced with a "you know let her" (line 18), son attributes shared knowledge about patient care to Gina while implicating her as aligned with medical procedures. By stating "you know let her< spend the nights at ho:me, .hh an' then take her into the hospital during the days for radi- ation", he demonstrates the taken-for-granted and unproblematic authority granted to medical staff, that is, professionals whose actions involve "let her" and "take her".

As son begins to close his elaboration of medical procedures for treating mom, "That's the next thing." (line 21) situates the described medical procedure (i.e., radiation for her legs) as an event within a series. The relevance of news updates are thereby substantiated as a routine consequence of closely monitoring mom's cancer journey. Inherent uncertainties of medical treatment are also made relevant. Unfolding events are constantly shifting and, as apparent in Excerpt 5 (above), even medical staff are reported as facing ongoing ambigu- ities throughout cancer care.

These omnipresent themes are further apparent as son closes his elaboration with "But I haven't talked to her yet. I have no idea." (lines 21-22). This is yet another display of son's terminating his reporting by repeating key words, in this case "talked" (lines 1-2), employed at the outset of this NDS (see Schegloff, 1998). It is also curious that son quali- fies the news he has updated, received from his dad, as valuable information that is never- theless removed from the actual source and scene: his mother. Thus, having delivered sev- eral details about mom's treatment and condition, he disclaims his knowledge with "I have no idea" (see Beach & Metzger, 1997). There is a possibility that what son has just report- ed is already outdated and thus inaccurate, a distinction that further exemplifies the predicament son, as family member and news-deliverer, is immersed within.

Perhaps not surprisingly, then, in (4→) Gina does not provide an assessment of news that son has just closed-down and disclaimed. Rather, beginning with "Well anyway", she shifts back to a specific moment and topic being discussed prior to her inquiring about son's mom (line 1).

Fundamentally, Excerpt 5 reveals how a troubling news delivery can create difficulties for both participants. Throughout, Gina displays being uncertain about whether and how to deal with son's news. In turn, son's delivery and own withholdings are shaped by her displayed ambiguities. Being in the cancer journey thus involves numerous courses of action, marked by shifting mixtures of good and bad news that must be addressed simulta- neously. Patients and family members alike are implicated in tracking different diagnostic, treatment, and relational trajectories in real time. In this instance mom may get to go home (but only at night), even though cancer is in her bones, which requires that she receive inpa- tient radiation treatment during the day. As we have seen, discerning whether or not (and when) to travel home is obviously troubling business. So too is the management of an estranged, yet seemingly friendly and long-term relationship, throughout the emergence of uncertain illness and family dilemmas.

INTEGRATING TEMPORAL
AND RELATIONAL FRAMEWORKS

This chapter has provided a temporal and relational framework for grounding and tracing several news updates, occurring in a period of two days, regarding mom's "stability". As son informed Gina, and dad informed son about mom's "stabilization", key features were revealed about how news and social relationships are reflexively constituted over time. Across these phone calls, it is possible to observe the changing face of news, on the cusp of interactional time and cumulatively, as health conditions, travel plans, and social relationships get progressively intertwined.

Suspending and Recreating "Obdurate Orderliness" in Everyday Life

Selected excerpts from four calls have been examined as a resource for understanding contingencies involved when monitoring and reporting on another's illness and arranging travel plans become recurring, predominant, and inherently ambiguous activities in everyday life. In Chapter 1 it was noted that the discussion of unpleasant issues pertaining to cancer may disrupt and violate traditional communication patterns (Gotcher, 1995). From the interactions examined in this chapter it is clear that bad and ambiguous news events may rupture and alter everyday life, dissolving the "obdurate orderliness" as observed by Maynard (1996, pp. 4-5). It is also apparent, however, that those involved in reporting and receiving such news devise ways of managing their relationships with one another and to the events being described. In most general terms, to the extent that speakers display limited knowledge about newsworthy events and construct the news as happening to others, they exhibit their "distance" to persons and their circumstances. And in the ways speakers demonstrate being affected by the news, including their ability and willingness to narrate about events being discussed, their "closeness" becomes apparent as primary and consequential figures caught up within the news being depicted.

This framework provides unique insight into how dad speaks with son, and in turn, how son updates Gina.[3] Beginning with call #3, son's conversation with mom and dad enabled him to directly hear and inquire about mom's condition and wishes, dad's orientations to troubling circumstances, and subsequently to deliver and update news about mom's treatment and diagnosis to Gina (who was somehow implicated in son's travel plans). As a primary family member for whom the news was consequential, son was engaged in altering his plans for traveling home to spend time with his mom and family before she died. Such decision making was shown to be contingent upon discerning the timing of mom's death, which is, inevitably, replete with uncertainties for medical professionals and family members alike.

The In-Flux and Delicate Character of Reportings and Responses

Such uncertainties were attended to by son as central features of his owning the experiences, frustrations, and fatigue he displayed and reported to Gina. The personal and professional quandary he was embroiled within, as a primary family member, was repeatedly established as a direct consequence of how he dealt with ambiguities regarding mom's treatment and the dying process she (and thus other family members) appeared to be enduring. On first glance it may appear incongruous that mom's "stability" represented both good and bad news for son. Yet this possibility was underscored as the volatility of mom's health status created ongoing and unresolved circumstances for son and dad (e.g., see Excerpt 2, lines 6-8, when dad states dad's "This >been a damn up an down an up an down.< I °ya know° ya- ya don't know whether to be p:le:ased or not ple$ased [$hah hh$]".)

Similarly, at times son's efforts to accurately report to Gina what medical staff had told him (and/or his dad and mom) appeared in conflict with his inclination to describe mom's treatments and outcomes optimistically. Taken as a whole, the in-flux character of son's reportings are visible manifestations of the instability associated with being affected as a primary figure in mom's cancer journey.

Just as son displayed the need for closure in the face of an equivocal health and travel situation, so did Gina orient to his news in delicate ways: as being affected by the news about mom, yet marking with appreciation and sympathy the dilemmas son was describing. When producing her assessments, Gina twice exhibited (with laughter and aspiration) not an insensitivity to mom's health problems, but an affiliation with son's family involvements. These dual orientations are perhaps reflective of the tenuous nature of dealing with any bad news received by a marital partner or significant other. As noted, Gina's own precarious status as son's recently divorced wife also creates a situation where she demonstrated shared knowledge and history, yet was "technically" no longer, a family member.[4]

Both son and Gina, in their own ways, exhibited being affected by mom's cancer. However, son did not formulate himself as a cancer patient (as did mom in Chapter 4), nor did Gina construct herself (but rather son) as the primary figure facing the consequences of mom's illness. Because these orientations emerged interactionally, problems arise when assuming that being in a cancer journey and being with another are mutually exclusive rather than delicately interwoven.[5] For example, at times both son and Gina revealed themselves as *being in* and thus adversely (although variably) affected by the news. Other moments involved Gina's attempts to be *with* son yet were receipted by him as an unwillingness to be *in* a closer relationship with Gina at this moment in time.

In these and other ways, problems may exist when news participants attempt to solicit, acknowledge, and/or avoid closeness with one another. Repeatedly, Gina provided displays of affection or sympathy that were neither reciprocated nor pursued by son. By closing down his news delivery following a sympathetic assessment by Gina, for example, son essentially declined Gina's invitation to disclose further details about his problems. He ignored these opportunities and the possibility of receiving additional commiseration from Gina. Whether these moments are reflective of an estranged relationship between Gina and son or not—as a recently divorced couple remaining in contact—they document how News Delivery Sequences are not simply content-driven but sensitive to the ongoing management of inherently *relational* boundaries and enactments.

A Solemn Reminder

The excerpts analyzed in this chapter function as solemn reminders that the future is inevitably uncertain. Even though it can now and retrospectively be surmised that speakers' assessments about mom's dying (i.e., at this juncture of her illness) were premature by five to six weeks, it is clear that cancer patients, family members, and medical professionals alike invest considerable time attempting to make "best guesses" about "what the future will hold"—and how to behave accordingly. Repeated inspections of these interactions provide revealing illustrations of the volatility of illness diagnoses, impacts on practical decision making and plans, and the interactional work involved in acting *as if* a family member's active dying was underway. Throughout, it is also clear that time, and illness, inevitably alters social relationships.

NOTES

1. There is an additional possibility here, namely, that son's explanation amounts to an accounting for something he has done (e.g., his orientation to the ringing phone or summons, and/or the manner in which he produced his immediately prior narrative for Gina). Following the descriptions

he offered to Gina (see Excerpt 1, 32-37) he eventually reports "'Cuz I am very wigged out.", and understandably so. This may add significantly to creating an interactional environment that was first, for them, replete with difficult and delicate moments.

2. Framed as a central feature of illness experiences, Babrow, Kasch, and Ford (1998) review alternative orientations to ways that "communication is thought to be essential to the construction, management, and resolution of uncertainty" (p.1). Although individual psychological models of uncertainty are most prominent, and the management of medical uncertainty is socioculturally and historically significant, limited contributions in the areas of linguistic and discourse analyses are noted. Atkinson (1984, 1995), for example, has examined how hematologists express and qualify degrees of uncertainty regarding the believability of various sources of information (e.g., clinical experience, published research).

3. Any inclination to artificially dichotomize "distance" and "closeness" is misleading, however, and too easily removed from actions co-enacted by news participants. In real time, as the analysis in this and related chapters reveal, any assessment of relational intimacy is barometric and mandates detailed consideration of often specific and subtle interactional features.

4. There are clearly other, salient ethnographic considerations not taken into consideration here. For example, details regarding Gina's prior and ongoing relationship with son's mom and dad are unknown, as are the exact contingencies surrounding her and son's divorce.

5. Although "laughing at" and "laughing with" have been clearly distinguished (see Glenn, 1995, 2003), moments involving being affected by news reveal orientations in which both deliverers and recipients of news appear to calibrate their closeness and distance to the person and/or events being described.

7

STATE OF READINESS

Figurative Expressions
and the Social Construction
of Emergency Preparedness

This phase of the family cancer journey is marked by a state of readiness for addressing mom's imminent, though unpredictable, death. What social actions comprise emergency preparedness? Below, first consider how son reconstructs for aunt his prior conversation with dad in call #12, when he was informed that because mom's condition had stabilized he should put his travel plans on hold (see Excerpt 2 in Chapter 6). In particular, notice the four contiguous figurative expressions (→) employed by both son and aunt:

1) SDCL: Malignancy #17:9

((Aunt had just stated that the family will need to "<u>pull</u> together",
and that "This is jus' gonna: <u>knock</u> us for a lo::op uh. =".))[1]

1		Aunt:	[But I- ↑<u>we</u> will <u>be</u> there,] and you will ↑<u>be</u> part of <u>it</u>, <and>
2			you will not be (.) pushed <u>aside</u> for ah for even a moment.
3		Son:	pt. .hhhh ↓Well what I <u>told</u> dad is I will- I will ↑<u>keep</u> things
4	→		(.) i::n as <u>much</u> ah state uh <u>readiness</u> as possible. =
5		Aunt:	= Ye[ap.]
6	→	Son:	[pt] And I'll ↑<u>keep</u> my lesson plans nice and °current°.
7		Aunt:	Yeap. =
8	→	Son:	= pt .hhh A:nd uh hhh .hhh (.) I'll jus' (.) ↑<u>do</u> what I need to
9			<u>do</u>.
10		Aunt:	= Yeap. (0.2) and (.hhh cough) if I- if I- (0.3)
11	→		>↑smell anything in the wind< ↓ o::r Dr. Wylie has anything
12			<u>further</u> (.) .hhh either your father or I will <u>ca::ll</u> and I will <u>back</u>
13			it up <al:way:s.> =
14		Son:	= ↓Okay. =
15		Aunt:	= O↓kay:. (.) Jus' like this call:.
16		Son:	Okay. =

This excerpt begins with aunt providing assurance to son that he will be included and not "pushed <u>aside</u>" (line 2) on the occasion of mom's death.[2] In response, son attempts to summarize (see Drew & Holt, 1998) for aunt that he will remain (as best possible) in a "state uh <u>readiness</u>" (line 2): a condition marked by being prepared for quick and efficient respon-

125

siveness to travel home should mom's health fail. Because son's actual conversations with dad did not include the descriptive phrase "state uh <u>readiness</u>", son has recruited this language on the spot to metaphorically depict for aunt his being prepared for prompt, speedy, and thus responsible action. With this expression he is not reporting to aunt the "empirical details" of talking with dad, but providing an overview of the gist, or bottom-line issues, emerging from what he reported to his dad during the prior phone call. Thus, son's indirect reporting of what he told dad also makes clear his assessment of, and thus position toward, the events he is reconstructing (see Beach, 2000b; Buttny, 1997, 1998; Drew & Holt, 1998; Holt, 2000; Schegloff, 2004). At a moment's notice, with few additional planning actions required, son's emergency readiness will allow him to be there for the family as well. His figurative expression, "state uh <u>readiness</u>", is therefore a primary resource for (a) communicating that assurance initially to dad and now to aunt, and (b) as disengaged or detached from the empirical details of talking with dad—a device for generically and more powerfully moving to close current topic (Drew & Holt, 1998; see below).

He next continues his topical summary by invoking two additional figurative/ metaphorical phrases, each adding impetus to his readiness and commitment to act promptly. First, with "↑<u>keep</u> my lesson plans nice and °current°" (line 4) he not only summarizes his prior telling, but further situates the reported trouble in the midst of teaching responsibilities: insuring that whoever might teach for him will, in his absence, have adequate lesson plans for instructing his students. Importantly, this transition—from a reporting of what he told dad, to a characterization of his lifeworld circumstances—makes possible that the concerns son raises emerge in a stepwise and seamless fashion (Drew & Holt, 1998; Holt & Drew, 2005; Jefferson, 1984b):

> These mechanisms are especially clear in pivotal transitions and perhaps particularly so in figurative pivotal changes in which the transition may take place over two turns: a figurative expression that summarizes the previous telling and has independent topical potential and a next turn that introduces a new but related matter by connecting it to the expression, so exploiting this independent topical potential. . . . The pivot forms a bridge, connecting to the previous matter but providing an opportunity to introduce a new one. (Holt & Drew, 2005, p. 56)

Second, in Excerpt 1 (lines 6-7, above) the next turn by son, and thus the new and relevant matter, is "= pt .hhh A:nd uh hhh .hhh (.) I'll jus' (.) ↑<u>do</u> what I need to <u>do</u>.". Produced with a preceding and aspirated sigh, and prosodic emphasis ("↑<u>do</u>, <u>do</u>"), son portrays a steadfast conviction to continue being vigilant: closely monitoring and being attentive to updated news about mom, literally at a moment's notice. This utterance is responsive to aunt's initial assurance (lines 1-2), further qualifying him as capable of doing his part to be there for the family just as they will be there and include him. It is in this particular sense that son's "I'll jus' (.) ↑<u>do</u> what I need to <u>do</u>." emerges gradually and seamlessly, yet *exploits* its independent topical potential: to reassert his commitment to the family through readiness and to remain sensitive to exigencies caused by cancer (see also Excerpt 19, below).

Throughout this exchange, aunt has agreed and aligned with son's reporting, a routine feature of "standard sequences" involving figurative expressions (Holt & Drew, 2005, p. 37). In lines 10-11, however, notice also her own and next-positioned figurative expression: "if I- if I- (0.3) >↑smell anything in the wind<". In this way, and again seamlessly, aunt responds to son's exhibited dedication by metaphorically summarizing her own vigilance. Within the animal kingdom, for example, scent is one primal survival instinct relied upon to ward off potential danger, commonly relied upon by members of a pack or family to forewarn and update others. This fourth figurative expression, across only seven lines of transcript (lines 4-11), exhibits aunt's ability to adapt such a primal resource to align herself with the preparedness and resolve conveyed by son. Finally, with "↓Okay." son next acknowledges aunt's continued reassurance, which she connects to "this call:" (line 15), and which son again affirms.

Including aunt's "gonna: <u>knock</u> us for a lo::op" and "it's ↑<u>still</u> gonna knock us for a lo:op" (see Footnote 1), a series of six figurative expressions emerged in a very brief peri-od of time. Their condensed recruitment by son and aunt, as summary assessments of their orientations to troubles surrounding mom's cancer, reveal that actions can be taken to maintain readiness, resolve, and to remain ever-watchful as emerging and inherently uncer-tain circumstances arise. An understanding of why *six figurative expressions* might be recruited, and in such a very short period of time, is further bolstered when recognizing that son and aunt attribute significant importance to these events in their lives (see also Footnote 5 and Excerpt 10, below). They simultaneously attempt to coordinate their plan-ning actions, commiserate about their dilemma, and evidence shared commitment to jour-neying through mom's cancer together. Grounded in familial relationships, a distinct social structure in enacted whereby son and aunt's figurative expressions are, in practice, metaphorical depictions of the mood and soul of the social worlds they inhabit.

Fundamental Social Actions Achieved Through Topic Transition and Closure

Returning to Excerpt 1 (above), the phone call then moves quickly to closing, not unex-pectedly, because figurative expressions routinely occur in environments involving both topical transition and closure. As Drew and Holt observed concerning

> discernable distribution in talk . . . determining whether the phenomenon has any regu-lar or recurrent position in sequences of talk . . . a very striking pattern emerged. In this pattern, following a turn in which a speaker produces a figurative expression, the co-par-ticipants briefly agree with one another, after which one or the other introduces a new topic of conversation. Hence, it appears that the use of a figurative expression is associ-ated with topic termination and transition to a new/next topic. (1998, p. 499)

Without exception, this topical pattern is confirmed in the analysis of 26 figurative expres-sions analyzed in this chapter. However, it has been noted that in the course of moving to close the call (following Excerpt 1, above) a number of *key social actions* are achieved: reciprocal offerings of assurance and ongoing commitment to closely monitor and keep one another informed of mom's condition. Figurative expressions (also referred to as fig-ures of speech) thus were recruited by son and aunt as primary resources for (a) evidenc-ing their shared emergency readiness, (b) supporting and comforting one another during this critical, and urgent, phase of the family cancer journey, and (c) movements toward top-ical (and in this case, phone call) closure.

It is the interactional work achieved through figurative expressions that the current chapter addresses most specifically (for a summary, see Figure 3 near the end of this chap-ter). In addition to facilitating topic transition and closure, family members manage their primary concerns through fundamental social actions including evidencing shared readi-ness, offering support and comfort and a host of related activities identified as numerous excerpts are analyzed below. For example, moments involving disagreement, disaffiliation, and lack of alignment (implicit and subtle, explicit and marked) were examined by Drew and Holt as instances revealing "the interactional functions of that object . . . the kinds of interactional 'problems' for which participants need to have solutions, and the way that this object is fitted to managing that task" (1998, p. 518). Certain of the instances examined in this chapter seem to fit these "disaffiliative" functional descriptions (e.g., see Footnotes 1 & 5, Excerpts 10, 12, & 13). But as revealed in following discussions, considerably more and diverse practices get recruited as speakers utilize figurative expressions.

This chapter, then, extends the above single case analysis (Excerpt 1, above) involving a series of contiguous figurative expressions. Also examined are additional and related interactional devices employed by family members when constructing emergency preparedness. A tracing will be provided of how *urgency* gets progressively built across phone conversations. Excerpts from calls #3-18 will be examined to reveal the generative conditions for handling emerging and changing (e.g., stabile yet ambiguous) illness circumstances. These basic patterns make clear how a language of readiness is embedded within identifiable sequences of practical action, comprised of specific practices for organizing and navigating through a precarious state of cancer-related affairs.

DISPLAYING AND RESPONDING TO URGENT READINESS

Analysis begins during call #3, triggering events (i.e., the ontogenesis) of this phase of the family crisis: Mom's discussion with son about life support, as well as excessive pain she is experiencing.[3] Just prior to Excerpt 2, son announced to dad that he would rather travel home now than wait for mom's memorial service:

2) SDCL: Malignancy #3:5

```
 1    Son:   hhh But ah (.) given my druthers I:'d come home now.
 2           (1.2)
 3    Dad:   Okay. (.) Let me talk to: ah: Auntie Carol, see about a plane
 4           ticket.        Don't ( 1.0 ) drive to the >airport< yet.
 5  →        [(But pack your bags).]
 6    Son:   [  No        but-  ] I will be here. (.) I'll stay home.
 7           Call me.
 8           (1.0 )
 9    Son:   Tell me what to do, when to do it. I will ah- .hh
10    Dad:   ( Okay [  I- )   ]
11    Son:          [As soon] as I know what and when (.) I will make the
12           arrangements on this end. (.) and- ah (0.2) and take care of it.
13           (1.0)
14    Dad:   Okay. I'll find out what I can do about a plane ticket if there's
15           a way to get ya know. =
```

Dad's figurative expression, "But pack your bags" (line 5)—the first of five instances referencing "bags" (analyzed below)—provides a summary of his previous "Don't (1.0) drive to the >airport< yet.". In response, son acknowledges yet initiates his readiness to spring into action. Marked with repeated and redundant phrases, son's pivotal elaboration (lines 6-12) is noticeably overbuilt: He exhibits an anxious orientation toward awaiting another phone call and being (more than) eager to receive updated information, make "arrangements", and "take care of it." (line 12). Although the emphasis son gives to his readiness is responsive to dad's "But pack your bags", his actions also reveal the intensity of his concerns as a new, independent, inherently troubling matter in its own right: He exudes a willingness and ability to do being ready to respond to news dad (or other family members) might deliver.

At this moment, dad's doorbell rings and for 46 seconds son awaits dad's return. Dad then states "Allright let me talk to Carol and find out what I do about plane tickets.". With

"Allright" dads brings closure to talk about Aunt Carol and the tickets, and son transitions by providing additional information about compassion fares (see Chapter 5).

Left hanging is the critical timing of son's decisions to travel home, addressed several minutes later in the same call:

3) SDCL: Malignancy #3:7-8

1	Son:	Okay. I- I've got a day at least I hope.
2	Dad:	Yep.
3	Son:	Okay.
4	Dad:	(I would think so.)
5 →	Son:	Allright **I'll stay by the phone.**
6	Dad:	Okay. =
7	Son:	= Let me know. Ca<u>ll</u> <u>grandma</u>. I just got off the phone with
8		her. She was gonna go take a nap. (.) <u>But</u> she doesn't have any
9		<u>clue</u> at this point (.) she might want to know.
10	Dad:	Yeah she saw her last night so.
11	Son:	Okay.

Hopefully (line 1), son queries about having "at least a day", a time-metric further establishing the urgency faced by this family. Though dad initially acknowledges that son's assessment is correct (line 2), he continues in line 4 with "(I would think so)". Dad's doubtful extension implies the inevitable uncertainty of events which cannot be controlled. In response, son manages this doubt with a familiar "Allright I'll stay by the phone." (line 5), which adds momentum toward closure of this phone call (occurring 22 lines later, following a brief story by son about mom's "<u>fake</u> guacamole" recipe). Although son's figurative "stay by the phone" expression may or may not be a literal portrayal of his plans,[4] son displays his recognition that being consistently accessible provided partial solutions to the volatile problems they are facing together. Notice also that son expresses concern that grandma be informed (lines 7-9), which dad can address knowingly and authoritatively as he reports seeing her last night (line 10).

Revisiting Calls to the Airlines

During son's subsequent calls to different airline representatives (Excerpts 4-8, below), it becomes apparent how son transforms his "a day at least I hope" into a series of descriptions informing agents about his family predicament. The temporal category of "tomorrow" becomes a critical resource as son attempts to balance uncertain plans, including his urgent but not immediate need to travel (i.e., on the next possible flight). In Excerpt 4, for example, son is faced with responding to AA's query in lines 1-2, specifically, what's his sense of "as soon as possible?":

4) SDCL: Malignancy #4:1

((AA = American Airlines))

1	AA:	↑Well let's check out. uh Do you wanna leave uh like leave as
2		soon as possible?
3 →	Son:	Yeah uh well tomorro:w I've got- I'm a teacher I've got some
4		<u>stuff</u> I have to do first thing in the morning, and .hh
5		conceivably (.) tomorrow afternoon. I'm- I'm waiting for one
6		more phone call before I'm:: sure, but I want to figure out what
7 →		I have to do (.) ah to **pull this off.** So-
8	AA:	Okay. Let me check just one second please.

His qualified answer begins with being busy in the morning, and shifts to a departure tomorrow afternoon as conceivable because he's awaiting a phone call. Even though he is not yet sure when he might depart, he informs the agent (lines 6-7) that his primary business is "to figure out what I have to do (.) ah to pull this off.". Just what the colloquial "ASAP=as soon as possible" means in practical terms, then, is contingently tied to son's unique circumstances. The metaphorical expression "pull this off" summarizes and embeds his efforts within a more complex series of events he is dealing with (e.g., calling different airlines, discerning when it is best to travel, awaiting phone calls, paying for the travel, arranging his classes, taking the dog to the kennel, etc.). Son is uniquely entitled to speak about his experiences, because no other person is fully aware of the tasks necessary to "pull this off". But before he can elaborate the upshot of his telling ("So-", line 7), the agent politely places son on hold as she checks for possible flights (and thereby officially moves to the business at hand). Her topical and transitional action treats son's figurative expression as contributing to a sequential environment conducive to transition/closure.

Soon thereafter, son once again emphasizes to the AA agent that he's not ready to book the flight until he receives not any, but "one more phone call":

5) SDCL: Malignancy #4:3

```
1   Son: Yea:h:. ↑Um at this point don't actually book this. I'm ah- I'm
2        like I said I'm waiting for one more phone call before I'm sure I
3        have to do this: to:morrow. I'm just trying to figure out if I
4        .hhh you know if I'm going to have to wire for some money
5        er: or what- what's involved = what kind of information are
6        you going to need?
```

Any actions to be taken "to:morrow" remain uncertain until he receives an update (likely from dad). He then makes known that the purpose for his call is to gain information about cost and related matters, details that if addressed now would later facilitate efficient travel.

Several calls later son speaks with another airline agent. He again makes the distinction between "tomorrow" and the qualifier "Maybe tomorrow afternoon" (lines 2 & 4, below), actions strikingly familiar with his prior discussion with AA (e.g., see Excerpt 4, lines 3 & 5):

6) SDCL: Malignancy #8:1

((CN = Continental Airlines))

```
1      CN:   Oka:y. Um how soon did you want to travel.=
2  →   Son:  =We:ll like to morro:w.
3      CN:   °Tomorrow°. Okay, just a [moment.
4  →   Son:                          [Maybe tomorrow afternoon.
5      CN:   Okay one moment?
```

Later in this same call, when speaking with a service manager for CN, son's not being "sure" (line 6) is restated for the third time (see Excerpt 5, line 2; Excerpt 4, line 6):

7) SDCL: Malignancy #8:2

((SM = Service Manager for CN))

```
1      SM:   Hello sir. My name is Pablo, I'm the customer (.) service
2            manager. How can I [help you.
3      Son:                     [Hi: well I- I'm tryin to find out
4            something. I just (.) r:eceived this wonderful phone call, that
```

5	it looks like my <u>mother's</u> gonna <u>die</u>. .hhh Uh- and I <u>need to:</u>,
6 →	<u>find o:ut</u>. They're gonna let me know for <u>sure</u> in the
7	morning, but I think I need to get back to [city] from [city].

And during his call to Southwest (SW), son's urgency is once again clearly stated (1→) in a manner that agent treats as qualifying for an "as soon as possible" status (2→). But in (3→) son, having previously mentioned that he is awaiting another phone call, attributes shared knowledge to agent about his inability to leave immediately. Positioned at the end of his utterance (line 10), the delicacy of son's dilemma is marked with laughter ("$ts[h$"), which agent acknowledges in overlap:

8) **Malignancy #9:1**

((SW = Southwest Airlines))

1	SW:	They may have ah- is it a <u>passion</u> fare or berevance fare.
2		Something like tha:[t. =
3	Son:	=[Yeah ah- there's a couple places that °will°
4		1→do this when (.) if I want to go for a funeral? But I'd just as
5		1→soon get there before she <u>dies</u> and [that's] =
6	SW:	[R:ight.]
7	Son:	1→= A matter of <u>days</u> at this point and um .hhh
8	SW:	2→You want to get [there as soon as possible.]
9	Son:	3→ [Ye: ah] But I can't- (.) you
10		know you know how it is. $ts[h$
11	SW:	[Ri:ght.

For son, then, it is an ongoing necessity to make clear for agents just what his needs are. The cases son has made for airline travel (see also Chapter 5) invoke some urgency regarding mom's dying, prompting two agents to respond by utilizing the category "as soon as possible" (AA in Excerpt 4, and SW in Excerpt 8, above), and another to query "how soon" son wants to leave (CN, Excerpt 6, above). Yet because son is awaiting updated news from home, he is unable (at the time of calling) to commit by reserving specific flights. His actions, therefore, are best understood as designed to gather information ensuring preparedness: to enhance the state of readiness necessary to travel in a timely (and relatively hassle-free) manner whenever he receives the phone call encouraging him to travel home (or not).

BAGS, LESSON PLANS, AND LISTS

The following five figurative expressions involving *bags* are examined in chronological order (see Figure 7.1).

Attention is drawn to how each is situated in the local, sequential environment in which such figurative expressions get utilized. Progressively, however, it is also apparent that, and how, such expressions get precisely tailored to prior news—*recalibrated* and adapted to the cumulative impact of trying to figure out how best to orient to mom's volatile health status.

The first reference to "But pack your bags," employed by dad in call #3 (prior to calling the airlines) and examined in Excerpt 2 (above), initiated a figurative expression characterizing readiness for subsequent actions (e.g., finalizing reservations, driving to the airport, and traveling home).

Call #3

Dad: Don't (1.0) drive to the >airport< yet. [(But **pack your bags**).]

↓

Call #10

Son: =Yeah well I would- I would probably not **unpack my <u>bag</u>** heh-

↓

Call #12

Son: =Yeah pt .hhhh <u>huh</u> <u>o:ka::y</u> (.) Well (.) pt I will- hh .hh I will
un<u>pack</u> my ba:g: hhh [.hh and I'll keep] my lesson plans current.

↓

Dad: [Uhright] (.) keep yu- your <u>list</u> up tuh date an >ya know<
leave the bag where ya know where it is.

↓

Call #18

Son: =A:nd ba:sically what they said i:s .hhh
<u>keep</u> you're le:sson pla:ns <u>current:,</u> a:n <u>don't</u> <u>unpa:ck</u> <u>your</u> **ba:g** comple:tely.=

Figure 7.1. Serial References to "Bags/Bag" Across Four Phone Calls.

Below, aunt overviews the "chance" that following doctor's "rounds in the morning" (lines 2-3), mom will once again receive morphine pills (line 10):

9) SDCL: Malignancy #10:6

```
 1      Aunt:  Uh hmm Okay. (.) Alright ahm by- I would- (.) the way
 2             <normally> things work with Dr. Wylie is she makes rounds
 3             in the morning.
 4      Son:   Um hmm. Yeah that's what dad said.=
 5      Aunt:  =And we should have s:ome clue (.) <if this is> (.) an- and ya
 6             know there is the chance now I don't know what (.) how
 7             well of a chance it is. =
 8      Son:   = Um hum.
 9      Aunt:  But there is the chance that this is a (.) matter of putting her
10             back on decadro:n (.) giving her morphine pi:lls.
11      Son:   [Um hmm.]
12      Aunt:  [>  Blah   ] blah blah blah blah,< (.) and we've got (0.8) more
13             time. (.) What kind of time. >I don't know.< I don't know
14             what kind of time. At this point I would say it's not a hell of
15             a lot. =
16  →   Son:   = Yeah well I would- I would probably not unpack my bag
17             heh-[ hh ]
18      Aunt:      [No.] Don't do that. =
19      Son:   = Yeah.
20      Aunt:  You're right. Ahh but what we'll do is we'll make sure that
21             we <get to you in the morning.>
22      Son:   Yeah bear in mind that there's a two hour time difference.=
23      Aunt:  Yeah [I know.]
```

In line 11 aunt's "Blah blah blah blah blah" portrays these procedures and treatment decisions as altogether routine—more of the same and perhaps (at least in part) previously discussed—thus explicitly treated as *not* the primary topic for this present discussion. She next transitions to the central issue: the uncertainty of time remaining with mom (lines 13-15).[5]

Her description shifts from "we've got (0.8) more time" to a series of "I"-centered state-ments of doubt prior to her personal, uncertain assessment.

Son's response to mom's appraisal is also situated in his own ("I/my") circumstances. In contrast with dad's original usage "but pack your bags", son's figurative expression—"prob-ably not unpack my bag" (line 16)—reveals that dad's urging was somehow attended to. Son's expression is carried over from dad's initial utterance yet adapted (both temporally and lexi-cally) to the contingencies of this specific interactional moment. A shift in tense has occurred from an action needing to be done to packing already completed and not to be undone. It cannot be determined, of course, whether son actually had his bags packed or just reported them that way. As the packed bag indicates, however, his readiness is summarily represented and speaks to what he is entitled to address: being prepared for uncertain and unwelcome travel, an orientation punctuated by his final laugh token "heh-" (line 17). And again, this fig-urative expression occurs in an environment of topical transition. In lines 20-23, attention is given to the next morning and the time difference that needs to be taken into account.

Revisiting Figurative Expressions in a Series

Two calls later, dad informs son that because mom has stabilized it would be best for him not to travel home as planned (see Excerpt 2, Chapter 6). With uncertainty, dad also spec-ulates that mom has "at least a month." to live.[6] Similar to the series of metaphorical refer-ences previously examined in Excerpt 1 (above), what follows is another remarkable series of five figurative expressions occurring between lines 4-17. Across a span of only 15 sec-onds of actual talk, the importance given to describing and coping with mom's cancer is once again evident:

```
10)  SDCL: Malignancy #12:7-8
      1      Dad:   = She looks and she said >We:ll okay. So we got uh few more
      2             tumors here we can radiate those that'll slow those down.
      3  →          Then the next ones pop up ya know this is like-< .hhh trying
      4             to squash mushrooms in a rainstorm. Eh ya know those
      5             suckers just keep popping up eventually you're gonna lose
      6             but who knows what eventually is. =
      7  → Son:    = Yeah pt .hhhh huh o:ka::y (.) Well (.) pt I will- hh .hh I will
      8             unpack my ba:g: hhh [.hh and I'll keep] my lesson plans =
      9      Dad:                       [  Ye::p (    ) ]
      10            = current.
      11     Son:   [ hhhhhh] .hh
      12  → Dad:   [Uhright] (.) keep yu- your list up tuh date an >ya know<
      13            leave the bag where ya know where it is.
      14     Son:   Yeah. hhh pt Okay. hhh [.hh  ]
      15     Dad:                          [Tha ]t's the best I can tell ya at the
      16  →        moment? <I told ya life's a bitch.>
      17     Son:   Yeah ri- $hhhh .hh hh .hh$
      18  → Dad:   No rose garden.
      19     Son:   No. hhhh pt O:kay (.) <Well> (.) keep me posted.
      20            (0.6)
      21     Dad:   O↑kay.
      22     Son:   Thanks pop.
      23     Dad:   Ahhrighty Doug see ya later. =
      24     Son:   = Bah bye.
      25     Dad:   °Bye.°
```

This excerpt begins with dad's reporting of what the doctor had stated (see also Chapters 8 & 9): As tumors were identified, they would be radiated to "slow <u>those</u> down." (line 2). Dad then shifts away from reporting what the doctor had stated, to his own characterization of "the <u>next</u> ones pop up ya know this is like-< trying to squash <u>mush</u>rooms in a rainstorm." (lines 3-4). This visually alluring analogy addresses the ultimate futility of doctors' proposed radiation—treatments that might "slow down" but not effectively eliminate the spread of tumors. In essence, tumor growth in mom's body is likened to a wet (and likely dark) natural environment conducive to growing mushrooms. In lines 5-7, dad's utterance has three distinctive yet conjoined features: (a) He shifts back from mushrooms to tumors by describing the latter as "<u>suck</u>ers just keep <u>pop</u>ping up"; (b) The upshot of such growth is tantamount to a loss of the battle for mom's life, that is, "eventually you're gonna lose."; and (c) With "but <u>who</u> knows what <u>even</u>tually is.=", an inherently vague prognosis is emphasized.

Prefaced by agreement and affirmation (line 7), son's figurative expression is recipient designed as a tailored summary of dad's prior description. He addresses both the uncertainty raised by dad as well as the inevitability of mom's loss: "Well (.) pt I will- hh .hh I will un<u>pack</u> my ba:g: hhh [.hh and I'll keep] my lesson plans current.". Son's response begins reflectively, exhibiting a mixture of tiredness and frustration, then moves to "I will un<u>pack</u> my ba:g:". This expression reveals how dad's just prior update caused son to downgrade his readiness position from that reported when speaking with aunt in call #10 (Excerpt 2, above): "= Yeah well I would- I would probably not un<u>pack</u> my bag heh-[hh]". Yet, given dad's uncertain prognosis, son will also "keep my lesson plans current." (line 8) so as to maintain adequate preparedness. However, this mitigated position is only partially affirmed by dad. In line 11, he first encourages son to "keep yu- your <u>list</u> up tuh date.", an alternative mode of readiness in that both "lesson plans current" and "<u>list</u> up tuh date" denote being organized by attending to details facilitating quick, efficient, and responsible action (i.e., should the need arise to cover son's classes so he can leave town). Further, "<u>list</u>" can include a wider variety of tasks needing to be done for preparedness (e.g., board the dog, take care of the apartment, etc.) than only attending to "lesson plans".

Dad's next "leave the bag where ya know where it is" (lines 11-12) corrects son's reference to unpacking his bag (lines 7-8), alerting him to maintain a relatively high state of readiness. Although there is indeed ambiguity about how long mom will live, her dying looms on the horizon and could arrive even sooner than expected. Despite mom's most recent stabilization, son is thus forewarned by dad to not be caught off-guard, an effort designed to insure intersubjective understandings (see Schegloff, 1992) about how to best remain vigilant and efficient in achieving the desired goal of facing mom's death together.

And with his closing "<I told ya life's a <u>bitch</u>.>…<u>No</u> <i>rose</i> garden." (lines 15, 17) dad aptly summarizes not only the difficulties they have been discussing together, but a father's ongoing reminders to a son that life is filled with a series of challenges that are not easily managed. Indeed, this is yet another poignant and somber phone closing, achieved through expressions finely calibrated to the dire state of affairs they are caught up within.

Reconstructing Dad's Expression

The final instance of a figurative expression involving <i>bag</i> appears below (previously analyzed in Chapter 6, Excerpt 3). As noted earlier, son is now reporting two concurrent events to Gina: how actions taken by unspecified medical personnel ("the:y've") have resulted in mom once again becoming "<u>sta</u>:bilized" (line 2), and consequently an upshot of his prior conversation with dad in call #12 (see Excerpt 10, above) about his ongoing need for readiness:

11) **SDCL: Malignancy #18:2**

```
 1    Gina:   What's up?
 2    Son:    We:ll (.) the:y've sta:bilized 'er again.=A:nd ba:sically
 3  →         what they said i:s .hhh keep you're le:sson pla:ns
 4            current:, a:n don't unpa:ck your ba:g comple:tely.=But-
 5            (.) I don't need ta sho:w up: quite ↑(ch)yet.=So:=
 6    Gina:   = < O:h my G(h)o::d. >
 7            (0.3)
 8    Gina:   You poor thi::ng. hhh
 9            (0.4)
10    Son:    pt So tha:t's:=↑really all I can tell ya.
```

As before, son's figurative expression is altered to accommodate not just news provided by dad, but son's own orientations to worldly matters (e.g., teaching) he is preoccupied with. Though he attributes his ".hhh keep you're le:sson pla:ns current:," to "what they said", from Excerpt 10 (above) it is clear that dad's actual expression was "keep yu- your list up tuh date.". Son thus retained his repeated use and emphasis on "lesson plans" rather than "lists" in his reporting (see Excerpts 1 & 10, above). What dad actually stated was treated as "dispensable" by son (see Schegloff, 2004) in favor of retaining the gist of dad's encouragement: to remain ready to act upon short notice. Once again, however, son alters how he refers to *bag* and thereby constructs his figurative expression as an outcome of dad's prior actions. Earlier it was described how son's responsive and downgraded "I will unpack my ba:g:" was countered by dad's "leave the bag where ya know where it is." Six phone calls later, during call #18 with Gina, son's version of dad's correction was "a:n don't unpa:ck your ba:g comple:tely. .=But- (.) I don't need ta sho:w up: quite ↑(ch)yet." (lines 4-5). He has reported what is, for all practical purposes, a reasonably accurate version of dad's position—even though he retained his own "unpa:ck" language. And son has also (and importantly) provided the essence of dad's call for vigilance. With "quite ↑(ch)yet.", son addresses the delay, but also the inevitability of soon making a trip home for mom's funeral.

It is this presentiment that triggers Gina's immediate next "= < O:h my G(h)o::d. >" and following "You poor thi::ng. hhh" (lines 6-8; see also Excerpt 3, Chapter 6). As described in Chapter 6, her responses are carefully tailored to the shifting and troubling circumstances son has encapsulated. However, rather than address her surprise or even offering of sympathy, in line 10 son moves to transition and close with "So tha:t's:=↑really all I can tell ya" (a continuation of what he apparently did not complete with his earlier "=So:=" in line 5). It is thus evident that son's figurative expression (lines 3-4) was employed *en route* to transition and closure on matters about which he has little more to say.

LANGUAGE OF READINESS

The ongoing impact of entering into, and residing within a state of readiness, is further apparent in the following expressions (see Figure 7.2). Below, son utilizes two figurative expressions when responding to his aunt:

12) **SDCL: Malignancy #10:4**

((Prior to this excerpt, son and aunt had been discussing problems with mom becoming addicted to morphine. Below, Aunt shifts off of the topic of morphine and back again to son's travel plans.))

```
 1    Aunt:   Ahh:: (.) the the point  is that eh-(( Background noise ))
 2  →         Right this very second,(.) <the best that I can determine,>
```

3   (.) <u>you</u> <u>don't</u> need to come home = >certainly <u>not</u>< <u>tonight</u>.
4   [[At least what] I can see and what I can do.
5   1→ Son: [.hhh <u>NO</u>. I-] I- I eh- eh- **The way I got things set up right**
6   **now** I should be there tomorrow evening.
7   Aunt: Okay.
8   2→ Son: **That's- that's the way I've got it in motion.** I got the feeling
9   from <u>dad</u> that it wasn't <u>come</u> home to:<u>night</u>.(.) .hh =

As aunt summarizes the "<u>point</u>" of her position on son's travel arrangements, the phrase "Right this <u>very second</u>" (line 2) makes clear that events dictate precise timing and planning. Her momentary best-assessment and recommendation, a form of advice-giving (Beach, 1996; Heritage & Sefi, 1992) that son not travel home "<u>tonight</u>" mitigates (but only slightly) a portrayal of urgency for being with mom before she dies. Son next concurs with aunt's position (lines 5-9) by utilizing two figurative expressions, further summarizing yet extending aunt's offering in key ways. He portrays himself as being fully aware and in control of his decisions and actions—first with "The way I got things set up right now" (1→), and next with "That's- that's the way I've got it in motion." (2→).[7] Particularly, "set up" and "in motion" depict a series of ongoing and preparatory actions, enacted by son and thus very much anchored in his own lifeworld experiences. He further evidences that he is not only organized, but directly informed by dad that it was best not to come home tonight —a more direct and authoritative source than aunt for receiving news and making subsequent decisions.

Son's figurative expressions also initiate topical closure, in that his plans are characterized as definitive (though volatile, see Footnote 6) and anchored in his knowledge about unfolding and shifting events. While son aligns with his aunt's recommendation and advice by citing his personal efforts and knowledge, he also makes clear that the travel matters addressed by her were already taken care of. This is the case even though aunt is mom's sister, an integral part of the family who lives in the same city as mom and dad (son's original home town). Son's figurative expressions, revealing ongoing attention and readiness to travel only when it is best to do so, are thus employed by him as resources for managing and asserting his rights and boundaries as an independent son in this family system (see Heritage & Raymond, 2005; Raymond & Heritage, 2006; Chapter 10). In a slightly disaffiliative way, son thereby re-establishes and maintains his social identity in the very midst

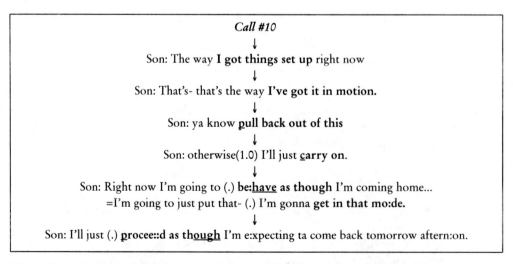

Call #10
↓
Son: The way **I got things set up** right now
↓
Son: That's- that's the way **I've got it in motion.**
↓
Son: ya know **pull back out of this**
↓
Son: otherwise(1.0) I'll just <u>c</u>arry on.
↓
Son: Right now I'm going to (.) be:<u>have</u> as though I'm coming home...
=I'm going to just put that- (.) I'm gonna **get in that mo:de.**
↓
Son: I'll just (.) **procee::d as though** I'm e:xpecting ta come back tomorrow aftern:on.

Figure 7.2. *Expressions Depicting Son's Reported and Anticipated Lines of Action.*

of these trying circumstances. This is achieved, in part, by son's authoritatively making known that (and how) he possesses unique entitlement to act upon and report his actions.

Yet several minutes later, in call #10, son actually invites aunt's involvement by requesting an update from her "just as soon as you can" (lines 5-6):

13) SDCL: Malignancy #10:9

1	Son:	U::hm (.) Yeah basically I said (.) et- earlier when I talked to
2		dad to just .hhh ummm (0.7) to call me if I shouldn't come
3		back.
4	Aunt:	[Yeah.]
5	Son:	[pt But] ummm, pt ya know if ya can (.) let me know either
6		way I gue:ss (.) as just as s<u>oon</u> as you can.
7	Aunt:	I think- I think for <u>y</u>our own (0.3) <me::ntalness.>
8	Son:	Um hm. =
9	Aunt:	= I think >to get a call either way< [is- is] =
10	Son:	[Ye::ah.]
11	Aunt:	= the way to do it. =
12	Son:	= Ye::ah.
13	Aunt:	That wa:y y̲ou're <<u>not</u> confu:sed.>
14 →	Son:	Um hm. pt **Right now I'm going to (.) be:<u>have</u> as though**
15		**I'm coming home.**
16	Aunt:	Yeah. =
17 →	Son:	= I'm going to just put that (.) **I'm gonna get in that mo:de.**
18		.hhh (.) A:nd ya know if you wan<u>na</u> (.) gi:ve me a pleasant
19		surprise tomorrow an tell me other wise (.) <u>fine</u>.

This is followed by an offering of concern by aunt (lines 7-13) for son to receive calls, both for his "<me::ntalness.>" and to minimize his confusion. This offering, though not a recommendation or advice as previously examined (see Excerpt 9, above), is once again receipted by son with two expressions (lines 14-18): "Right now I'm going to be:have as though I'm coming home." and "I'm gonna get in that mo:de.". With these utterances, he continues to assert the primacy of *his* planned actions. Despite aunt's prior stated concern for son's mental health and possible confusion, son further pursues an independent and authoritative demeanor of readiness.

It would seem reasonable to conclude that, knowingly or not, son's independent actions may provide some sense of stability in the midst of external events he cannot fully control. This is only speculation, of course, and cannot be discerned from the talk alone. But by reporting that he has a plan of action cued up—in a "mo:de"—he declares himself as being in a position to manage these events reasonably and responsibly. Son also displays a recognition that "a pleasant surprise tomorrow" (lines 18-19) may occur, and with his next and emphasized "<u>fine</u>" makes clear that he is capable of accepting whatever news comes his way—news that can only be anticipated on at this juncture of time. (Though not included in Excerpt 13 [above], he next initiates a stepwise movement toward topical transition by discussing how "funny" he will feel if he doesn't come home, and his "<u>wonder</u>ful feeling" that it may be "<u>t</u>oo late ta even squeeze her hand and have her know I'm there ya know.").

Several minutes later, aunt once again describes her own inherent uncertainty when prognosing mom's condition (lines 1-2)—doubt that may be (at least partially) remedied by what seems to be an omnipresent need to talk with the doctor (see Chapters 8 & 9) to receive valuable information:[8]

14) SDCL: Malignancy #10:13

```
 1      Aunt:    I- I me:an I just don't know (.) I don't know what ta te:ll
 2               you about it. All I can say is tomorrow morning we'll talk to
 3               Doctor Wylie an (.) she sh:ould be able to give us so:me-
 4   →           so:me path.
 5      Son:     Umhm.
 6   →  Aunt:    And it could be a:: ve:ry short pa:th <I [don't ] know.>
 7      Son:                                          [Ye:ah.]
 8   →  Son:     .hhh We:ll (.) like I said. (.) I'll just (.) procee::d as though
 9               I'm e:xpecting ta come back tomorrow afterno:on. (.) And
10               you call me (.) a- as so:on as you poss:ibly can and let me
11               know one way or another.
12      Aunt:    Oka:y.
13      Son:     And I will just adjust th:ings on my end accordingly.
14      Aunt:    Ye::ah. At- at the latest I will call you at ten which is no:on
15               yo:ur time. =
16      Son:     = Ye::ah.
17      Aunt:    That's at the latest.
18      Son:     O:kay.
19      Aunt:    Tha:t way you at least know. =
```

Each of the figurative expressions above occur en route to phone call closing (see Endnote 7).[9] Aunt's visual references to "so:me path and "a:: ve:ry short pa:th" (lines 4 & 6) portray a viable way through terrain aunt is not familiar with. The doctor "should" be able to provide a sense of guidance and direction, but also some grounded sense of prognostic time (i.e., shorter and longer paths are associated with how long mom might have to live).

It is in the face of this uncertainty, indeed as a way of managing such doubt, that son reasserts a stable line of action with ".hhh We:ll (.) like I said, (.) I'll just (.) procee::d as though I'm e:xpecting ta come back tomorrow afterno:on." (lines 8-9). This is not a disaffiliative action (Pomerantz, 1984a), but a reporting of an ongoing plan son has enacted as responsive to mom's crisis. Though he will await a phone call to the contrary and adjust his plans "accordingly" (line 13), he once again reports that his anticipated line of action will remain in effect unless he hears otherwise. As with Excerpt 10 (above), where son's "behave as though → get in that mode" occurs following mom's concern with son's "mentalness/confusion"—but with a caveat that son is open to "a pleasant surprise tomorrow" that may alter his plans—so too is a similar practice recruited here: Son's "procee::d as though" addresses, yet mitigates the impact of, mom's prior uncertainty. His orientation is subject to change, however, because receiving a phone call may occasion a necessary shift in priorities (i.e., staying home vs. traveling to be with mom and family).

Summary: Maintaining a Sense of Chronic Urgency

One way to summarize the analysis thus far is to suggest that in everyday life there are periods of time when bags are packed and unpacked, lesson plans are kept current, and family members are constantly staying by the phone to keep one another posted and remain accessible to updated news. Plans get set up, put into motion, and persons behave in a particular mode—as though one line of action or another will soon be enacted, but it is not known which or exactly when such actions might be necessary. In short, unfolding events are subject to change at a moment's notice depending on which phone call is received. These influx activities are indicative of not just a state of readiness, but a chronic sense of urgency.

Plans and actions get designed and redesigned in order to maintain the ability to respond efficiently to whatever events threaten (or in other ways alter) an otherwise healthy status quo.

As Maynard (2003) has clearly shown, both good and bad news events can disrupt the routine patterns of everyday life. Awaiting and receiving news about a mother's readiness to deliver her unborn child, for example, can trigger a host of actions by family members close enough to be somehow involved in the delivery. So too can an unexpected call, that a laboring mother is (prematurely) headed to the hospital, cause others to reprioritize their daily schedules. As discussed in Chapter 3, it is in marked contrast to routine everyday affairs, when events do *not* rupture a world we so easily take for granted and a benign order reigns (see Maynard, 2003), that a state of chronic urgency is marked by high readiness for (often unwanted) circumstances. Such periods of time are recognizable by their in-flux character, attending confusion, and even panic about events.

In the previous Chapter 6 (Excerpt 2), for example, it may be recalled that despite the considerable efforts invested to arrange son's travel plans, he was actually instructed by dad to "stay there" and await yet further news about mom's volatile condition. In Excerpt 15 (below), son answers a call from his recently separated wife who calls not to discuss mom's illness per se, but rather traveling to visit with son and his family during this difficult time. Notice how Gina, in lines 2 & 4, draws specific attention to her sense of son's troubled state of affairs:

15) **SDCL: Malignancy #13:1**

```
1      Son:    Hello, Doug he[re
2   →  Gina:            [(°It's°) me again.=[    I    ] know you=
3      Son:                                  [°H(h)i.°]
4   →  Gina:  =prob(ably) panic [every time the phone rings.
5      Son:               [.hhh<Y(h)es: I do:.> hh .hh
```

In the midst of continued crises, then, phone calls can trigger not just anxious reactions but the possibility of "panic" (see also Excerpt 16, below). At the outset of call #13 Gina claims the likelihood that son's orientation toward even receiving a call can be stress-inducing—which, in line 5, son quickly and emphatically confirms. In overlap, immediately following the word "panic", and before Gina's "every time the phone rings.", son claims entitlement to an experience he clearly owns. And he does so without knowing for sure that Gina is referring to "phone rings". Independently, then, son affirms that his accumulated involvement in often highly impactful (and at times emotionally charged) phone calls has created a residual state of "panic"—a condition that Gina knowingly attributes as a probability, given her understanding (from prior calls with him) of what son is enduring.

This is not to say, however, that Gina's recognition of son's probable "panic" occasions further empathic consideration and support. Immediately following son's ".hhh<Y(h)es: I do:.> hh .hh", Gina continues:

16) **SDCL: Malignancy #13: 1**

```
1      Son:               [.hhh<Y(h)es: I do:.> hh .hh
2                 [((Breathing hard.))]
3      Gina:   [ We:ll ↑I  need  ta- ] I need ta:: °s°-sort this ou:t.
4                 =So I need to talk to ta:lk to yo:u (.) about (.)
5                 >what I'm (gunna) s:ay to your parents.<
6                 (0.2)
7      Gina:   ↑Oka::y.
8      Son:    (hh)A(w)right.
```

Her concerns are clearly more focused on what she is going to say to son's parents than on the "panic" he just confirmed. Following a (0.2) pause, Gina's marked "↑Oka::y." seeks son's go-ahead to elaborate, which son's "(hh)A(w)right." provides.

At the closing of this call #13, son states "talk to ya tonight.", confirming the ongoing need to stay in close contact about urgent family matters. Son's subsequent call to Gina that evening, however, further reveals the volatility of planning for travel:

17) SDCL: Malignancy #14:1

((Response to greeting on phone answering machine))

```
1     Son:    pt ↑Hi::, this is <Dou:g:> (.)I'd like to leave a message
2             for Gina pt .hh u::h I'm not coming [.......
3                                               [((call waiting
4             clicks))
5             (1.0)
6     Son:    ↓S:o, (0.5) hu:m:: (0.5) doh- you don't need to call me
7             back. <I'll just> (.) write cha a letter letcha know what's
8             going on, but I won't be there (.) hhh u:h at least not
9             quite yet.  ↑Okay. Thanks bye.
```

In a short period of time, likely as a result of talking with his dad, son decided not to travel home to be with mom and his family—an occasion where he would also be visiting with Gina. As son states "I won't be there (.) hhh u:h at least not quite yet." (lines 8-9), his cancellation is not treated as final but only a postponement: an inevitable recognition of mom's dying at some unknown time in the near future.

INFORMING OTHERS OF POSTPONED READINESS: COUNSELING, KENNELS, AND AUNT

Further calls by son to update others about his altered travel plans—including a counseling center, a kennel, and eventually his aunt—are enacted in a very short period of time. Though figurative expressions per se do not occur during these calls, their inclusion here further substantiates the ongoing interactional work involved when navigating through aftershocks of son's decision to cancel travel plans. As will become clear, however, each call is designed for the unique background and circumstances son shares with those he is addressing. Specifically, son treats recipients not just on the basis of what they know, but by what they are entitled to know about mom's illness, his state of affairs, and overall family cancer dilemma. Examined chronologically, the following three calls also reveal increased personalization through son's disclosure and enacted demeanor.

The Counseling Center

In the first call to a counseling center, son begins by describing how his normal appointment became altered because "something came up" (line 5):

18) SDCL: Malignancy #15:1

((C=Counseling Receptionist; C2=Counseling Receptionist 2))

((Approximately 10 seconds of phone ringing))

```
1     C:      <°A second-°> Counseling center can I help you.
2  →  Son:    pt .hhh Yes. Hi. ↑I have uh normally got ah appointment
```

```
 3                   scheduled with ((name)).
 4         C:        Uum [ hmm.  ]
 5    →    Son:           [pt .hh ] uh And I had >something come up that caused
 6                   me to call an cancel it.< pt .hhh hh And the something has
 7                   gone away now. So I'd  like to (.) put it back.
 8                   .h[hh  pt .hhh  $hhhh$ $hh$]
 9         C:           [Okay let me transfer you.]
10                   I'm gonna put ya through to (.) her office hold on. =
11         Son:      = Alright.
12                       .
13                       . ((Approximately 4 seconds of phone ringing))
14                       .
15         C2:       Counseling center.
16    →    Son:       pt .hh ↑ Hi. um pt I normally have an appointment, (.) with
17                   <((name)) > (.) on Wednesdays at ten a'clock.
18         C2:       Um hm. =
19    →    Son:      = .hhh And I had >something come up that caused me to think
20                   I was going to have to leave town immediately, and I called
21                   an' cancelled the appointment. .hhh And then this thing
22                   didn't happen. (.) .hhh So I'm ↑still here in town. (.) .h[hh]
23         C2:                                                              [Do] ya
24                   wanna speak with ↑((name))?
25         Son:      .hh- uh- Is she available. =
26         C2:       = Hold on just a second. =
27         Son:      = Alright. Thank you.
28                       .
29                       . ((Series of 16 blips with 1.0 sec. in between, background noise
30                       . of papers shuffling and breathing))
31         C2:       ↑I'm sorry she's not back there right now. Wouldja ↑like to
32                   leave a message?
33    →    Son:      pt hhh ↑Well jus- jus- go ahead an:: (.) put me back down for
34                   my regular appointment. I- (.) >like I said,< I had cancelled the
35                   appointment: ↓ and then it turns out I don't really need to so if=
36         C2:       = Wh[en is it scheduled for]
37         Son:         [ .hhhhh   hhhhh  ] It's Wednesday mornings ten
38                   o'clock.
```

As son continues, he states "And the something has gone away now. So I'd like to (.) put it back." (lines 6-7). The vague reference to "something" is twice recruited by son to gloss the urgency occasioned by mom's cancer. In the manner son produces his explanation, he withholds providing details to a receptionist/call-taker—essentially, a third party son treats as unknown, distant, and fulfilling a role (i.e., of receptionist) not entitled to further disclosure. Left hanging is what "something" depicts, just as "gone away now" remains unelaborated by a narrative son could have, but did not, extend. Upon completion of his utterance, notice also that son, through laughter (line 8), displays resistance to the troubles he has indirectly reported. In this way, son exhibits his ability to manage the circumstance he is in as though he is (more or less) back to the normal state of affairs prompting his original appointment. And while C's initial response overlapped with son's laughing (line 9), she repeats her recognition and willingness to insure a basic yet important understanding: that she takes son's vague yet reported troubles seriously, in a troubles-receptive manner (see Glenn, 2003; Jefferson, 1984b), en route to transferring son to another receptionist who might assist him.

Later, akin to speaking with another airline representative following transfer (see Excerpt 19, Chapter 5), son presents his problem for the second time to a different recep-tionist. The comparisons between lines 2-8 and lines 16-22 reveal a striking resemblance. Son invokes "normally" to characterize his usual appointment, shifts to "something come up" as an indirect reference to troubles, then ends with "And then this thing didn't <u>hap</u>-pen." (rather than "And the something has gone <u>away</u> now."). In the second narrative, son inserts "to think I was going to have to leave <u>town</u> immediately" (lines 19-20), and later "So I'm ↑<u>still</u> <u>here</u> in town.". These are slightly more elaborated descriptions of his actions, which, understandably, further legitimate his need to reschedule the cancelled appointment for a (second) call-taker—a person treated as though she is in a better position to grant son's request (thus meriting his fuller explanation). And when C2 reports that the coun-selor is not in, asking if son would like to leave a message (lines 31-32), son reveals that it is the rescheduled appointment he seeks by more specifically requesting his "regular appointment".

Although there is certainly more to say about son's call to the counselor's office, atten-tion has been drawn to son's indirect methods for twice reporting his troubles—unspeci-fied events causing his routine of normal, regular appointments to be cancelled. Son achieves his work without mentioning the inevitable recurrence of these troubles in the future, namely, that mom's prognosis appears to be terminal. This absence of future-refer-ence contrasts markedly with his following call to the kennels to discuss his dog's board-ing, a more clear-cut instance of the interactional work involved in demonstrating post-poned readiness.

The Kennel

At the outset of his call to the kennels, son speculates that he believes he may have spoken with the same person yesterday (line 5). With "Uh huh.", K next seems to confirm his iden-tification (which is more clearly evidenced in line 13):

19) SDCL: Malignancy #16:1

((K = Kennel receptionist))

1	K:	Teltone ↑Kennels. =
2	Son:	= pt ↑<u>Hi:</u>. (.) I called yesterday about, bringing uh <u>do:</u>g out
3		there today.
4	K:	Uh [huh.]
5	Son:	[pt h]hh U:hm: uh I- I think I may have even <u>talk</u>ed to you.
6	K:	Uh huh?
7 →	Son:	pt .hhh Uh ↑Well it <u>turns</u> out, that I don't need to leave in
8		quite the <<u>pani:c:</u>> (.) that I <u>thought</u> I was gonna need to leave
9		in. W[e've go]tta ah very temporary reprieve and =
10	K:	[O k a y.]
11	Son:	= I ↑<u>didn't</u> know if you were <<u>ho:l:</u>ding a spot> (.) .hhh or
12		anything like that fer me. .hhh =
13	K:	= I was ↑just <u>expect</u>ing ya: [so I me]an =
14	Son:	[Okay.]
15	K:	= °Ya know,° tha- that's fine[( ) jus'] give me =
16	Son:	[We:l:l]
17	K:	= a c[all.]
18 →	Son:	[I- I'm] ↑<u>sure</u> its gonna happen in the ↑<u>near</u> future. hh =
19	K:	= Okay. =

```
20  →   Son:    = But it isn't necessarily gonna happen <today.> And I thought
21              if you ↑were holding a spot I didn't want'cha to <continue>
22              .hh[h uh holding] it.=
23      K:         [ ( Alright ) ]
24  →   Son:    =For right now I will- (.) .hh I will keep your number right
25              handy because (.) when it ↑does happen uhh <ya know.>
26      K:      Um hm. =
27  →   Son:    = pt But this >ya know how these things are ya
28              n[ever kn]ow n- in =
29      K:       [ Yeah. ]
30  →   Son:    = The middle of the night they tell ya one thing an' in the
31              morning they tell ya another.< .h[hhhh]h =
32      K:                                        [ Okay.]
33      Son:    = Hum but-(.) so- (.) pt I wanted to thank ya though for being
34              very helpful.
35      K:      Oh that's fi[ ::ne. ]
36  →   Son:               [ A:nd ] uh (.) I will-
37              (0.2)
38      K:      Jus' gim[ me  a ca:ll. ]
39  →   Son:           [Keep-  keep] -your number here a::nd I- it's nice
40              that'chur °open when you're open° so: =
41      K:      = O[ kay. ]
42  →   Son:       [ Whe]n I do need it I'll- I'll be out.
43      K:      Okay. =
44  →   Son:    = .hhh When I come (.) ↑what do I need to bring for my dog:.
```

What occurs next (lines 7-8), however, is particularly relevant to describing how a language of readiness gets implemented over time. Son carries over the word "panic" from Gina's earlier usage (in Excerpt 12, above). He adapts it here to the particular contingencies of the problem, that is, how to explain to K that when he previously enlisted their assistance he was in a panic mode from which there is now a "very temporary reprieve" (line 9). With "very temporary reprieve"—signifying a pardon or delay in some foreboding future event—it is as though the floodgates of disclosure have been opened in son's call to the kennels. When speaking with receptionists at the counselor's office, son was indirect and withholding about his family crisis. Here, and in marked contrast, son repeatedly portrays how he remains in a state of extreme readiness for events he has been preparing for (e.g., see Footnote 7). His orientation, however, stands in sharp contrast to K's actions. For example, as son describes that he was concerned that the kennel might be "<ho:l:ding a spot>" for him (line 11), K moves to bring closure to the matter with "that's fine ( ) jus' give me a call." (lines 15-16; see also 35 & 38). Yet he restates that it's likely to occur "in the ↑ near future", though not necessarily today (lines 18 & 20), before once again telling K what "I thought" about her holding a kennel for his dog. In response, K's "Alright" (line 23) again attempts to finalize this discussion, revealing that she is considerably less concerned than son about his cancellation.

Son also portrays the kennels as a priority resource throughout what promises to be a short, intense, yet uncertain future. At different moments he emphasizes the inevitability of needing the kennels when traveling to be with mom and family (see lines 24-25, 33-42), specifying that he will "keep your number right handy" (lines 24-25), an offering of thanks (lines 33-34), and a related "[Keep- keep] -your number here a::nd I- its nice that'chur °open when you're open° so: =". (lines 39-40). Moreover, throughout these actions, son solicits K's special understanding about events that have transpired (e.g., receiving conflicting phone calls from family members). Similar to moments when son invited compassion from airline representatives (e.g., see Chapter 5, Excerpt 22), son discloses the volatility of events in his life in an attempt to get K aligned with the dilemma he is facing (lines 27-32).

When examining notably different demeanors enacted by son when calling the counselor's office and kennels simply to cancel appointments, it is curious that son would be withholding with the former and pursue more personal and vulnerable matters with the latter. Although it is apparent that son had spoken with the same receptionist at the kennels previously (Excerpt 16, lines 5-6, 13), and that prior established relationship might account for his more informal manner, additional explanations might be offered. For example, his counseling needs may be treated by son as matters to be shared only with "the counselor" and not receptionists. Further, it is understandable that son might work to *not* come off as incessant, troubled, or otherwise in need of keeping their number handy. For example, he does not thank the counselor's office for being there, nor that he is assured in knowing they are open and flexible to assist him in this difficult period of time. In short, exhibiting such actions to counselor's receptionists might indicate, to them, that son indeed requires more urgent support and help than son seeks to portray. Their response could amount to classifying son as a particularly "troubled" patient necessitating more special assistance.

With K's receptionist, however, son needn't be as concerned about coming off as deeply embroiled in a state of readiness, thankful and even soliciting of K's understanding of what son is going through. He is, after all, calling on behalf of *his dog*. Being a responsible pet owner implies a relational commitment to a partner, the importance of which should not be underestimated because unremitting care is expected and even rewarded (i.e., by kennels and "vets"). And it should not be overlooked that K represents a care provider: understanding of pet owners' needs, invested in developing trusting relationships, capable of and receptive to hearing about reasons why the clients make (and cancel) reservations for their pets. Perhaps even more simply, it makes good sense to be overly concerned with maintaining good relations with a kennel. Owners who love their pets cannot and will not tolerate leaving them uncared for in times of absence, including family emergencies.

The Aunt

The final call to be analyzed in this chapter is received by son shortly following his calls to the counseling center and kennels. The opening few minutes appears below. Numerous contrasts with son's prior two calls are evident throughout (e.g., the obvious relational history evident in son's talking with his aunt rather than receptionists, the kinds of knowledge and experience son and aunt invoke in the midst of son's reporting). Unique opportunities are provided to compare son's reportings with actual moments from past referenced events, and the first of three stories about mom's "cigarettes" (see also Chapter 11) is told by son.

Undoing News

Lines 1-11 can be parsed as an opening News Delivery Sequence (NDS). Immediately following son's answer, Aunt queries son about dad in line 2:

20) **SDCL: Malignancy #17:1-2**

1	Son:	↑Hello. Doug here.
2INI→	Aunt:	Did your dad call?
3 1→	Son:	Yes he did.
4 2→	Aunt:	↑<u>O</u>kay a:nd-
5 1→	Son:	And I'm <u>un</u>doing.
6 2→	Aunt:	You're <u>un</u>doing.

```
  7 3→    Son:    Ye[ah. he-]
  8 2→    Aunt:     [ Ya ] talked to Dr. ↑Wy:lie.
  9 3→    Son:    ↑Yeah he said don't come home yet.
 10   10 4→       (1.0)
 11 4→    Aunt:   .hhh (.) O:↑kay.
 12               (0.2)
 13       Son:    .hhh ↑S:o (.) I'm wh- th- that you sound >puzzled by that.< =
 14       Aunt:   = U:h (.) ↑honey.
 15       Son:    = hhh [.hhh]
 16       Aunt:         [ $Hu]h $ No ↑I'm not <puz:zl:ed.> I- ↑I have not talked
 17               to Dr. Wylie. ↑I haven't talked to your dad.
 18       Son:    Oh::kay. =
 19       Aunt:   = I sent 'em in (.) °ya know.° =
 20       Son:    = ↑Yeah he jus' called me <like- like> (.) thirty seconds
 21               a[g o.]
 22       Aunt:   [<We]: :ll> (.) [ I- the lin ]e was busy.
 23       Son:                    [ Ah minute.]
 24       Aunt:   An' I was hoping that was him, so: =
 25       Son:    = Yeah.|=
 26       Aunt:   = I wanted to make sure I said I would get to you at ten
 27               a'clock. °However° (.) I wanted to make sure that >↑he had
 28               done it <cause I had instructed 'em last night ((mimic voice))
 29               ↑NO LATER THAN TEN, =
 30       Son:    = Yeah. .hh [ Huh. ]
 31       Aunt:              [An' I th]ought ↑well. =
 32       Son:    = ↑Yeah. ↓Well (.) he called and he said >↑don't come yet.<
 33               (0.7)
 34       Son:    .hhh      So I've (.) .h[h cal-  ]
 35       Aunt:                          [What'd-] did Dr. Wylie ↑say to him (.) >do
 36               ya know?<
 37               (0.6)
 38       Son:    No not <really.> hh u:m hhh (.) Ya know that they were gonna
 39               radiate these tumors in her le:g and that- they were gonna put
 40               'er on ↑pill form morphine (.) .hhh after a while. n::n .hhh u::h
 41               (0.4)
 42       Son:    An'that was about it. An' that there no >there wasn't quite the
 43               immediate danger they thought there was last ni:ght an' that's
 44               basically,< .hhhh a:ll::.
 45               (1.0)
 46       Son:    ↓Ya know dad said °ya know° last night (.) .hhh <it was one
 47               way an'> this morning she's m- .hh givin' 'em hell for
 48               forgettin' her cigarettes (.) ya know. pt hh An' so $hhh hhh
 49               hh .hhh$ =
 50       Aunt:   = Okay. So she was much better this m[orning.]
 51       Son:                                         [Ye: ah.] Much better
 52               apparently.
```

It is without identification that aunt's "Did your dad call?" (line 2) moves directly to not just any, but particular business at hand. And without hesitation, son affirms (but does not elaborate on) her query in the next utterance. This streamlined phone opening—including identification, recognition, and direct movement to unexplicated first topic—is possible only because of their relational history. This includes call # 10, only one day earlier, in which considerable efforts were made to create the understanding that aunt would call son "tomorrow" (e.g., see Excerpt #11, above; Footnote 7). From son's announced "I'm <u>undoing</u>.", and aunt's next "You're <u>undoing</u>.", there is apparently no need to specify *what* was undone. It is mutually understood that son's travel plans have been postponed. In lieu of a need to elaborate what was left unstated, however, aunt's repeated (and prosodically resonant) "<u>undoing</u>" exhibits some surprise (see prior discussions of "modified repeats" in Chapter 4; Stivers, 2005). And just as son begins to elaborate his news in line 7, aunt's "Dr. ↑Wylie." anticipates what son was next going to state: "he said don't come home yet." (line 9).

At the outset of this call, then, precise co-orientations to these shared moments reveal how speakers closely monitor and rely upon an *architecture of intersubjectivity* (Heritage, 1984b) to achieve shared understandings. That these moments are consequential for son and aunt is evident not only from the serial exchanges examined across numerous phone calls, but also aunt's delayed and intoned "O:↑kay." (line 11). As I have noted elsewhere, this utterance shares features indicative of

> a series of interactional environments within which speakers prosodically rely on "okays"—for example, "O:<u>:ka:::y</u>?", "↑<u>Ok:a::y</u>.", or simply "Kay?,"—to display that something is "not okay": that some prior actions are heard and understood to be somehow incongruous with "okay producer's" position toward those actions . . . stances are enacted that treat prior actions discrepantly: as perplexing, inappropriate, or even as grounds for mistrust and incredulity. (Beach, 2002c, p. 1)

Working Through Puzzlement and Embellishment

It is not coincidental, then, that son next responds with ".hhh ↑<u>S:o</u> (.) I'm wh- th- that you sound >puzzled by that.< =" (line 13), drawing attention to aunt's apparent perplexity and seeking some explanation for this reaction. With an endearing "↑honey." (line 14), aunt proceeds and with delicate laughter ("$Hu]h $) declines being puzzled by stating she has insufficient knowledge: She has not spoken with the doctor nor son's dad (lines 16–17). In this way she discounts her claim to authoritatively assess son's updated "<u>undoing</u>" news, thus minimizing not her right to know, but an inability to counter son's news with information drawn from her own experience (e.g., from speaking directly with the doctor or dad). It is this information that son next provides to authenticate his decision not to travel, and he does so by reporting an extreme case. Though he informs aunt that his dad called thirty seconds → a minute ago (lines 20, 23), it was at the outset of call #12 that son actually received the news "Stay there." (See Chapter 6, Excerpt 2). Since that call, son has been involved in four additional phone calls (see Timeline, Chapter 2): a call from Gina, a phone message he left to inform her he wasn't coming home ("at least not quite yet"), a call to reschedule his counseling appointment, and a call to cancel his Kennels reservation.

Could son could not have forgotten that these calls recently occurred? Not likely. What is more compelling is that son's reporting of having (literally) just received dad's call is designed to provide aunt with a sense of familial importance by being "in the loop." She was portrayed as the first to have received "the news" following call #12 between dad and son, and therefore is led to believe she is as close as possible to the scene and action. From this action it is clear that son gives priority to situating aunt as a primary and consequential family member, even at the expense of the factual basis of emerging events and phone calls. Because he had previously and recently made arrangements and agreed to keep in close contact with her about his travel plans—and perhaps for reasons well beyond what can be speculated upon here—she is constructed as *the first to know even though she was not.*

Embellishments such as this are exceedingly common in everyday life. It is often impossible to know the exact ordering of events as others report them, and just how we (as recipients) fit into the overall scheme of activities. Different reasons (e.g., relational, familial, and political) motivate the altering of chronology and timing. Though typically unstated, such reasons influence the organization of narratives offering particular, and not necessarily factual reconstructions, of (alleged) past events (e.g., see Atkinson & Drew, 1979; Beach, 1985; Bennett & Feldman, 1981;). What is clear, and evident in aunt's subsequent utterances, is that she responds as though she has been closely monitoring and involved—on the very front line of emerging circumstances (e.g., reporting a line being busy in line 22, "ho<u>p</u>ing that was <u>him</u>" in line 24, and with emphasis a restatement of her commitment to make sure she would call son by ten o'clock to inform him that she had "<u>instructed</u>" dad to call "↑<u>NO LATER THAN TEN</u>,=" in lines 26-29). In these and other ways aunt exhibits active monitoring and concern indicative of the primary familial status son has afforded her. Through sons's actions, she is made to believe, and acts the role, of a key player in ongoing decision making and planning occasioned by mom's ongoing illness.

Reporting Mom's Condition

It is before aunt can further report her thoughts (line 31) that son again states what he had earlier announced on line 9, namely, dad's stating "don't <u>come</u> yet." (line 32). With ".hhh So I've (.) .hh [cal-]" (line 34). Just as son appears to begin reporting his prior calls (e.g., to the counseling center and kennels), aunt queries about what the doctor told dad (lines 35-36). Her query triggered an elaborated response by son about dad's summary of mom's condition (lines 38-49). It is interesting and useful to compare son's reporting with dad's actual narrative from the earlier call #12:

21) **SDCL: Malignancy #12:1**

1	Dad: >Ya know, the trip was gonna come <u>about</u>.< It's just that ya
2	know (.) i:<u>f</u> ya wanna come this week, this is <u>not</u> gonna be an
3	e:n:d week kinda thing, . hhh <So:::.> (.) your mother's answer
4	was na::h stay there. Ya know she's- she is <u>much</u> <u>better</u> this
5	morning. She °is uh completely <u>lucid</u> or- seems to be° the few
6	>minutes I've had to <u>talk</u> to her 'cause I talked to <u>her</u> talked to
7	the <u>doctor</u>< (.) .hhh uh- The <u>tum</u>ors in her <u>legs</u> they're gonna
8	xra::y and scan or whatever tom<u>morr</u>ow they're gonna scan
9	the <u>hip</u> to see why <u>that</u> hurts. They're changing around uh
10	(0.6) the thyroid stuff 'cause she's cranked up too <u>high</u>. (.)
11	.hhh They had <u>her</u> on u::h (0.4) <u>morphine</u> all night on uh ya
12	know one uh these drip system >whatever the hell< s:o <<u>that</u>
13	<u>cal:med down</u>> some of this. So she got outta ><u>bed</u> on her
14	<u>own</u>< this morning. = She went to the <u>bathroom</u> so- .hhh

Upon inspection, son's descriptions (again, lines 38-49)—from tumors → morphine → less immediate danger—closely parallel basic issues addressed in dad's original narrative. But two primary contrasts are apparent: (a) Dad mentioned mom being much better and basically out of immediate danger first, whereas that was stated last in son's reporting; and (b) Obviously, son did not reconstruct as many details as dad originally stated (e.g., about mom being more lucid, pain in her hip, mom's thyroid, or the drip system administering the morphine). Additionally, in lines 46-49, son reports an event involving mom's "givin' 'em <u>hell</u> for forgettin' her cigarettes" that, as analyzed more closely in Chapter 11, did not occur during call #12 until over one minute later. Whereas son treated this incident as important enough to include in his summary to aunt, she did not treat it as interesting or relevant: A shift is made away from cigarettes and back to mom being "<u>much</u> better".

IT'S ALL PART OF THE GAME

The final instance brings us back to the primary emphasis of this chapter: understanding how family members co-produce a state of readiness, and in so doing, rely on figurative expressions to characterize their circumstances. At the outset of this chapter (Excerpt 1, above), attention was drawn to how son explicitly invoked the phrase "state uh readiness" to depict his ability to act quickly and efficiently should he need to travel home to be with mom and family. This expression preceded son's "keep my lesson plans current" and "do what I have to do", as well as aunt's "smell anything in the wind"—all of which exhibit a high state of alertness, anchored in a close and collaborative monitoring of mom's changing health status (and thus family's readiness).

The excerpt below occurred approximately three minutes prior to Excerpt 1. Son requests that he be kept informed in the case of "<u>any</u> (0.6) significant <u>change</u>" (line 1). Aunt responds by endearingly insuring son with "Honey, [you] will be the >f:ir:st (.) person< (.) I call." (lines 4, 6). Should changes occur, their joint actions further evidence a need to be ready for action:

22) SDCL: Malignancy #17: 5

```
1        Son:   If ↑there's- if there's any (0.6) significant change in
2               information.
3               (0.2)
4        Aunt:  Honey, =
5        Son:   = Let me know. [hhh]
6        Aunt:               [you] will be the >f:ir:st (.) person< (.) I call.
7        Son:   ↑O:kay.
8        Aunt:  O↑ka:y ?
9        Son:   pt A:nd in the meantime, (.) .hhh I have a bunch uh $phone
10              calls to ma[ke   now.$   ]
11       Aunt:            [I know. I'm-] sorry sw[eet heart.   ]
12       Son:                              [.hh Th- oh-] ↑that's a:ll ri:ght
13   →          it's all- all part of the ga:me. =
14   →   Aunt:  = Ya know a- and I- I know that- doesn't n- necessarily make
15              this any better but it's just as- (.) JUST as confusing here.
16       Son:   Mm hm:.
17   →   Aunt:  It- (.) y- <you may think> that because we're sitting here
18              looking at it (0.2) that it is (.) <eas::ier.> =
19   →   Son:   = Oh n:o [I- I know >I know<] it's just =
20       Aunt:          [ (          )     ]
21   →   Son:   = ↑All it is is different. (.).h[h Dad] and I were = ((continues))
```

As son next begins to move to closure because he has phone calls to make, aunt shows compassion for son's predicament with "I'm-] sorry sw[eet heart.]" (line 11). In recognition that it is not aunt's fault, but a consequence of simply being an involved family member, son responds with ".hh Th- oh- ↑that's a:ll ri:ght it's <u>all</u>- all part of the ga:me. =." (lines 12-13). This is a particularly apt figurative expression, summarizing both his obligations as a family member *and* likening life's troubles to participating in a game: a series of activities enacted (in this sense) not as sport, amusement, or play for its own sake, but as being willing to address a challenge and "toe the mark" as a responsible team member. This figurative expression is also a sequence closing assessment (see Jefferson, 1981, 1993), thus contributing to closure of this topic.

And difficult though it may be for son, with "it's just as- (.) JUST as confusing here." (line 15), aunt addresses what son implies by offering yet further condolence. By responding to son's figurative expression in this way, aunt explicitly recognizes (lines 14-15) that it may not lighten son's load. Her actions do share the burden. But importantly, and in a slightly disaffiliative manner, aunt also asserts rights to experiencing her share of the family dilemma. She therefore extends discussion about the topic, not facilitating the closure son initiated, by emphasizing that it's difficult on everyone, not just the son. Indeed, aunt continues by attributing to son that he might be thinking it is easier for them than him (lines 17-18). This is a rather bold assertion that, essentially, challenges son's prior "all part of the ga:me" position—a stance aunt herself had just commiserated with. With some surprise and recognition that aunt would assume that he thinks it is "eas::ier" for them, his oh-prefaced and next "= Oh n:o [I- I know >I know<] it's just =" (line 19) clearly aligns with and defers to aunt's correction. And aunt continues by further emphasizing that "= ↑All it is is different." (line 21).

In the very midst of expressing and commiserating about son's troubles, therefore, aunt makes clear that he is not alone in being adversely impacted by mom's cancer diagnosis and treatment. A fine line thus exists between commiserating with another and asserting one's rights to the very dilemmas another may be treating as claiming (more or less) exclusively as their own (see Chapter 10). Although it may at first glance appear to be contradictory to have competing stances to shared difficulties, moments such as these are exceedingly normal. In earlier work (Beach, 1996) on a grandmother-granddaughter conversation involving bulimia, for example, inherent problems were revealed involving caregiving. Not the least of these problems involved how speakers provide and withhold commiseration about what another treats as meaningful, relevant, and uniquely tied to their own circumstances. In Excerpt 22 (above), aunt's shift from being concerned about son, while also asserting her rights to equal consideration for ongoing troubles as a primary family member, reveals her propensity to caring for others but not at the expense of receiving "her fair due". This delicate balance, routinely negotiated and managed by family members facing illness dilemmas, appears to be *just part of the game*.

Improvising Scripts, Plans, and Language Games

In the midst of addressing urgent family matters, well-organized scripts and plans need to be constructed. Yet, as apparent in this chapter and throughout the Malignancy corpus, there is a simultaneous need to *improvise* social actions as responses to contingencies that cannot be fully anticipated in advance. Such is the primordial nature of not just evolving illness, but indeed interactionally negotiated alternatives for addressing all social interactions. Across urgent occasions and phases of social life behaving responsibly, in a timely and reasonable fashion, and in a manner that works for all (or nearly all) involved parties, remains a primary focus and thus locus of social actions. These collaborations reveal how individuals may and do assert their primary rights to make individual decisions as well as receive adequate acknowledgment for their efforts. At the same time, it appears that priority is given to exhibiting sensitivity to others' individual needs. As these fundamental matters get managed across multiple phone calls, involving different members, the finely interwoven, historically connected, and constantly evolving nature of "family"-over-time gets revealed.

SUMMARIZING THE INTERACTIONAL WORK
OF FIGURATIVE EXPRESSIONS

The interactional work achieved through 26 (previously examined) figurative expressions is summarized in Figure 7.3.

FIGURATIVE EXPRESSION	EXCERPT#/ CALL#	INTERACTIONAL WORK DISPLAYED
Aunt: gonna: <u>knock</u> us for a lo::op	(Note 1)	need to work together, brace for, & deal with mom's dying/death[T]
Aunt: it's ↑<u>still</u> gonna knock us for a lo:op	(Note 1)	repeated figurative expression in pursuit of withheld affiliation by son[T,D]
Son: state uh <u>readiness</u>	1/17	quick & efficient action; *being there* for family[T]
Son: ↑<u>keep</u> my lesson plans nice and current	1/17	anchoring trouble in lifeworld experience; summarizes prior telling & independent topical potential[T]
Son: ↑<u>do</u> what I need to <u>do</u>	1/17	new relevant matter; steadfast conviction; reasserts family commitment[T]
Aunt: ↑smell anything in the wind	1/17	vigilance & reassurance about timely updates[T]
Dad: But pack your bags	2/3	encourages son to attain readiness for likely action[T]
Son: I'll stay by the phone	3/3, also Note 6	remaining accessible during volatile times[T]
Son: pull this off	4/4	embeds efforts to travel within complex series of events[T]
Son: probably not unpack my <u>bag</u>	9/10	continued readiness to address emerging contingencies[T]
Dad: <u>educated</u> crystal ball	Note 5	references doctor's inability to accurately foresee the future, and disagrees with son's assessment[T,D]
Dad: trying to squash <u>mush</u>rooms in a rainstorm	10/12	analogy addresses futility of doctor's proposed treatment[T]
Son: un<u>pack</u> my ba:g: hhh [.hh and I'll keep] my lesson plans current	10/12	frustrated willingness to downgrade readiness yet remain vigilant[T]
Dad: keep yu- your <u>list</u> up tuh date an >ya know< leave the bag where it is	10/12	corrects son's downgraded and proposes alternative readiness; asserts primary knowledge of events [T,D]
Dad: I told ya life's a <u>bitch</u>… <u>No rose</u> garden	10/12	summary of earlier topics and reminder of life's challenges[T]
Son: <u>keep</u> you're le:sson pla:ns <u>current:</u>, a:n <u>don't</u> <u>unpa:ck your ba:g</u> comple:tely	11/18	reports and retains reasonably accurate version of dad's prior correction[T]
Aunt: Right this <u>very</u> <u>second</u>	12/10	momentary best-assessment of the need for precise timing/planning[T]
Son: The way I got things set up right now	12/10	reports being organized and in control of ongoing decisions/actions; asserts rights as informed and independent family member[T,D]

Son: That's- that's the way I've got it in motion	12/10	reports being organized and in control of ongoing decisions/actions; asserts rights as informed and independent family member[T,D]
Son: pull back out of this	Note 6	reversing his plans to travel[T]
Son: I'll just carry on	Note 6	commitment to move forward with current plans[T]
Son: Right now I'm going to (.) be:have as though I'm coming home	13/10	asserts primacy of planned actions; readiness & stability in the midst of uncontrollable external events[T,D]
Son: I'm gonna get in that mo:de	13/10	asserts primacy of planned actions; readiness & stability in the midst of uncontrollable external events[T,D]
Aunt: so:me path/a:: ve:ry short pa:th		visually refers to doctor's (possibly helpful) prognosis[T]
Son: I'll just (.) procee::d as though	14/10	reports anticipated (though changeable) line of action[T]
Son: it's all- all part of the ga:me	22/17	summarizes family obligations and willingness to "toe the mark" ; Aunt (recipient) asserts rights to experience her share of the family dilemma[T,D]

Listed In Order of Analysis

[T] = Topical Transition & Closure; [D] = Disagreement, Disaffiliation, and/or Lack of Alignment

Figure 7.3. *Interactional Work Achieved Across 26 Figurative Expressions.*

These 26 figurative expressions, listed by order of analysis, make clear that without exception this collection of moments unequivocally supports prior observations about how figures of speech are employed in sequential environments involving topical transition and closure (i.e., Drew & Holt, 1988, 1998; Holt & Drew, 2005). It is also apparent, however, that such expressions are recruited by speakers to achieve diverse kinds of (previously unexamined) interactional involvements. In most general terms, the interactional work summarized in Figure 7.3 might be also be categorized into the following three modes of social action: *Readiness, resolve,* and *cancer impacts, references,* and *prognosis.* Importantly, as visualized below, these overlapping categories are neither mutually exclusive nor dichotomous (see Figure 7.4).

Any given expression may simultaneously function across more than a single mode of action. For example, "↑do what I need to do" reflects resolve, makes readiness possible, while also exhibiting the impacts of being decisive as an upshot of cancer in the family. Similarly, "I'll stay by the phone" displays resolve, ongoing impacts from the need to closely monitor the family situation, as well as being a prerequisite for readiness, that is, to hear and respond to updated news. In these and related instances, therefore, the tendency to attribute singular pragmatic functions to multifunctional expressions must be avoided.

In Figure 7.4 it is also apparent that 8 of the 26 figurative expressions occurred in disagreeable/disaffiliative environments, involving at least some degree of withheld alignment or counterpositioning by one or both speakers. Both pursuit of response and disagreement with another's position are exceedingly normal and frequently studied social actions in everyday life (e.g., see Pomerantz, 1984a, 1984b). But such actions have only minimally been associated with the employment of figurative expressions (see Drew & Holt, 1988).

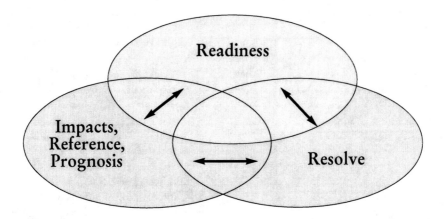

READINESS	RESOLVE	IMPACTS, REFERENCE, PROGNOSIS
• state uh <u>readiness</u>	• pull this off	• gonna: <u>knock</u> us for a lo::op
• ↑<u>keep</u> my lesson plans nice and °current°	• ↑<u>do</u> what I need to <u>do</u>	• it's ↑<u>still</u> gonna knock us for a lo:op
• ↑smell anything in the wind	• The way I got things set up right now	• <u>educated</u> crystal ball
• I'll stay by the phone	• That's- that's the way I've got it in motion	• trying to squash <u>mush</u>rooms in a rainstorm
• But pack your bags	• pull back out of this	• I told ya life's a <u>bitch</u>… <u>No</u> <u>rose</u> garden
• probably not unpack my <u>bag</u>	• I'll just carry on	• so:me <u>path</u>/a:: ve:ry short pa:th
• un<u>pack</u> my ba:g: hhh [.hh and I'll keep] my lesson plans current	• Right now I'm going to (.) be:<u>have</u> as though I'm coming home	
• keep yu- your <u>list</u> up tuh date an >ya know< leave the gag where it is	• I'm gonna get in that mo:de	
• <u>keep</u> you're le:sson pla:ns current:, a:n <u>don't</u> <u>unpa:ck</u> <u>your</u> <u>ba:g</u> comple:tely	• I'll just (.) <u>procee</u>::d as though	
• Right this <u>very</u> <u>second</u>	• it's <u>all</u>- all part of the ga:me	

Figure 7.3. *Generalized and Concentric Modes of Social Action.*

Each instance is interesting in its own right, and the collection as a whole is certainly deserving of more detailed inquiry. Working from the top of Figure 4, for example, the first[T,D] moment reveals how aunt repeated her expression in pursuit of son's withheld response. Later, dad disagrees with son's assessment of the doctor's prognostic ability. Equally routine, though certainly less understood, are the remaining six[T,D] figurative expressions involving how dad, son, and aunt assert their own rights and access to knowledge—as "epistemic" claims to authority, devices for legitimating their actions, and, indeed, when substantiating their roles as primary and thus consequential family members. For example, when dad corrects son's move to unpack his bag, son twice references his organized and independent ability to be decisive, and twice asserts the primacy of his planned actions (i.e., as a resource for remaining ready and stable during ambiguous times). Through these actions, fundamental rights to know and act upon their knowledge are asserted. And as son continues to demonstrate his own family obligation with his final "it's all- all part of the ga:me," aunt's response makes patently clear that her epistemic status should not be discounted. She asserts herself as equally involved in mom's and the families' unfolding illness drama, and thus as a central family member not to be taken lightly in the face of son's repeated references to his own burdens. As further examined in Chapter 10, "epistemics" should increasingly be understood as omnipresent tensions between speakers, routinely negotiated and managed in ways revealing just how interactional participants stake out and defend their own personal boundaries and territories in everyday affairs.

Taken together, each figurative expression examined above, and the varied other moments examined throughout this chapter, comprise the generative conditions and practices for springing into action: launching, embarking upon, and constantly rearranging trajectories of response readiness. The specific language employed, on the brink of emerging moments and as carried over from prior events (e.g., bags, panic) reflects the often critical and impactful nature of constructing and adapting to an "on hold" status in the face of an inherently uncertain (though seemingly probable) future. Also relevant are efforts made to *undo* prior arranged plans, as with son's calls to the counselor's office and kennels, when only a "temporary reprieve" has occurred: Son continues to need their services as mom's health fails. Indeed, as son initiates and receives calls from dad, his aunt, and Gina, it appears that within sequential environments involving a state of readiness, considerable efforts are invested to insure that continued and anticipated trouble can be adequately managed. These interactional and inherently collaborative efforts are one central feature of functioning family systems.

NOTES

1. Below aunt appeals for the need to "pull together.", and confidently offers reassurance that "we really will.". Her actions summarize and begin to close a prior topic focusing on how devastating mom's death will be for her, dad, and son (see Excerpts 8 & 9, Chapter 11). Following son's agreement and confirmation, Aunt Carol's first "gonna: knock us for a lo::op" (1→) provides a reason for the need to work together to brace for and actually deal with the impact of mom's dying and eventual death:

SDCL: Malignancy #17:8

Aunt:	°Ya know° we're gonna <a:ll> have to pull together.
	(0.4)
Aunt:	An' we really will.
	(0.2)
Son:	↓Ye:ah. =
Aunt:	1→ = This is jus' gonna: knock us for a lo::op uh. =
Son:	=$Hhh [hh hh hh$]

Aunt: [Even thou]gh we've been (0.2) ↑w<u>ai</u>ting for <u>these</u>
          2→ days it's ↑<u>still</u> gonna knock us for a lo:op.
Son: ↓Ye:ahh.
         (0.6)
Son: pt hh[hhh hhhh   hhhh hhhh hh] hh

This is a curious moment, in that she simultaneously exhibits a strong resistance to mom's looming death, yet also receptiveness to talking about and addressing the considerable troubles she describes. Son's response is equally curious, in that his aspirated laughter displays being "discriminating in terms of whose trouble this is proposed to be" (Jefferson, 1984b, p. 360). This is not to say that son is not also impacted by mom's cancer, but that his laughter reveals an orientation toward discerning how Aunt Carol's proposed "<u>knock</u> us for a lo::op" might impact him differently than her. From son's response, it is not clear that he fully agrees or identifies with her assessment. Consequently, in overlap Aunt Carol elaborates how, despite the waiting that has been endured, "it's ↑<u>still</u> gonna knock us for a lo:op" (2→). Her repeat of this figurative expression treats son's prior aspirated laughter as somehow withholding the affiliation (see Beach, 1996; Drew & Holt, 1988) with her initial and inclusionary "<u>knock</u> us for a lo:op". Thus, Aunt Carol recruits her figurative expression to once again pursue son's alignment (see Pomerantz, 1984a). It is only then that son provides "↓Ye:ahh.", followed by a long aspiration evidencing that the troubles being faced—and the manner in which Aunt is articulating foreseeable impacts—are, indeed, impactful *for him* as well as Aunt. The topic is then shifted to "[But I- ↑<u>we</u> will <u>be</u> there,]" as Aunt continues in Excerpt 1.

2. It is not clear whether aunt is referring to son's being absent (i.e., long distance) as a problem requiring extra effort to include him and/or to some other part of the family history.

3. Just prior to the Excerpt below, mom has just informed son that she does not want life support. Here, in mom's first utterance (1→), she displays difficulty talking about what "If U get there?" means, namely, being on the brink of death when a decision must be made about utilizing life support or not. This excerpt draws to close (3→) as she further evidences difficulty talking about what she doesn't know, because "I've not done it.". In between these two difficult moments, mom describes the intensity of the pain she is experiencing, and reports to son that she told dad she does not want the pain to continue:

SDCL: Malignancy #3:1-2

Mom: 1→   If I get there? (1.1) and (1.7) they are not um (1.2) I don't know how
               to say it. pt .h
Son: How 'bout just the quickest way.
Mom: It's hard for me to <u>ta:</u>lk. =
Son: = Ok:ay.
          (1.5) ((music playing in background throughout rest of call))
Mom: 2→   Um (1.3) °↑the <u>pain</u> is ju<u>st</u> (1.2) <u>unreal</u>°.
Son: Okay.
Mom: 2→   There's <u>no</u> way. (.) I <u>can't</u> go on.
Son: Okay.
Mom: 2→   So: (1.0) I said to dad, maybe I'm being te:rribly naive?,
               but (.) I want them to stop the pain.
Son: [Ok:ay.]
Mom: 1→   [(Now-)] now if: a::- (1.5) if they can do that you know I can sit there for five or
               ten days an' (.) I <u>d</u>on't know. I mean I just don't know. I'm- (.) I've not done it.
               = So I don't know.
Son: Okay. =

Throughout this exchange, son's repeated "Okay's." display his close monitoring, but withholds commenting on involving experiences and difficulties only mom can adequately address: pain and preferences for eliminating discomfort.

4. At the time of this recording (1989), prior to the advent of cell phones, it was necessary to "stay by the phone" to insure being contacted by others. Phones employed by family members were connected to their bases by cords (short and long), constraining even the areas where conversations occurred.

5. Notice that aunt finalizes her uncertain report by stating "At this point I would say it's not a <u>hell</u> of a lot. =." Earlier it was noted that moments of invoking the deity (e.g., God, Jesus, Holy Christ) appeared to be employed by speakers in troubling moments that could not be controlled. In this instance, aunt's reference to and emphasis with "<u>hell</u>" associates mom's lack of time with a (negative, dark, possibly evil) source—the opposite of "heaven". Other instances, analyzed throughout the "Malignancy corpus," appear to be organized in similar fashion.

6. Following dad's attempt to offer a prognosis for mom son claims to know, and sarcastically offers, that the doctor will not be helpful in confirming or disconfirming dad's assessment (lines 6-7):

SDCL: Malignancy #12:7

```
 1   Dad:  I- it may wind up bein' over the Christmas holidays or
 2         somethin'. I- >ya know< I don't know I- I- in my mind
 3         I can't (0.6) visualize this goin' past the end of the year,
 4         but lookin' at her to↑day I say puhchuuuu gotta be at
 5         least a month.
 6   Son:  Hmkay. pt .hhhh Well yeah and I know Dr. Wylie will
 7         never say anything in particular right.
 8         So- [hhhhh $huh ch$]
 9   Dad:     [We:::ll  ya know] she doesn't have any- >ya know< she's
10→           only got an educated cr[ystal ball] =
11   Son:                          [ pt Sure.  ]
```

In response, however, dad rationally explains doctor's inability to know for sure how long mom has to live: "she's only got an <u>e</u>ducated cr[ystal ball] =" (line 10). Although dad's figurative expression summarizes son's prior depiction, he also disagrees with his assessment, defending the fact that despite formal education and training the future cannot accurately be foreseen. Son's "Sure." (line 11) offers agreement with the contrary and slightly disaffiliative position dad is taking, but due to overlap not "crystal ball". And although the topical potential of "crystal ball"—and most generally, predicting the future—is considerable, it does not get pursued by dad as he shifts back to what the doctor reported about mom's tumors. His trajectory, evident in the series of figurative expressions in Excerpt 10, is evidently more than sufficient to be given priority at the expense of any further elaboration on "crystal ball" (at least at this juncture).

7. Yet such plans and actions are subject to change. Only minutes later, as son updates aunt about his plans tomorrow, she further advises him "An- and then >stay home.<" (1→):

SDCL: Malignancy #10:8

```
 1        S:     = We:ll. pt I just may (1.0) go: through and get somebody to
 2               take my class tomorrow anyway. Ummm (2.0) pt a::nd .hhh
 3               because I don't know that there is any I- don't- I  can't
 4               imagine you could get the information fast enough for me
 5               to- to stop <doing that> if I'm going to do it.
 6        Aunt:  Yeah go ahead and do that.
 7        Son:   Ye::ah.
 8   1→   Aunt:  An- and then >stay home.<
 9   2→   Son:   Ye::ah an I'll just stay b- by the phone. (.) I'll take the lesson
10               plans over tomorrow and if I find out that I can (.) .hhh ya
11               know pull back out of this then I will.
12        Aunt:  [°Ye]::ah°.
13        Son:   [pt ] A::hh (.) A:nd a- all I will have lost is one day teaching
```

14   and that's not a big deal.
15   Aunt: Ri:ght.
16 3→   Son: Ummm otherwi:se (1.0) **I'll just <u>c</u>arry on.**
17   Aunt: Um hmm.

Son's readiness is evident in his response, as he once again references his staying by the phone and making "lesson plans" available (2→). He next qualifies with "<u>p</u>ull back out of this" (line 11), a figurative expression in which "this" refers to all the plans currently being negotiated and managed. Should pulling back not be possible, "otherwi:se (1.0) I'll just <u>c</u>arry on."—where "carry on" depicts and summarizes the ongoing and processual nature of moving forward with currently formulated plans. When referring to both canceling and maintaining plans, then, these figurative expressions were invoked by son to encapsulate that and how he is caught up within a volatile, but closely monitored, line of action. It is following both expressions that topic is shifted—not to a new topic, but as son once again summarizes his request that dad call him if he shouldn't come back.

8. Here aunt makes clear that although she does not know how to assess mom's prognosis, the doctor becomes a resource for providing a "path" through illness. Such "paths" are not always easily recognized, however, and change with the terrain. In mountaineering terms, this reminds me of the practice of "bushwacking"—veering off the designated, hard-to-recognize, or absent trail—which may or may not lead to desired destinations. The effort typically requires more effort, however, and often with risk of getting lost.

9. The remainder of this phone call appears below and will be particularly useful as a resource when subsequent excerpts are analyzed—son's call to the kennel (Excerpt #16), and during his subsequent discussion with his aunt (Excerpt #17):

SDCL: Malignancy #10: 13-14

Son: = Tha:t gi:ves me time ta [ge:t the <u>dog</u> an-]
Aunt: [And say   ] I don't know a <u>DAMN</u>
        thing [anymore.]
Son: [Ye::ah.] Ye::ah. [.hhh]
Aunt: [$Ya kn]:ow (.) now we'll make that
        decision when that time [comes.]
Son: [Yeah.] The one th:ing that <u>I</u> ca:n't re:ally
        do is ta:ke the dog to the ke:nnel (.) .hh until I kn:ow. So that'll give
        me ti:me to take the dog to the kennel and get to the airport and get
        on the plane.
Aunt: Ye::ah. Ye[ah.] =
Son: [So.]
Aunt: = I will- I will (.) with: <u>any</u> lu:ck at <u>all</u> I will get to you
        befo:re then.
Son: pt Oka:y.
Aunt: Oka:y.
Son: .hhh We:::ll ti:ll <u>then</u> .hh
Aunt: Till then <u>my</u> dear.
Son: →Ha:ng in there.
Aunt:→<u>I</u>:'m hanging.
Son: Oka:y.
Aunt:→I have no <u>cho:</u>ice.
Son: Thanks for the call.
Aunt: Oka:y hon:ey. >I'll talk to you tomo:rrow.<
Son: <u>A</u>lright. >Bye bye.<
Aunt: Bye.

What I will address here are the arrowed (→) utterances, near the call closing, initiated by son's "Ha:ng in there." (see also Excerpt 14 and Endnote 3 in Chapter 13). This colloquial expression is typically (a) invoked in everyday interaction at or near call topical closure, phone call closings, and/or physical departure immediately prior to termination of a conversation, (b) regarding prior discussion topics that are troubling in nature, and (c) as an attempt to encourage and perhaps even facilitate troubled others' abilities to cope with specific events and/or circumstances. With aunt's "I:'m hanging.", she not only treats son's figurative expression as meaningful and relevant, but as the very activity in which she is engaged: coping, as best possible, with ongoing and uncertain events surrounding mom's (her sister's) critical illness caused by cancer. Further, with her next "I have no cho:ice.", she introduces (once again) the element of necessarily dealing, as best one can, with unwanted and challenging circumstances (the "deck life deals you", as I have heard it stated before). This moment might usefully be contrasted with mom's utterance "My only hope- I mean (.) my only choice.", examined more closely in Chapter 4/Excerpt 7.

There is one additional and possible *poetic* observation that might be forwarded. Is it only coincidental that in such difficult times the terms "hang/hanging" are recruited? One literal meaning, of course, involves dealing "with a noose around one's neck". But who knows? Is that stretching it too far (excuse the pun)? In an earlier paper on 'poetics' (Beach, 1993a), I referred to a quote from Sacks's (1992) lectures that also seems apt here:

> Well, who knows? Noticing it, you get the possibility of investigating it. Laughing it off in the first instance, or not even allowing yourself to notice it, of course it becomes impossible to find out whether there is anything to it. (271)

IV

REPORTING ON AND ASSESSING MEDICAL CARE

8

"SO WHAT'D THE DOCTOR HAVE TO SAY"

Lay Reportings About Doctors, Medical Staff, and Technical Procedures

Patients and family members routinely summarize for one another, and for others, what doctors and other medical experts have told them about cancer diagnosis, treatment, and prognosis. These reportings are typically provided by *lay persons* throughout their cancer journeys.[1] Although cancer patients and their family members may indeed be experts in their own professions, in the vast majority of cases those embroiled in cancer care lack sufficient knowledge and expertise to render anything but ordinary, commonsense versions of their illness circumstances.

These frequent and commonsensical renderings are innately interesting. They reveal the diverse and important roles attributed to doctors and medical staff throughout cancer care, including stances taken toward medical experts' routine activities. They also reveal how lay persons are interactionally involved in attempting to comprehend and report basic understandings of often foreign technical and biomedical terminology, coordinate decision making about ambiguous health matters, and simultaneously manage unfolding events in their lives that might not otherwise (or so it would appear) be related to cancer.

How does this interactional work get organized? What implications arise for laying bare the interwoven character of lay-medical relationships? What insights might be generated from examination of a large collection of moments wherein family members report on the work of doctors and medical staff? In short, how do family members refer to non-present medical authorities, and what consequences might these references have for family members working through cancer?

This chapter samples from a collection of well over 100 instances across the 61 Malignancy phone calls, 35 of which involve explicit references to "doctors" and the remainder "they/they're/they've" references to medical staff. Although the primary focus is on the systematic deployment of referring to "doctors", dozens of related "they/they're/they've" references (and their interplay) will also be directly examined. There are two primary issues that will be addressed across "doctor" and "they/they're/they've" references. The first, which is the focus of this chapter, involves how family members routinely reference nonpresent doctors and medical staff. Attention is given to speakers' constructions of utterances in which these references occur, how they get designed for particular recipients, their overall sequential position, the activities achieved through these deployments, and recipients' orientations to what they treated as meaningful about prior utterances. The second primary concern involves assessing (critiquing and praising) doctors, taken up in more detail in the following Chapter 9.

REFERENCE TO NONPRESENT PERSONS

As a backdrop for this and the ensuing chapter, it will be useful to provide a brief overview of Sacks and Schegloff's (1979) initial paper focusing on reference to persons, as well as Schegloff's (1996c) extended sketch of a partial systematics for referring to persons. These writings, anchored in Sacks's (1992) varied *Lectures on Conversation*, provide a preliminary framework for understanding person-reference as a complex set of interactionally organized social actions.

Written in 1973, but not published until 1979, Sacks and Schegloff proposed two basic preferences evident in the social organization of conversations involving person-reference: (a) *Minimization* by using a single reference form to a person (e.g., "Aunt: [What'd-] did **Doctor** (name) ↑say to him (.) do ya know?<"), even though any number of ways of referring to a specific individual could be employed; (b) *Recipient design*, to facilitate (if possible) recipients' abilities to recognize the person being referred to as somehow known in common (e.g., as with "**Doctor** (name)" above. As conversation unfolds, so doing allows recipients to rely on this recognition when seeking to affirm, and expand upon, current knowledge about persons, events, and/or circumstances. Put simply, "If recognition is possible, try to achieve it" (p. 18).

The identification of minimization and recipient design, recurrently employed and thus sufficiently patterned to be characterized as a "preference", only begins to address how a vast set of devices are employed by speakers to aid recognition when referring to persons. One set of examples, considered by Sacks and Schegloff (1979), involves moments when speakers assert recognition through sequences involving *try-markers* (e.g., referring to a name followed with an upward intonation and/or pause, as with "the uhm tch **Fords**?, Uh Mrs. Holmes Ford, You know uh//the the cellist?", p. 19). These attempts to assert and seek recognition often trigger responses, and thus sequences, which affirm recognition ("Oh yes.") or treat as unrecognized (e.g., "Who?") the person being referenced (e.g., see Beach, 2006).

Nearly 20 years later, Schegloff (1996c) examined "the place of the utterance in the larger sequence structure in which it occurs and its interactional preoccupations . . . some of the systematic resources informing, constraining, and being deployed" (p. 438). A primary concern, evident in the data Schegloff analyzed, might be summarized as follows: Is more than *referring* being done by speakers, and if so, how do recipients analyze and respond as though "referring has carried with it other practices and outcomes as well?" (p. 439). These questions figure centrally in the following analysis, where a variety of moments are drawn from diverse phone calls among family members. Although these moments are similar because speakers repeatedly refer to doctors and medical staff, they will be shown to be uniquely adapted to particular problems and circumstanced faced together by family members. As Schegloff (1996c) observed:

> An important point in all of this is that various reference outcomes may be the product of practices and choices made on other than reference-related grounds . . . different forms of person reference can embody practices for implementing a range of *different other activities*. . . . It remains the case that these will be marked forms which will be understood to be doing other than simple reference. They invite a recipient/hearer to examine them for what they are doing *other* than simple reference to speaker or recipient; they are marked usages. (p. 449; italics added)

A Framework for Examining Family Member's References to Medical Experts

The questions most relevant to the present analysis are as follows:

- For *these* family members, conversationally engaged throughout *this* Malignancy phone call series, what might these *"different other activities"* (described by Schegloff) be comprised of?
- What "interactional preoccupations" persist and how are references to nonpresent medical experts situated in the midst of family members' ongoing attempts to monitor (and if possible, respond appropriately) to mom's cancer?

At the outset, a general framework for responding to these queries can be delineated. As family members work together to refer to and construct lay understandings of doctors, medical staff, and technology, a predominant but not surprising pattern of communication is identified: Biomedical and technical details are routinely reported objectively, often anonymously, and in the midst of ongoing uncertainty. Throughout these interactions, family members reveal their *lay* status by (a) referring to, reporting on, objectifying, and assessing the talk and actions of doctors' and anonymous medical experts' (i.e., "they"), (b) exhibiting a lack of knowledge about numerous and ambiguous matters (e.g., technical procedures, treatments, and the passage of time), and (c) displaying related and diverse orientations to emergent troubles comprising a families journey through cancer (e.g., ongoing attempts to understand the management of pain and medication).[2]

There is also an essential paradox at work across the moments analyzed in this chapter: Although family members exhibit intimate stances and involvements through their reportings, they remain subordinate to the very technical matters being described and explained. As lay persons, those reporting and responding to updates are not capable of capturing the full range of biomedical/technical concerns: the type and characteristics of the cancer involved (e.g., location(s), stage, aggressiveness/spreading), procedures (and their impacts) for assessing and treating the cancer (e.g., biopsies, bone scans, surgery, radiation and chemotherapy), and bottom-line attempts to predict experts' abilities to halt cancer's development and seek remission (and if so, for how long, or if not, what if any implications arise for dying and death). Inevitably, only basic versions of events or procedures are depicted. However, whatever gets communicated forms the basis of family members' understandings, at least until new information is provided by medical professionals. In some cases information is provided by others as well, including friends claiming experience or knowledge about events or procedures (e.g., see lines 15-20 in Excerpt 4, below). The cycle of passing on and making sense of updated news then continues.

INITIAL REPORTINGS ABOUT MEDICAL STAFF AND DOCTORS

Analysis begins by examining how references to "they" and "doctor" (boldface below) get routinely constructed by family members. As initially examined in Chapter 3, analysis begins by returning to excerpts drawn from the opening moments of call #1. These were the first identified instances of "they" and "doctor", occurring within the first four minutes of the initial dad-son phone call. A case study of these moments is followed by examination of a larger (whenever possible, chronological) collection across the Malignancy calls.

In call #1, the transition from phone call opening to the business at hand (news about mom's biopsy results) appears below:

1) **SDCL: Malignancy #1:1-2 (S=son; D-dad)**

```
1      Son:   What's up.
2             (0.6)
3  →   Dad:   pt(hh) They ca:me ba:ck with the::: hh needle biopsy
4             results, or at least in part:.
5      Son:   °Mm hm:°
6      Dad:   .hh The tum:or:: that is the:: uh adrenal gla:nd
7             tumor tests positive.=It is: malignant.
```

In response to son's "What's up.", treated next by dad as a direct solicitation of news about mom (i.e., an itemized news inquiry, Button & Casey, 1985; Maynard, 1997), dad's utterance (lines 3-4, 6-7) is best understood as itself embedded in an unfolding sequence of critical, conversational activities.

First, dad's announcement of the news begins with "They" (line 3), a third person plural pronoun. It is not inconsequential that dad initiates his reporting in this manner. By deploying "They", dad distinguishes the referred persons from "we". As Sacks (1992) noted:

> "We" excludes "they" and "they" excludes "we." . . . And if you have a statement of the "Y do X" form, then those plural pronouns are usable. If you're not a member of Y you can say "They do (or did) X." . . . The instruction that "we" or "they" would be treated as giving, would be "find the categorical"—not necessarily a *mentioned* categorical. (pp. 250, 570, 574; italics added)

As the utterance unfolds, the categorical import of dad's "They" reference is clear: Actions were performed by anonymous and skilled medical professionals, capable of accomplishing technical biopsy procedures, including interpreting the results of those procedures. That "They ca:me ba:ck" with awaited information, assumably from "removed and unseen" labs and clinical settings (see Beach, 2002a, p. 286), places family members in a position as recipients of news they themselves ('We') were incapable of producing.

And it was the *news* that dad gave priority to, in stark contrast with the need to clarify just who "They/they" might be. In this way, the outcome of those procedures, embodying a third person plural pronoun, was treated by dad as considerably more important than revealing or describing the identities of anonymous, though apparently skilled and trustworthy, medical professionals. In this important sense, dad's single references to "They/they" adhere to the preference for *miminization*. His references also, though differently than might be expected, adhere to the preference for *recipient design*: Dad facilitated son's recognition of "They/they", but only in a manner sufficient for son to link the role of medical experts and subsequent (reportable) cancer diagnosis. What was known in common by dad and son thus had less to do with exactly who "They/they" might be and more with the circumstances they confronted, together, regarding cancer news about mom's condition.

In turn, son collaborates with dad's orientation to not making person reference a priority. He does not inquire about who "They/they" might be and he does not, then-and-there, pursue a remedy for dad's repeated references. Rather, son subordinates the need for such information in favor of the trajectory dad is pursuing: delivering bad news that mom's tumor was diagnosed as "malignant" (line 7).

There are, then, at least three distinct and simultaneous levels of *subordination* impacting how dad and son begin to announce and respond to bad cancer news: (a) As family members, dad and son ('We') could not perform procedures that medical experts ("They/they") routinely do. Nor could dad and son dictate where the tests were conducted or when the results would be available; (b) Choices were made by dad and son to not elaborate who "They/they" might be, information less relevant than what dad (as speaker) was moving next to specify to son (as willing recipient); (c) It is apparent that dad's utterance, prefaced by "They/they" as a person-reference, was itself only a part of an unfolding sequence tailored to deliver and respond to what eventuates as bad cancer news. The related and unfolding conversational activities—of moving to the news (line 1), delaying (line 2) and announcing biomedical features of the news (lines 3-7), monitoring yet withholding commentary on news son treated as not yet fully announced (with "°Mm hm:°", line 5)—work together to reveal that the interactional preoccupations exhibited by dad and son transcend orientations where referring alone was being accomplished. Indeed, it was these different activities that were treated as a primary concern by two involved family members.

In Excerpt 1 (above) dad and son exhibit their *lay* status as persons embroiled in delivering and receiving bad cancer news. These activities are more encompassing than "referring to persons" which, as noted, neither dad nor son orient to as *the* primary matter to be addressed. This single excerpt only begins to reveal how dad and son interactionally inhabit a world replete with technical and thus difficult to understand matters, procedures replete with uncertainty. For example, as dad describes "the::: hh needle biopsy results," (lines 3-4) he begins with an extended and stretched "the:::". Understood as an attempt to search for a description that was not immediately forthcoming, dad further demonstrates his 'We' vs. 'They' status. Though dad's search did yield "needle biopsy results,", it is nevertheless clear that he is attempting to describe technical terminology about medical procedures—depictions adopted and carried over from whatever doctors (and/or other medical staff) had utilized when dad was initially informed. (See also dad's stretches/searches as he subsequently attempts to describe "tum:or:: that is the:: uh adrenal gla:nd tumor" in lines 6-7). Dad is, then, reporting what others reported to him. At the same time, dad and son also confront an inherently uncertain future (only a glimpse of which is provided in this instance). With "or at least in part:." (line 4), dad qualifies his announcement as incomplete and thus uncertain, contingent upon subsequent results.

Several moments later, following son's request for clarification about mom's kidney, dad's repeated attempts to describe mom's "results" (a) remain anonymous (e.g., "They"), (b) are comprised of technical terminology (e.g., "testing positive", and (c) are repeatedly marked with different modes of uncertainty (e.g., "I don't know", "I guess", "That one they do not have the results on"):

2) SDCL: Malignancy #1:2

```
 1      Dad:   [ May-] (.) ma:ybe I'm not saying it right. .hhh There
 2   →         is- I don't kno:w that there is a tumor there. They
 3              nee:dle biopsied the adrenal gla::nd.=
 4      Son:   = O:°[kay.°]
 5   → Dad:         [I gue]ss °that's what I should say° .hhh and tha:t
 6              one came back testing positive.
 7      Son:   Mm:k(h)a:y.
 8   → Dad:   pthh They di:d u:hh double needle biopsy of the (0.2)
 9   →         lu:ng. .hh That one they do no:t have the results on.
10              (0.6)
11      Son:   °Je:[sus.°]
```

Dad's three references to "They/they" all preface technical activities either performed by anonymous medical staff (lines 2 & 8) or awaiting results from a needle biopsy (line 9). Each reference also occurs in the midst of continued uncertainty and ambiguity. Dad's recognizes that he may not be "saying it right" (line 1), and with "I don't kno:w" (line 2) next claims insufficient knowledge about the tumor (see Beach & Metzger, 1997; Metzger & Beach, 1996). Subsequently, it is reported that "they" do not yet have results about the lung (line 9).

As with Excerpt 1 (above), across these three "they" references in Excerpt 2 there is no attempt by either speaker to treat referring as the primary activity being addressed. Rather, other and different focal activities are being achieved. As speaker, dad acknowledges the possible incorrectness of his prior announcement about the "adrenal gla::nd" (lines 1-6), then proceeds to announce new news about the "lu:ng" (lines 8-9). In so doing, prior to announcing a technical term ("double needle biopsy" in line 8), dad once again hesitates and searches with "di:d u:hh". In response, as initially observed in Chapter 3, it is while dad repeatedly attempts to provide a more detailed and accurate update that son's voice breaks while uttering "Mm:k(h)a:y.". This is followed by quietly offering a hearably emotional, even sorrowful assessment via "°Je:[sus.°]". In these ways, son progressively displays increasing and affective recognition of the unequivocally bad nature of the news he is assimilating. This news has been constructed in an environment of anonymous references to medical staff, attempts to report technical details, uncertain and ambiguous descriptions of the circumstances they are facing.

It is these types of conversational activities—dad's acknowledging incorrectness, searching for and announcing biomedical terminology, and in response, son's displaying audibly emotional responses as assimilations of bad news—that repeated references to "they" are encapsulated within. It is not that dad's references to "They/they" are inconsequential. These references allow speakers to frame activities and events as conducted by anonymous though official medical staff. The exact identities and capacities of these persons are left unarticulated. Whether dad even knew who these persons were, and/or their job titles/descriptions, is a matter of speculation. Attempts to clarify such details, however, were passed by in favor of the central work dad focused on: updating son about mom's condition.

Referring to "the Doctor": An Authoritative Yet Anonymous Reporting

Immediately following Excerpts 1 & 2 (above), the reference term "doctor" appears for the first time in the phone call corpus:

3) SDCL: Malignancy #1: 2-3

```
 1  Son:   °Je:[sus.°]
 2 → Dad:      [pt .h]h So: the doctor was in there tonight about (.)
 3             sevenish. .hhhh And he said ba:sically that >ya know< ye:s
 4             she has a malignant tu:m- um she has a mali:gnancy <i:n the:
 5             adrenal gland.> = He said .hhhh (0.2) basically the adre:nal
 6             gla:nd <does not become ca:ncerous> in and of itself. = It
 7             comes from some place else. = °So he said.° .hhh
 8             [ Mo:st likely the  lu:ng     ] =
 9  Son:   [°So it's an assumption then.° ]
10  Dad:   = is also malignant.= That's where it sta:rted.
11  Son:   (°Wo[ w) o]kay.° =
```

On line 2, dad summarizes by making reference to "the doctor". He excludes a specific name, proceeding instead to report being "in there tonight". Apparently, doctor was engaged in what is typically understood to be conducting rounds: checking in on patients and their condition, discussing circumstances with family members, and conferring with other medical staff about diagnosis and treatment.

In line 2, dad summarizes the doctor's schedule and then begins to report what "he said ba:sically", an instruction for son to hear that dad's reporting is neither exact nor complete. A number of features comprising dad's reporting are noticeable and significant:

- Beginning with a confirming "ye:s" on line 3, dad reports versions of doctor's speaking in progress. The doctor is portrayed as responding to a prior question, or in some other manner extending an ongoing discussion.
- Dad's voice exudes a "business as usual" authoritative tone and manner throughout his reporting. With "he said", dad repeatedly (lines 3, 5, 7) attributes his information as originating from the doctor.
- In line 4 he repairs "malignant tu:m-", thereby avoiding stating "tumor". This repair appears to be an upshot of a clarification addressed only moments before: As examined in Chapter 3, when son questioned whether there was a tumor in the adrenal gland, dad stated he didn't know for sure but that the gland had been "nee:dle biopsied".
- Emerging from dad's repair was his version of "she has a mali:gnancy <i:n the: adrenal gland.>", an attempt to describe what a needle biopsy might reveal. It is with a slowed (< >), staccato-sounding voice, that dad reenacts how the doctor treated "the: adrenal gland" with emphasis—a voice designed to underscore the importance of making clear that the adrenal gland "<does not become ca:ncerous> in and of itself.". Both the rate and delivery of dad's speaking are marked instances of an authoritative tone and manner.
- On line 8, as dad continues by reporting that "= It comes from some place else. = °So he said.°", it is (to this point) left for the son to provide an upshot of his understanding, which he does with "°So it's an assumption then.°" (line 9). In this way son reflectively and hopefully treats dad's reported findings as speculative, thus less serious.
- Yet in overlap, dad's "[Mo:st likely the lu:ng] = is also malignant.= That's where it sta:rted." (line 10)—though it still leaves implicit any explanation or proposal that "lung cancer" may be the root of mom's illness—essentially contradicts son's speculation.
- And finally, with "(°Wo[w) o]kay.°" (line 11) son quietly affirms what dad's elaboration did not make explicit. It is with surprised resignation that son displays his recognition that any cancer starting in the lung is serious: It has already spread, a fact that son's response treats knowingly as foreboding danger.

The details noted above, from the first reporting by dad of what the doctor "said", highlight the following three features: (a) Although dad's report is drawn from more extended discussions with "the doctor" expert earlier that day, his talk is also sensitive to moments occurring with son just prior to this report (i.e., "malignant tu:m-" in line 4); (b) Though the doctor remains unnamed, repeated and progressive efforts are made by dad to take an official, authoritative position by informing son of what "the doctor" stated. Yet dad refrains from stating directly that mom has "lung cancer", or the seriousness of such a diagnosis; (c) Consequently, son provides his own interpretation in line 9, a somewhat hopeful but fleeting assessment that is immediately overridden by son's knowing "(°Wo[w) o]kay.°" in line 11.

As Drew (1984) has noted, reportings are curious in that they "are cautious ways of proceeding" (p. 147). Analysis of diverse speakers, topics, and circumstances have revealed that speakers avoid (or at least minimize) rejection by portraying an "official position" designed to objectify and provide reasonable versions of circumstances. Speakers may also withhold stating direct proposals or in other ways avoid stating facts in ways that might lead to rejection (or overreactions). It is left for recipients, then, to discern just what the significance or upshots might be for their future plans and lives in general (e.g., see Schegloff, 1988).

As evident in Excerpt 3 (above), the actions by dad and son are essentially aligned with Drew's (1984) observations. There is a strong resemblance between his findings and the "official position" that dad has constructed in the prior excerpts. The objective rationale dad has provided is a resourceful practice for reporting on mom's circumstances. And by not stating directly the upshot of mom's condition, dad leaves it for son to realize the seriousness of her diagnosis.

Cautious Reportings: The Dialectics of Authority vs. Uncertainty

With the present interactions, attention is drawn to how family members, as unofficial medical experts, report on and make sense of a doctor's informed insights about a loved one's condition. It is noteworthy that "the doctor" is portrayed by dad as definitive, an authority that remains unchallenged throughout Excerpt 3 (above). Yet the doctor is not omnipotent. Dad does report that the doctor stated ""[Mo:st likely the lu:ng] = is also malignant.= That's where it sta:rted." (line 10)". Thus the doctor is also awaiting further test results, and without this information is characterized as not willing (and/or able) to move from "probability to fact".

These rather peculiar and seemingly dichotomous positions—authoritative versus unknowing—continue to be interwoven as the conversation from Excerpt 3 gets extended. In Excerpt 4 (below), 11 subsequent usages of "They/they" are apparent in dad's utterances. Following dad's more explicit summary on line 2 (above), his reporting shifts from the perspective of what the "doctor/he said" to how "they" not only lack knowledge, but are uncertain about ongoing treatment (lines 3-4):

4) SDCL: Malignancy #1: 3-4

```
  1     Dad:        [pt .hh]
  2     Dad:        = And so it has go:ne from the lung to the adrenal gland. .hhhh
  3 →               No:w they do <no:t know what ki::nd? They do no:t know
  4 →               what they will do: as a course of treatment.> .hhh u:m I did
  5                 a::sk I said you know in ca:ses like this I said wou- (0.2)
  6 →               would you know would the:y ex:pect to do su:rgery on this.
  7                 = And °he said° .hh no. (.) pt [Fo::r several reasons.]
  8     Son:                                       [(Is this) for chemoth]er:apy? a:nd =
  9 → Dad:          = .hh Ye:ah they would- he said, they would choose to do (.) .hh
 10                 radiation and chemotherapy.
 11                 (0.4)
 12     Son:        [°O]kay.°
 13     Dad:        [ pt]  And in- .hh uh:m (.) ta:lkin' to him he said you know
 14 →               if it's in more than one place they normally <do:n't try:> and
 15                 do anything surgically. = And in talkin' to .hh Ja:n la:ter and
 16                 in (.) several other discussions about, >you know< ho:w
 17                 they treat this, .hhh uhm °pt° sur:gery is a la:st option
```

```
18                because it's °.hh° it's des:tructive to the bo:dy and hard to
19                recover from. .hhh A:nd also it tends to spre::ad:, more than
20                (0.4) giving you the option of remo:ving it.
21 →              [ .hh ] So: they can't do be:tter, =
22      Son:      [°Mm:°]
23      Dad:      = .hhh with- with ve:ry specific, °.hh° a:iming or however the
24 →    heck they do: the- (.) the radiation stuff. =
25      Son:      = [°O:kay.°]
26      Dad:      = [ °.hh° A:]nd- and then give her the che:motherapy.
27      Son:          °Hm[m:]°
28 →    Dad:            [pt ] .hh So:, (.) the pla::n from here is <they will do::,
29                (.) a bo:ne sca:n tomorrow.> .hhh A:nd from what I understand
30                she will just get a:: sho:t, which should be no big deal. pt .hh
31 →              And a couple glasses of stuff to drink. .hhh And then they
32                will take her do:wn, .hh and do the <bo:ne> sca:n. >I: don't
33                know whether< that's done by x:ray or (.) cat scan. But in
34                either case, .hh <that's not inva:sive> like some of the rest
35                of this stuff. >So that shouldn't hurt her.<
36                .hhh [ h h h h h h     ]
37      Son:           [How did she fa:re] through these pr[ocesses].
```

This shift involves an inclusive and anonymous "they", representing groups of individuals working as a medical team to diagnose and determine treatment options. Clearly, doctors do not work alone in search of healing outcomes for cancer patients, a fact acknowledged through dad's repeated "they" references and an indirect reference to interacting with a doctor.

First (lines 4-7), dad shifts back from "they" by reporting his asking of a question to a doctor—a query marked by dysfluency (e.g., word repeats, cut-offs, pauses). In line 5, dad states "I said you know in ca:ses like this I said wou- (0.2) would you know would **the:y** ex:pect to so su:rgery on this.". One regular environment where patients have been shown to be dysfluent, for example, is when asking questions, making requests, and/or reporting events to doctors (Beach & Mandelbaum, 2005; Beach et al., 2004; Gill, 1998; Gill, Halkowski, & Roberts, 2001; Jones & Beach, 2005; Stivers & Heritage, 2001). One explanation for these dysfluencies, reflected in speech and action, is that patients treat particular topics as *delicate* matters. A related explanation is that patients routinely defer to medical authority, especially (but not exclusively) when asking questions or otherwise taking positions they may not be knowledgeable about, and/or that could be regarded by doctors as challenging their expertise. In the case of dad's reconstruction of a question to the doctor in lines 4-7 (above), the matter at hand (i.e., surgical options) is understandably a delicate topic, just as dad's query positions himself as not being knowledgeable on courses of treatment (thus deferring to the doctor's medical authority).

Second, in the midst of dad's reconstructed question to the doctor it becomes clear, with a generic "**the:y**" (line 6), that dad recognizes the doctor may be informed about but not necessarily an expert in, nor primary decision maker about, surgical options.

Third, immediately following dad's query, doctor's initial response is reported as "= And °he said° .hh no." (line 7). Dad's version of doctor's "no." is hearably direct, definitive, and uttered without hesitation—a capsulized version of reported authority-in-action.

Fourth, as dad next continues to report the doctor's "(.) pt [Fo::r several reasons.]", it is in overlap that son once again provides the reasons for why surgery might not be considered (line 8): "[(Is this for chemoth]er:apy a:nd =". And it is only then that dad states what had previously been implied, namely, "= .hh Ye:ah **they** would- he said, **they** would choose to do (.) .hh radiation and chemotherapy." lines 9-10).

Fifth, in so doing, dad again attributes to the doctor ("he said") the use of the terms **"they/they"**, suggesting that the doctor himself reported that s/he is working with a team of variously skilled medical experts in caring for mom. These generic references continue throughout Excerpt 3 (above, lines 14, 21, 24, 28, 31). As dad continues reporting what the doctor said in lines 13-15, another reference to **"they"** confirms that this doctor works with others who contribute in making decisions and implementing treatment options. Further information about why surgery is not a viable option was apparently gleaned from talking with "Ja:n" (a family friend, line 15), which dad also reports to son. What follows is a series of four additional **"they"** (lines 21-31) references, all involving anonymous medical staff involved in administering radiation, chemotherapy, and a bone scan.

Finally, from Excerpt 4 (above) a distinction can be made between information obtained from others and reported by dad (e.g., about surgery, radiation and chemotherapy, and a bone scan), and dad's own sense and understanding of those procedures. In these instances, dad comes off as more knowledgeable when reporting what others have told him.

In marked contrast, the following moments reveal the limitations of dad's own *lay* understandings as dad attempts to summarize ("So") the implications of his prior reportings. In Excerpt 5, with dad's "however the heck **they** do: the- (.) the radiation stuff. =", he exhibits an inability to fully grasp technical details (e.g., "a:iming") with decidedly lay terms such as "heck and stuff":

5) SDCL: Malignancy #1:3

```
    21     Dad:  [  .hh  ] So: they can't do be:tter, =
    22     Son:  [°Mm:° ]
    23  →  Dad:  = .hhh with- with ve:ry specific, °.hh° a:iming or however
    24  →        the heck they do: the- (.) the radiation stuff. =
```

And in Excerpt 6, dad vacillates between what he does and does not know. When describing plans for a bone scan, dad's "A:nd from what I understand" frames his report as incomplete: The shot she will get (line 30), which "should be no big deal.", and the liquids she will drink ("stuff", line 31), reflect uncertainty:

6) SDCL: Malignancy #1:4

```
    28     Dad:     [pt ] .hh So:, (.) the pla::n from here is <they will do::, (.)
    29  →           a bo:ne sca:n tomorrow.> .hhh A:nd from what I understand
    30  →           she will just get a:: sho:t, which should be no big deal.
    31           And a couple glasses of stuff to drink. .hhh And then they
    32  →           will take her do:wn, .hh and do the <bo:ne> sca:n. >I: don't
    33  →           know whether< that's done by x:ray or (.) cat scan. But in
    34           either case, .hh <that's not inva:sive> like some of the rest
    35  →           of this stuff. >So that shouldn't hurt her.< .hhh [ h h h h h h  ]
```

With ">I: don't know whether< that's done by x:ray or (.) cat scan." (lines 31-32), dad specifically claims insufficient knowledge (see Beach & Metzger, 1997). This gives way to what he does know ("<that's not inva:sive>", line 34) which, through slowed staccato delivery and emphasis, is audibly and visibly another instance of a direct reporting. Though excerpted from a longer conversation dad had with the doctor, "<that's not inva:sive>" is stated authoritatively. But in the next moments, dad's "stuff" and "shouldn't" once again reveal the inherent ambiguity embedded in dad's own reportings. These juxtaposed instances further confirm how, as noted above, dad's portrayal of more knowledgeable positions are rooted in reenacting what he heard from others (e.g., the doctor). These reported actions stand in marked contrast with the doubt and uncertainty arising from dad's lay inability to fully understand procedures, treatments, and events. Analysis is now extended to a collection of excerpts revealing additional and diverse features evident across routine reportings about "doctors".

THE SHAPE OF ROUTINE "DOCTOR" REPORTINGS

There are numerous additional instances in which "doctors" are routinely reported on by family members. Below, three more specific and distinct types of involvements are examined: (a) reporting on routine matters (e.g., processing papers/requests, scheduling, location, and prescribing medications), (b) reporting about talking with doctors (and medical staff) as experts on procedures and treatment (similar to Excerpt 4, above), (c) reporting on doctors as resources for hope.

Reporting on Routine Yet Critically Important Matters

On numerous occasions family members either involve doctors in, and/or report about, their doctors' involvement in care. These matters often address what family members treat as critical issues: life support, prognosis, how a doctor's scheduled visit and assessment of mom's condition impacts travel plans, how a doctor's location impacts family driving time and quality of care provided, and how providing routine medications can be problematic for family members.

Decisions and Actions Regarding Life Support

In the following excerpt, mom informs son that she has provided two different doctors with her written intention to not be placed on "life support". This is the first set of moments where doctors are referenced by name:

7) SDCL: Malignancy #3:1

```
   1      Son:   Life support or not huh::? =
   2      Mom:   = Now I have up until this point?
   3      Son:   Hmm huh .hhh
   4      Mom:   Said none I mean I have done it in my will.
   5             ( 1.0 )
   6  →   Mom:   I have given that ah paper to Doctor (name 1)?
   7             ( 1.0 )
   8  →   Mom:   Given one to Doctor (name 2)?
   9             ( 1.0 )
  10      Mom:   And it has been my issue all along. I don't want to be
  11             put on life support? >My mother was and I didn't like
  12             it.< =
  13      Son:   = Hmm huh.
```

In lines 6 & 8, though mom mentions the names of both doctors, son does not provide responses. Nor does mom treat his lack of uptake as noticeably absent or otherwise troubling. Why might this be the case? Simply because it does not appear that mom references two doctors and their names to evoke or confirm their identification by son. Nor is she soliciting son's opinion or advice about a decision already enacted. Rather, as discussed in Chapter 4, it is mom's claimed right to make choices about her own life support, enacted here as she simply appears to be informing son of the actions she has taken: "I ha_ve_ done _it_ in my U" (line 4), and has provided "that ah paper" (lines 6-8) to two doctors. With "ah" mom evidences a slight search, but one that does not yield the specific name of the document. (This practice is similar to dad's, noted previously, as he searches prior to stating technical/biomedical terminology or procedures.) Further identification of either or both doctors is therefore treated as less relevant than the fact that two medical authorities, apparently selected by mom (which is sufficient on its own merits), were officially informed. And by referencing not only two doctors, but their names, mom announces that the position she has taken toward life support is indeed official. The interactional work she is performing thus involves not only informing son of the stance she has taken, but legitimating the finality of her position through written notification of two medical authorities. This is sound reasoning: without the doctors' receipt and subsequent distribution of mom's wishes to medical staff, these important documents would likely not be attended to at times of critical decision making.[3]

During these moments between a mom and her son, these serious matters literally involve details about how life and death will be managed. Referring to doctors is a critical part of these discussions. Though mentioned by name, it is apparent that these two doctors are constructed as institutionally relevant only insofar as they are officially informed parties, authoritatively capable of (and accountably held responsible for) ensuring that mom's wishes be carried into practice. By reporting to son the decisions and actions she has taken regarding life support, mom treats son as a consequential family member entitled to know about, and if necessary act upon and enforce, what mom has put forth as being in her best interests. Though such actions and enforcement are not explicitly stated, they are implied through mom's informing son about her preferences.

Impacts of Prognosis on Son's Travel Plans

In Excerpt 8 (below), occurring following calls #4-9 to the airlines (see Chapter 5), son had just summarized to aunt (a flight attendant) that the information she had provided about "compassion fares" was inaccurate. He then transitions to summarizing his travel itinerary to visit mom. His plans, however, are tied to what the doctor might say not only about mom's condition, but how long she might have to live:

8) SDCL: Malignancy #10:6

1	Son:	[.hhh] Yeah I- I called about six places .hhh and hh th- the
2		details would be u:h I would leave <u>here</u> two twenty my
3		time go through Phoenix end up there five thirty your <u>t</u>ime.
4	Aunt:	Uh hmm Okay. (.) Alright um by- I would- (.) the <u>way</u>
5 →		< normally > things work with **Doctor** (name) is she makes
6		rounds in the morning.
7	Son:	Um hmm. Yeah that's what dad said.=
8	Aunt:	=And we should have <u>s:</u>ome clue (.) < <u>if this is</u> > (.) an- and
9		ya know there is the <u>ch</u>ance now I don't know what (.) how
10		well of a chance it is. =
11	Son:	= Um hum.
12	Aunt:	But there is the chance that this is a (.) matter of <u>putting</u> her
13		back on decadro<u>:n</u> (.) giving her morphine <u>pi:</u>lls.
14	Son:	[Um hmm.]
15 →	Aunt:	[> Blah] blah blah blah blah, < (.) And we've got (0.8)
16		more time. (.) What kind of time. > I don't know. < I don't
17		know what kind of time. At this point I would say it's not a
18		<u>hell</u> of a lot. =

Recognizing that son's travel plans are dependent upon doctor's assessment of mom's health status (see Chapters 5 & 6), in lines 4-6 aunt reports that "Doctor (name)" normally makes "rounds in the morning." (line 6). Her reference to the doctor by name displays her familiarity, but also (though not necessarily) that this doctor is also known by son. By claiming this ability to cite the doctor by name, aunt situates herself as an involved family member knowledgeable about both the doctor and schedule. In response, however, son informs aunt that he had already been updated by dad. In this way son does not invalidate, but rather minimizes the impact aunt's informing might have.

This is yet another instance of *social epistemics*, in which laying out the territory of personal knowledge (related here to the business of family travel and illness) is shown to be anchored in "who knows what" about ongoing circumstances. In this family, in which son is calling long distance and aunt is actually in the town where mom and dad reside, each speaker makes available to the other that they are centrally involved in mom's care and illness—each having resources for getting and staying updated about her condition. It is these and related interactional preoccupation, with travel itineraries and exhibiting being informed about the doctor's schedule, that make further identification of the already named and referenced doctor (line 5) less relevant here and now. Reference to the nonpresent doctor accompanies but does not dictate the concerns or topics addressed, namely: Who knows more about the doctor's schedule, is thus in a better position to assess impacts on son's travel and, consequently, is more centrally involved in the family business of dealing with predicaments occasioned by mom's illness? How these and related matters get interactionally organized further reveal the social epistemics of family relationships.

When aunt continues in line 8, she makes inclusive reference to "we" having some information to rely on that may be helpful for finalizing son's travel plans. As her utterance unfolds, distinctions between "we", "doctor", and "I" are apparent. She exhibits difficulty shifting from what "we" might know about schedules and travel plans, to actually describing treatment procedures (known by doctors). Evident in her searching, pausing, and cutting off a word on line 8, followed by an "I don't know" qualification in line 9, she demonstrates being incapable of describing just how a doctor might prescribe medications for mom's condition. Once again, a speaker comes off as more capable of reporting on what she has heard or observed (i.e., about the doctor's rounds in the morning) than on talking about specific, biomedical details. In this case, aunt is trying to providing some insight about the use of prescriptions she knows little about: "the chance...a chance" of "putting her back on decadro:n (.) giving her morphine pi:lls." (lines 12-13).

Rather than continue to describe these chances or medications, however, aunt immediately and quickly states "> Blah blah blah blah blah, <" (line 15). But how are these repeated "blahs" being employed, specifically, why these here?

Consider, first, the following contrasting instance: An advertisement for Chevy Trailblazers that appeared on the rear cover of *Time* magazine (July 15, 2002). A photo included the front seat interior, including instrumentation, of their new SUV. The attending caption was as follows:

> Bigger, wider, more luxurious.
> All of the blah, blah, blah.
> None of the blah.

Through these "blahs", advertisers attempted to illustrate that their new SUV does not deserve to be advertised in the typical fashion. As a result, "None of the blah" denotes a vehicle worthy of something different—an out of the ordinary experience that is *not* routine, boring, or subject to overused descriptions.

Aunt's description is similar. Her actions stand in marked contrast to providing more information about mom's medical circumstances. She exhibits a refusal to attempt offering further descriptions of medications, not only because she does not fully understand them, but also by treating further details about technical matters as trivial and insignificant when considering what is at stake: an uncertain and potentially terminal prognosis, about mom's chances to live or die in the near future and beyond (see also Excerpt 21, below). It is these concerns that aunt addresses next by focusing on "What kind of time." (line 16) mom might have. She raises these serious issues doubtfully, twice repeating "I don't know" before offering her opinion: "At this point I would say it's not a hell of a lot.=" (lines 17-18). The term "hell" is used by aunt to depict that mom might not have long to live, associating such a probability not with "heaven" but its more dreaded counterpart. These are the bottom-line concerns aunt moves away from "blah" to address. Matters of prognosis are much more important for mom and family members, especially when contrasted with further and routine reportings of medical staffs' treatment/medication procedures—only short-term solutions to long-term (potentially terminal) problems.

During son's very next phone call #11, in line 1 Gina requests a news update. She queries about a call "they" made, which is subsequently described by son (lines 4-12). At the outset of his elaboration, son confirms that he did receive a call (from his aunt in Excerpt 8, above, though this is unstated). He then immediately references a "doctor" visiting mom this morning (line 4):

9) SDCL: Malignancy #11:2-3

1	Gina:	( ) Did they call you last night?
2	Son:	Yeah.
3		(1.5)
4 →	Son:	Yeah. We::- uhm- (.) an' pt she's gotta- .hhh a **doctor**
5		who's gonna see her this morning, but (.) you know (.) the
6		ti:me difference an everything. .hhh uhm pt Th- they won't
7		(.) kno::w anything for a little whi:le yet. So it's kinda
8		puts me in an awkward spot ↑here. 'Cuz ge:ez I >ya know<
9		pt .hh I got everything arranged to go::, and .hh >ya know<
10		got somebody to pick up the ma:il, and got somebody to
11		take my classes and all that. And if I end up sta:ying
12		I'll (0.2) f- feel a little weir:d. But- .hhh uhm =

As son continues he makes clear that the doctor's identity is, once again, subordinate to the more pressing matter: that the family ("they" in line 6) is awaiting information from the doctor, and until that occurs, there is little or no news to report about mom's changing condition and, thus, son's travel plans. The families' reliance on the doctor's visit, as an expert providing an assessment the family needs to assess mom's wellness, is treated by son as important yet altogether routine. It is taken for granted by son that Gina knows that the family cannot evaluate mom's condition without assistance from a medical expert. The family is therefore dependent not only on another's knowledgeable opinion, but also the doctor's scheduling.

Given "the ti:me difference an everything." (lines 5-6) that son mentions, this dependence is not inconsequential. In lines 7-13, son elaborates by describing that since he has "everything arranged to go::" he'll "f- feel a little weir:d." if he stays. This dilemma (addressed in considerably more detail in Chapters 5 & 6)—of being on the cusp of traveling home, but awaiting information arising from a doctor's scheduled visit—reveals a stark contrast between doctors and family members. For the doctor, a scheduled visit with a patient is routine, likely one in a series for any given period of time on any given day. Even though the doctor may be aware that the outcome of the visit is consequential for others' plans (travel and otherwise), and is concerned about their lives, s/he can only inform the family and offer advice. It is up to the family to make decisions, to directly experience and manage the dilemmas brought on by such circumstances.

For son in Excerpt 9 (above), this quandary is capsulized with "'Cuz ge:ez" in line 8. Here "ge:ez" is a derivative of "Jesus" and thus invoking the deity: Son is embroiled in yet another troubling predicament he obviously seeks remedy for, yet he does not control the doctor's medical evaluation and scheduling. Any emerging solution arises only as an outcome of "a **doctor** who's gonna see her <u>this</u> <u>morning</u>," (lines 4-5), and it is the outcome of the doctor's visit and assessment that is consequential, not who the doctor is per se. Son's otherwise benign reference to the doctor is potentially of monumental importance to mom's life and, though less vital, son's decision to travel home before his mother's death or, despite his considerable efforts, stay where he is (which as Chapter 6 reveals, is what eventually occurs).

Hospital Location and Quality of Care

The reporting below focuses on which hospital mom is being treated in, and the importance of their doctor's location to that hospital. When son queries "Is it a <u>cancer</u> hospital." (line 6), he is informed by dad that it is not, but that their doctor is "<u>right</u> across the street" (line 10). The first four references to "Doctor + (name)", in lines 8-17, focus on a specific doctor's affiliation with a hospital and its location:

10) SDCL: Malignancy #25:8-9

1	Dad:	↑Yeah. And it's a (.) real <u>nice</u> little hospital? It's not a big
2		(1.2) mausoleum like (.) (<u>name</u> of hospital) is. = > Over here it's
3		a < o:ne sto:rry spread arou:nd little thing like (city)
4		Tennessee was.
5	Son:	Um hm. (.) Is it a <u>cancer</u> hospital.
6	Dad:	No (.) not necessarily. =
7	Son:	= Oh okay. <u>How</u> come she's in that one is that just the one
8 →		**Doctor** (name) works out of or [some:thing.]
9 →	Dad:	[Yep.] **Doctor** (name)
10		<u>right</u> across the street
11	Son:	Oh okay. (.) Well that's handy.
12 →	Dad:	She works- (.) **Doctor** (name) works out of <u>either</u> of the (name)
13		hospitals. uh (.) This one or the one tha:t's i:n (city).
14	Son:	<u>Huh.</u> =
15	Dad:	= [But th]a:t's a tougher one for us to get to. =
16	Son:	[Okay.]
17 →	Dad:	= >And as I said **Doctor** (name) office< is right <u>smack</u> across
18		the street. You could <u>walk</u> over and you know it's five
19		hundred feet away.
20	Son:	<u>Okay</u>. (.) Well that works huh.
21	Dad:	°Yeah.° (name of hospital) was such a colossal (.) bitch the last
22		time she was in it because she couldn't get (.) people to take
23		care of [ya and] =
24	Son:	[Uhmhm.]
25 →	Dad:	= °a whole bunch of other stuff.° >We couldn't< and **Doctor**
26		(name) said ya know ya- you you're welcome to <u>go</u> to (<u>name</u>
27		of hospital) but I'll have to work with the local oncologist there
28		and I'll just do it by <u>pho:ne</u> and °I: don't want to get into that.° =
29	Son:	= Uhmhm::::, (.) not at this stage in the game

```
30                 [that doesn't-]
31    Dad:    [   No::::   ] she likes the doctor the doctor does good
32             things       for he:r that she can't.
33             (The hell with it [ya know.]) =
34    Son:                     [  Yeah.  ]
35    Dad:    = we'll drive so she can be comfortable.
36    Son:    °Okay.°
```

The last hospital mom was treated in is described as a "colossal (.) bitch" (line 21): It was too big (lines 1-2), offered poor care (lines 21-22), and "= °A whole bunch of other stuff.°" (line 25). Next, dad reported (with some dysfluency, i.e., "ya know ya- you you're welcome", line 26) that the doctor stated the family is welcome to work with another hospital. Yet a preference is stated to avoid working with an "oncologist" by phone, an arrangement that neither son nor dad would like. Following son's agreement and alignment with doctor's position (lines 29-30), dad aligns further by upgrading with "the doctor the doctor does good things for he:r that she can't." (lines 31-32)—clearly, a positive endorsement and assessment of medical competence (see also the next Chapter 9).

It is not just the location, then, but a particular (named) doctor's offering of quality care that motivates dad to follow doctor's recommendation: "we'll drive so she can be comfortable." (line 35). Once again, a routine reporting—in this case about the location of a doctor and hospital—is rooted in critically important matters: enhancing mom's care and comfort, matters well worth the time and effort to ensure. It is important that through the naming of a doctor, dad and son unequivocally know who is being referred to. More critically, however, this doctor is not only strategically positioned due to location, but also (apparently) skilled in providing personal care. Convenience and comfort are intertwined with—indeed constitute—the identity attributed to this doctor. As Schegloff (1996c) observed, marked outcomes of referring to a nonpresent person invite involvements across "a range of *different other activities*" (p. 449; italics added).

Routine Problems with Administering Medications

A final instance of a routine reporting, about dad's troubling experience administering medication to mom, appears below:

11) **SDCL: Malignancy #36:5**

```
1    Dad:    And then we came home hh and ah (0.2) e:::h she spends a
2             lot of time sleeping or at least dozing partially because of
3             the medication etcetra.
4    Son:    Sure.
5    Dad:    I kinda screwed up the medication on Friday because (.)
6  →          doctor wrote out the whole set of instructions on all the pills
7             that she takes and how often and all that stuff. .hh I don't
8             know I guess in my mind I hadn't thought it through too
9             well but she said yiknow .hh particular pain medicine
10            should be three times a day
11   Son:    Mm [hm.
12   Dad:       [Y'know fine breakfast lunch and supper.
13   Son:    O:h so you didn't have anything to go through the night
14            with.
15   Dad:    Yeah [ (    ) ] =
16   Son:         [Oops.]
17   Dad:    = Took y'know like the best shot at and missed.
```

```
18    Son:    Mm hm.
19    Dad:    Four or five o clock in the morning everything hurt like hell
20            and she's frantic and all that kind of business (.) So I gave
21            her a coupla pain pills and then (.) that calmed her down a
22            little but it still hurt. An' then Saturday morning there was
23            u:h gal who does .hh kind of a visiting nurse but this was an
24            introduction and (.) so forth the hospice stuff.
```

As dad extends his story about being home, and the impacts of mom's medication, he announces that he "screwed up the medication on Friday"—not because doctor's written or verbal instructions about pain pills were wrong, but because dad reports not having "thought it through too well" (lines 5-10). Here again, the doctor's name and identity is less relevant than dad's revealing of the mistake he made: not giving mom sufficient pain medicine. Before dad reveals his oversight as the punchline for his story, son articulates the problem: "O:h so you didn't have anything to go through the night with." (lines 13-14). With "= Took y'know like the best shot at and missed." (line 17), dad confesses that it was indeed his misunderstanding, then proceeds to elaborate what son had assumed: that early in the morning mom was hurting and frantic, and although giving her a "coupla pain pills" helped, mom remained in pain.

Of course, dad did not intentionally fail to provide mom with her evening medication. His was an honest mistake, the likes of which are well known to any individual or family bearing caregiving responsibilities across diverse illnesses—an error skilled professionals, such as hospice staff, are much less likely to make. It is perhaps not coincidental, then, that immediately following dad's confession and elaboration of mom's discomfort, the next triggered topic involved a "visiting nurse" marking the onset of hospice care.

When do References to Doctors Occur?

From the excerpts examined above, it can be seen that when "doctors" have been referenced by family members, such actions are initiated by a speaker (i.e., without being asked a question),

12) SDCL: Malignancy #1: 2

```
1    Son:    °Je:[sus.°]
2  → Dad:       [pt .h]h So: the doctor was in there tonight about (.)
3            sevenish. .hhhh And he said ba:sically ((continues))
```

13) SDCL: Malignancy #10:6

```
1    Son:    [.hhh ] Yeah I- I called about six places .hhh and hh th- the
2            details would be u:h I would leave here two twenty my
3            time go through Phoenix end up there five thirty your time.
4    Aunt:   Uh hmm Okay. (.) Alright um by- I would- (.) the way
5  →         < normally > things work with Doctor (name) is she makes
6            rounds in the morning.
```

produced as responsive to a question that may or may not have been directly pursuing information about doctors,

14) SDCL: Malignancy #3:1

```
1  → Son:    Life support or not huh::? =
2    Mom:    = Now I have up until this point?
3    Son:    Hmm huh .hhh
```

4   Mom: Said none I mean I ha<u>ve</u> done it in my <u>will</u>.
5   (1.0)
6   →   Mom: I have given that ah paper to **Doctor** (name 1)?
7   (1.0)
8   →   Mom: Given one to **Doctor** (name 2)?

15) **SDCL: Malignancy #11:2-3**

1   →   Gayle: (   ) Did they <u>call</u> you <u>last</u> night?
2   Son: Yeah.
3   (1.5)
4   →   Son: Yeah. We::- uhm- (.) an' pt she's gotta- .hhh a **doctor**
5   who's gonna see her <u>this</u> <u>morning</u>, but (.) you know

or, in contrast, as part of a follow-up question seeking clarification—in this instance, about doctor's location:

16) **SDCL: Malignancy #23:8-9**

5   →   Son: Um hm. (.) Is it a <u>cancer</u> hospital.
6   Dad: No (.) not necessarily. =
7   Son: = Oh okay. <u>How</u> come she's in that one is that just the one
8   →   **Doctor** (name) works out of or [some:thing.]
9   → Dad: [Yep.   ] **Doctor** (name)
10   <u>right</u> across the street

This basic pattern is confirmed across additional instances below: Reports of talking with the doctor, including what the doctor "said" (Excerpts 17-19, below), are either initiated during a speaker's elaboration or when responding to others' direct or indirect queries about the doctor (Excerpts 20-22). Each set of moments, examined chronologically (i.e., call #'s 12→16→25→36→38) reveal yet additional insights about how family members cumulatively portray involvement of doctors and medical staff throughout cancer care.

Reports About Talking with the Doctor

Excerpt 17 (below) occurs following a defining moment when dad informed son that, despite their preparations, he needn't travel home because mom's condition had stabilized (examined in Excerpt 2, Chapter 6). As dad shifts from updating son about mom's improvement (lines 3-6), to reporting that he had "talked to the doctor." (lines 6-7), the topic immediately shifts to technical matters and anonymous medical staff (lines 7-13):

17) **SDCL: Malignancy #12:1**

((Immediately following dad informing son to "Stay there."))

1   Dad: >Ya know, the trip was gonna come <u>about</u>.< It's just that ya
2   know (.) i<u>:f</u> ya wanna come this week, this is <u>not</u> gonna be an
3   e:<u>n:d</u> week kinda thing. . hhh <So:::,> (.) your mother's answer
4   was na::h stay there. Ya know she's- she is <u>much</u> <u>better</u> this
5   morning. She °is uh completely <u>lucid</u> or- seems to be° the few
6   →   >minutes I've had to <u>talk</u> to her 'cause I talked to <u>her</u> talked to
7   →   the **doctor**.< (.) .hhh uh- The <u>tumors</u> in her <u>legs</u> **they're** gonna
8   →   xra::y and scan or whatever tom<u>mor</u>row they're gonna scan
9   →   the <u>hip</u> to see why <u>that</u> hurts. **They're** changing around uh

```
10            (0.4) the thyroid stuff 'cause she's cranked up too high. (.)
11 →          .hhh They had her on u::h (0.4) morphine all night on uh ya
12            know one uh these drip system >whatever the hell.< S:o <that
13            calmed down> some of this. So she got outta >bed on her
14            own< this morning. = She went to the bathroom so- .hhh
15    Son:    Mmm hm. 'Kay. =
```

From dad's reporting, the doctor depicted how a variety of potential problems are going to be addressed with a team of professionals. Each listing of a bodily description—"tumors in her legs", "hip", "thyroid"—are to be treated by anonymous medical staff ("they're/they") with a variety of procedures (e.g., "xra::y", "scan", "changing around"). It was "They" (line 11) that had mom on morphine all night, even though dad's next "S:o <that calmed down> some of this." (lines 12-13) resembles the prosody (i.e., slow staccato rate, emphasis) of enacting doctor's authoritative voice. In this way, dad's reporting reflects a seamless shift from his summary of doctor's depictions of the actions of a medical team, to reported speech of actual language the doctor employed to characterize a reduction in pain.

Throughout dad's extended narrative, two prominent and previously identified features are also apparent. These actions further demonstrate dad's lay orientation to increasingly familiar, yet continually foreign, medical protocol. First, when describing each technical procedure, dad again searches (with stretching of the voice, as with "xra::y" in line 8), including the use of filled and actual pauses as with "uh (0.4) the thyroid stuff" (line 10) and "u::h (0.4) morphine" (line 11). These searches and hesitations exhibit routine difficulties describing what dad does not have the technical expertise to assess: resources doctor and medical staff will use for the pursuit, not necessarily of remission for mom's cancer, but reduction of pain. Second, in the midst of describing procedures and treatment options, dad's language (i.e., "whatever" and "stuff") reveals an inability to more accurately depict events. With "xra::y and scan or *whatever*" (line 8), "the thyroid *stuff*" (line 10), and "drip system >*whatever* the hell<" (line 12), dad is dismissive and generic as he exhibits the limits of his own stock of knowledge.

Approximately one minute later in call #12, son seeks more specific information from dad about what the doctor said:

18) SDCL: Malignancy #12:3

```
 1 → Son:   Yeah. hhh .hhh heah .hh So what'd the doctor have to say
 2           specifically anything. =
 3    Dad:   = We:ll. (0.2) Th- the thyroid is too high, the pa:in: is
 4           tremendous and it will just slowly keep accumulating. They
 5           will leave her o:n (0.6) u::h the morphine stuff. But it will be
 6           pill form instead of this drip system and they will just keep
 7           the pain under control.
 8           (1.0)
 9    Son:   Okay. [      .hh hhh hhhh hhh hh ]
10    Dad:          [Uh >ya know< beyond th]at I don't have any more
11           answers at the moment.
```

In responding to son's itemized news inquiry (INI, see Chapter 3), dad both summarizes what he had previously stated (in Excerpt 17, above) and provides additional (new) information: Mom's pain is now characterized as "tremendous" (line 4) and expected to slowly increase, and morphine will be administered in pill form rather than the drip system to control her pain (lines 6-7). His announcement is organized as a three-part list (Jefferson, 1990; Sacks, 1992), replete with extreme-case depictions (e.g., "too high,", "tremendous";

Edwards, 2000; Pomerantz, 1986), and offers little apparent hope for a reduction in mom's discomfort. This second reporting, prompted by son, provides a capsulized and even more serious assessment of mom's pain, which can only be managed rather than eliminated.

The medically proposed solution, to "leave her o:n (0.6) u::h the morphine stuff" (line 5), is once again attributed not to the "doctor" but to "they"—another recognition that it is not doctors who administer morphine to patients, but nurses and related medical staff. Dad's utterance is also delivered as a result of obvious searching ("o:n (0.6) u::h"), marked by stretched vowels and a pause (see Goodwin, 1987), for what and how to characterize "the morphine stuff". Together, dad's searching and generic reference to "stuff" further reveal his *lay* orientation to treatment and medications he possesses limited information about.

There is a marked difference, therefore, in reporting what the doctor has said—an apparent outcome of speaking with the doctor directly—and dad's offering of his own (*lay*) depictions of treatment/drug options managed by anonymous staff. As mom's cancer progresses, family members make specific distinctions between types of morphine pills and "drips". But in Excerpt 18 (above), "stuff" is recruited by dad in a general manner, revealing his inability to further specify details about medication. The source of dad's difficulty is unknown: Did the doctor not mention details about morphine options? Did discussions not occur with staff dispensing the drugs? Is dad tired after a long day and unable to retrieve such technical information? These questions remain. What is evident from these moments is that dad's second reporting of what the doctor had told him was marked with fewer interactional dysfluencies than his searching for information about morphine treatments.

It is this bad news, following a (1.0) pause, that occasions son's resigned and troubled "Okay. + [aspirated sigh]" (line 9). And "beyond that" (line 10), it is significant that dad states *not* that he has nothing more to say, but "I don't have any more answers at the moment." (lines 10-11). By so doing, dad addresses the fact that he treated son's pursuit of more specific information from the doctor as seeking not just an overview, but bottom-line "answers" about mom's condition. As it turns out, these "answers" appear unequivocal and not encouraging. The valence of this news further accounts for how a position could be taken that son's "Okay. + [aspirated sigh]" (line 9) is not underdeveloped, but specifically tailored to dad's prior, ambiguous, and less than heartening news—a response exhibiting both the impact *and* affective significance of dad's prior update.

Reporting on Dad's Report

As examined previously (see Excerpt 2, Chapter 6), within a day but four calls later when speaking with his aunt, son reconstructs being informed by dad to "Stay there.", portrayed here as ">↑don't come yet.<" (line 1):

19) SDCL: Malignancy #16:2

```
 1    Son:   = ↑Yeah. ↓Well (.) he called and he said >↑don't come yet.<
 2           (0.7)
 3    Son:   .hhh          So I've (.) .h[ h  cal-  ]
 4  → Aunt:                              [What'd-] did Doctor (name) ↑say to him (.)
 5           >do ya know?<
 6           (0.6)
 7  → Son:   No not <really.> hh u:m hhh (.) Ya know that they were gonna
 8  →        radiate these tumors in her le:g and that- they were gonna put
 9           'er on ↑pill form morphine (.) .hhh after a while. 'N::n .hhh
10           u::h (0.4) an' that was about it. An' that there no >there
11  →        wasn't quite the immediate danger they thought there was
12           last ni:ght and that's basically,< .hhhh a:ll::.
```

In line 4, aunt's response to son's informing was to inquire about what it was that "**Doctor** (name)" said to "him" (dad). By referring to the doctor's name, aunt displays specific knowledge about *whom* dad must have spoken with as a basis for informing son that he should remain home. She also demonstrates her ability to identify a primary resource for explaining the cancellation of son's trip to come home, and to be with mom and family prior to her (assumably impending) death. Though son begins with "<u>No</u> not really.>" in line 7, he proceeds to provide his own capsulized version of dad's earlier reportings (Excerpts 17 & 18, above).[4] His reporting leaves unstated much of what dad earlier reported. Yet what he highlights are *integrations* of dad's two attempts to describe mom's condition and proposed treatments: "<u>tu</u>mors in her le:g" (line 8) and "↑<u>pill</u> form morphine" (line 9) are drawn, respectively, from dad's first and second reportings. Son then concludes by explicitly stating that there was less "im<u>me</u>diate <u>danger</u>" than the prior evening.

As with dad, son's overview of what the "doctor" said to dad relied heavily on repeated references to "they" (lines 7, 8, & 11): anonymous medical staff conducting the radiation, administering the morphine, and assessing the danger of mom's condition. Again, it is not that the "doctor" is blamed as failing to be involved in these actions and decisions. Rather, son shows recognition that the "doctor" works with a team of professionals, utilizing different but needed expertise to offer responsible cancer care. It is the tasks performed by these individuals that is given priority by son, not their specific identities, and thus their anonymity is not treated as problematic. Instead, through "they" a category of members are invoked whose anonymity releases, for son, the responsibility of needing to provide a more specific sense of social structure. Son therefore eliminates the necessity to articulate a set of local contexts, that is, circumstances within which the disclosure of individual (named) identities would be critical for depicting key aspects of mom's care and prognosis.

Seeking Balance and Sending Mom Home

Nine phone calls and several days later, following a series of *three* stories about dad and son's dogs, son shifts topics with another itemized news inquiry (INI, Excerpt 29, line 1, below) that does not specify concerns about mom. Yet in lines 3-4 dad (a) hears and treats son's query as addressing mom's condition, (b) announces that things are fine and under control, then (c) moves to report what the "<u>doctor</u> did say yesterday":

20) **SDCL: Malignancy #25:9**

```
 1    Son:   So everything else goin al<u>right</u>?
 2    Dad:   Ye:ah, seems to be. hhh u:mm (0.3) Yeah ↓things around here
 3  →        are doin <u>fine</u>. = That's all under control. .hh U:h <u>doctor</u> did say
 4           yesterday (0.5) what she was ↑<u>go:nna</u> try and do was t'get-
 5           get (mom/name) bala:<u>nced</u> out as well as she- she <u>ca:n</u> as far as
 6  →        this (.) she seems to have some kind of <u>infection</u> that **they're**
 7           periodically giving her (0.5) u:h intervenous: (.) antibiotics for.
 8           (1.0) And she said she would keep her <u>through</u> the weekend
 9  →        and then ↑<u>Monday</u> **they** will talk about maybe she can come
10           <u>home</u> for awhile.
11           (2.0)
12    Dad:   Then uh- we::ll I guess she didn't say for a while   I'm assuming
13           for a while, uh Monday or Monday afternoon or <u>Tuesday</u>.=
14    Son:   =Um hm.=
15    Dad:   =If- if she is <u>balanced</u> out as well as (.) can be expected
```

16   o:n the pain medicine to where she does not need any kind of
17   sh:ots.=She's now taking it in a (.) yucky tasting liquid form.
18 →   (1.5) But if (.) ya know if **we** can keep it <u>calmed</u> do:wn with
19 →   that then maybe you know **we** can deal with it here? = So she
20   may be comin home (.) Mon:<u>day</u> afternoon or <u>Tuesday</u>.
21 Son: Okay.

In lines 3-4, dad's sole reference to the doctor in this excerpt, he reports what "U:h **doctor** did say yesterday (0.5) what she was ↑<u>go:nna</u> try and do". Here it is seen that although dad did not reference doctor by name, he did invoke "she" as a pronoun (line 4) and thus provided adequate identification (i.e., as the sole female doctor primarily responsible for mom's care and treatment). In prior excerpts (e.g., 13, 16, 17) references are also made to this particular doctor, either explicitly by name (16) and/or "her/she".

The phrase "<u>balanced</u> out" is employed twice in this excerpt (lines 5 & 15), dad's depiction of how the doctor characterized attempts to address mom's infection and pain medication. Dad is able to specify that mom has "some kind of <u>infection</u> that they're periodically giving her (0.5) u:h intervenous: (.) antibiotics for." (lines 6-7). However, again in lay fashion, the kind of infection is left unstated, and the involvement of anonymous medical staff is described ("they're"). As with numerous prior moments, dad also pauses and searches prior to uttering the technical terminology for treatment.

It is treated as newsworthy that the doctor will "keep her" (line 9) for a few more days, and then allow mom to come "<u>home</u> for awhile" (line 10). This is apparent good news, embedded within an otherwise uncertain illness trajectory. Since "awhile" is not permanent, a need to return to the hospital when mom's condition worsens is implied. Until that time, the treatment goal is to get mom sufficiently stabilized to return home. As with "<u>bal-anced</u> out as well as (.) can be expected o:n the pain medicine" (line 15), it is clear that no perfect solution exists for controlling mom's pain. If "shots" can be avoided, and medication can be taken in liquid form (even though it is "yucky tasting", line 17), her move home can be facilitated.

Dad's language accommodates this transition from the hospital to home. Yet another contrast between "we" and "they" is deployed, but here indexing the location where mom's care will be provided (i.e., the hospital or home). He switches from "they/they're" (i.e., medical staff) to "we can keep it <u>calmed</u> do:wn" and "we can deal with it here?" (lines 18-19). It is unclear just who "we" refers to, but as with medical teams in the hospital, caregiving will apparently not be done by dad alone. It is plausible, of course, that a plan had been developed for caring for mom upon her return home. And if so, it is also likely that such a plan would not involve dad, who had a full-time job, as the only caregiver.

In Excerpt 17 (lines 12-13) dad previously stated "S:o <<u>that calmed down</u>> some of this.", an apparent reconstruction of the doctor's authoritative description that, by means of a morphine drip system, a treatment goal had been achieved. Here, in Excerpt 20 (lines 18-19), dad again makes reference to "<u>calmed</u> do:wn", emphasizing an ongoing priority that will be carried over from the hospital to managing home care. Clearly, regardless of the setting and providers, caring for mom remains a constant preoccupation and concern. And dad has evidently adapted the doctor's language, as primary caregiver in the hospital, to his speculation: If the pain medicine (implying morphine, but now in a "yucky tasting liquid form" in line 17) continues to "keep it <u>calmed</u> do:wn", "we can deal with it here" (line 19). The "it" in line 19 appears to index the ability to manage mom's pain sufficiently to keep her home. Of course, in-home medical experts will remain involved in providing instruction about how the morphine will be administered. Other tasks can be performed by family members, but only if the morphine is in liquid rather than drip form (which requires insertion of a needle).

Hospice Involvement: Ensuring Mom's Comfort at Home

That mom did in fact return home is evident in Excerpt 21 (below), a call occurring several days following call #25 (Excerpt 20, above). Following an extended phone opening discussing a variety of matters about son's life (e.g., problems with his phone recorder, equipment and activities at work), and a sensitive discussion about how tough it is for mom to be home,[5] in line 1 dad again reports what the "**Doctor** said":

21) SDCL: Malignancy #39:4-5

```
 1  →  Dad:   Doctor said you know take her home (.) handle her with
 2                hospice and she can be ther:e and know she probably like
 3                the surroundings better etcetra and she wasn't overly
 4                thrilled but .hh you know.
 5     Son:   Hmm.
 6     Dad:   But I brought her home (0.8) Frida:y. Let's see we left I
 7                dunno ten eleven o'clock I guess. .hh And they have
 8                elected to do radiation on both the upper and lower spine to
 9                try and reduce the tumors in there and see if they can (.)
10                make it any less painful for her.
11     Son:   Mm hm.
```

Dad reports an unnamed doctor's instructions to "take her home (.) handle her with hospice" (lines 1-2). It is not known, of course, whether "handle" was doctor's word or dad's. But it is clear that the doctor's recommendation involved hospice care. As discussed below, this is significant news (discussed below). It was also possibly bad news that, at least as dad reports it, gets rationalized with doctor's assessment that mom will "probably like the surroundings better etcetra" (lines 2-3). The first portion of this utterance, "probably like the surroundings better", is offered by dad as doctor's offering of some good news—a silver-lining or "bright side" (see Holt, 1993) balancing out the ending of in-hospital care. With "etcetra", however, dad does not report doctor's talk but displays an unwillingness to further summarize doctor's attempts to justify the decision to send mom home. As with Excerpt 8 (above), when aunt stated "Blah blah blah blah blah", she refused to provide additional descriptions of medications that, at the moment and in contrast to what really mattered, were treated as essentially unimportant. So too does dad, with "etcetra", gloss over any further "good" reasons to discharge mom that doctor may have provided. In this way, it is clear that what dad treated as consequential was not doctor's attempts to make the transition easier, but the bottom-line outcome: It will be tough to care for mom at home.

Apparently it was not just dad that was troubled by the doctor's announced decision. In lines 3-4, dad refers to mom when he next states "and she wasn't overly thrilled". As evident, patients and doctors don't always agree on what might be best for their care, and this is a normal feature of medical treatments (e.g., see Stivers, 2002). When hospital and hospice staff work with patients and family members to facilitate understanding and acceptance of the dying process, ongoing differences in opinion can (and will always continue) to unfold. Yet it remains a particular and primary goal of hospice care to enhance the quality of a patient's remaining time with family and significant others, including working through routine troubles and conflicts inherent in palliative care.

It is noteworthy that for the first time in the phone call corpus, "hospice" is reported as a viable caring resource. Normally, as hospice care is provided only during the last six weeks of a patient's life, the doctor's recommendation marks a significant development in the family cancer journey. A shift from curative to palliative care is occurring and a critical juncture is arrived at: It is realized, and acted upon, that because a disease is not curable, increasing and focused attention must be given to ensuring patient's comfort throughout the dying process. Yet even though the expectation of death looms, and the patient is beyond medical recovery, considerable and ongoing interactional work (e.g., regarding hope, acceptance, grief, and very practical matters of day-to-day care) occurs and is designed to organize the environment needed to progressively move toward, and beyond, death (e.g., see Kubler-Ross, 1969a, 1969b; Peräkylä, 1991).

As dad continues on line 7, he describes how "**they** have elected" to radiate the spine to reduce tumors, and "see if **they** can (.) make it any less painful for her." (lines 7-10). In each instance, "they" is inclusive of the doctor working in unison with medical staff. The word "elected" also attributes to the medical team a process of careful examination and decision making, yielding a choice or nomination giving priority to optimizing mom's comfort in the face of advancing (now clearly terminal) cancer (see also Excerpt 3, line 19, Chapter 9).[6]

In the final instance involving a routine reporting of "doctor", dad had just stated to son that "time is just takin' it's toll" (#38:10), including atrophy of mom's muscles. In lines 1-3 below, dad informs son that mom can still walk, though a wheelchair has been made available if needed. It is at this moment, in line 4, that son asks dad "What's the **doctor** saying these days.":

22) SDCL: Malignancy #38:11

```
 1    Dad:    As long as she can walk around y'know that's a little help.
 2            And there's a wheelchair here if we have to eventually get to
 3            the point where we wheel her around, but-
 4  → Son:    What's the doctor saying these days.
 5  → Dad:    We:ll doctor was outta town last week. She was gonna be in
 6  →         town Friday but not here, so she doesn't go see the doctor
 7            until (.) think the twenty first or twenty second somethin'
 8            like that. So,
 9    Son:    Hm.
10    Dad:    The hospice care nurse comes in twice a week, and she
11            yiknow checks her an' talks to her and that kind of business.
12            But um y'know they just basically are saying keep her
13            comfortable.
14    Son:    Hm. .hh That's not a very good sounding prognosis but-
15    Dad:    No- no there isn't a prognosis for this [  so  ] =
16    Son:                                            [Yeah.]
```

With reference to "the **doctor**" son shifts from dad's assessment of mom's condition, and what the future might hold, to seeking information by a medical expert: A known but unnamed person whom dad, with "We:ll **doctor**", next also fails to refer to by name. But as dad proceeds with "She", it becomes clear that referencing doctor's name is not needed when both speakers know and recognize who is being referred to. As has been repeatedly shown in this chapter, a pronoun is sufficient if and when shared knowledge exists about who the person being referenced is and his/her role in mom's care. Further, because the doctor was out of town and mom won't see her for some time, dad has little to report involving a provider who, at this point in time, has less to do with mom's care than does hospice.

In line 10, dad begins to summarize a nurse's "twice a week" hospice care as regular and routine. His "checks her an' talks to her and that kind of business.", occurring in line 11, is structured as a three-part list with a generalized list completer ("that kind of business", see Jefferson, 1990). This description leaves unspecified the exact medical tasks nurse performs, the kinds of conversations occurring with mom, and does not provide further details about the nurse's care. It is offered by dad as only a summarized version of events, treated now by dad as altogether routine. This stands in marked contrast with Excerpt 21 (above), where anticipated hospice care remained on the horizon. By stating "just basical-ly are saying keep her comfortable" (lines12-13), an understanding of a primary goal of hospice care is offered.

Son's uptake is "That's not a very good sounding prognosis but-" (line 14), an assess-ment voicing his recognition that attempts to cure mom have given way to caring for her comfort. Dad's response, "No- no there isn't a prognosis for this [so] =", which son next (and in overlap) agrees with, reflects a postprognosis orientation to managing mom's can-cer: Increasingly, whether or not mom will die is not an issue, but when and how.

Doctors as Resources for Hope

The final two excerpts in this chapter begin to exemplify complex relationships between doctors, hope, and in general "hope" as an interactional accomplishment (see also Chapters 12 and 13). The first excerpt (below) was initially and briefly discussed in Chapter 4 (Excerpt 7), when examining how son spoke with mom for the first time about the serious-ness of her bad cancer news. This set of moments marks the onset of one of the most dif-ficult and delicate discussions between family members in the entire Malignancy corpus:

23) SDCL: Malignancy#2:3

1	Mom:	So, (0.4) it's re::al °ba:d°.
2		(0.8)
3	Mom:	((sneezes))
4	Son:	pt .hh I guess.
5		(0.4)
6	Mom:	And uh: >I don't know what else to ↑tell you.<
7		(1.0)
8	Son:	.hh hhh Yeah. (0.2) um- ((hhhh)). Yeah, I don't know what to
9		say either.
10	Mom:	No there's nothing to say. >You just-< .hh I'll I'll wait to
11 →		talk to **Doctor** (name) today°= he's the cancer man and =
12	Son:	= Um hmm.=
13	Mom:	= see what he has to say, and (0.4) just keep goin' forward. I
14		mean (.) I might be real lucky in five years. It might just be
15		six months.

Mom's bottom-line assessment in line 1, "So, (0.4) it's re::al °ba:d°.", is followed by two extended pauses and her intervening "sneeze". Next, and not surprisingly, son's "I guess." (line 4) acknowledges but withholds commenting further on what his hearing about such bad, and possibly even fatal news, might amount to. As examined in Chapter 4, son can lit-erally only "guess" about technical matters he knows very little about. He is thus not in a position to claim *epistemic rights* and speak about these dire circumstances. And in the very next turn at talk, mom's ">I don't know what else to ↑tell you.<" gives rise to what son's earlier "I guess" left unstated: "I don't know what to say either." (lines 8-9; see Beach & Metzger, 1997). It appears that there is "nowhere else to go" (Jefferson 1984b, p. 191) in bringing this troubling diagnosis and prognosis to a close, which mom's "No there's noth-in to say." further emphasizes (Beach, 2003a).

Yet repeated displays of "hope" routinely emerge as the upshot of bad news and even despair, as with mom's "I'll I'll wait to talk to **Doctor** (name) today.= he's the cancer man". By referencing this doctor by name, and then operationally defining for son who this doctor is —"the cancer man"—the relative importance of the doctor's name pales in comparison to the expertise to diagnose and treat mom's cancer. In cases in which family members exhaust their resources for responding to a serious cancer diagnosis, it becomes clear that "Only the doctor has the expertise to announce any new, potentially good, and more or less definitive news regarding her acute medical condition" (Beach, 2003a, p. 183). One way to "manage optimism", then, is to faithfully move forward in hopes that the future may hold better rather than worse news, possibilities that only a cancer expert might elucidate. As portrayed in mom's subsequent "I mean I might be real lucky in five years. It might just be six months." (lines 13-15), however, considerable uncertainty remains: Even expertly trained doctors don't possess "educated crystal balls" revealing how the future might unfold (see Endnote 5, Chapter 7).

In Excerpt 8 (above), following a visit by a doctor who had yet to examine his mom "this morning", a moment was examined where son announced that he was awaiting news. Below, as dad twice reports mom's status as "about the same" (lines 1 & 16), his ability to update news for son is also pending a doctor's visit (lines 2-4):

22) SDCL: Malignancy#37:1-2

```
 1     Dad:    On this end about the same. hh Umm (0.2) should finally get
 2  →          a chance to talk to the doctor this morning. She has been out
 3             of town at a symposium or somethin' fo:r couple days. (.) So
 4             we haven't seen her since Friday.

               ((17 lines deleted where dad reports that mom "drifts",
                is less hostile but more "spacy", and had undergone
                another bone scan in the "nuclear medicine ward"))

 5     Dad:    Uh I had no idea of what they found, or what they were
 6  →          looking for 'cause there wasn't any of the doctors there
 7             yesterday, except ya know for emergency on call. So
 8             obviously I didn't see one of 'em.
 9             (1.2)
10  → Dad:     But I hope to fi- ((clears throat)) hope to find out this
11             morning so,
12     Son:    Umkay.
13     Dad:    Maybe I will learn some more.
14     Son:    But other than that looks as though things are relatively
15             status quo, huh. =
16     Dad:    = Yeah they're just about the same. U:m
```

Just as dad begins this excerpt by stating "should finally get a chance" to speak with the doctor, it is clear that family members regularly rely on the doctor's updates and, when absent, know and treat a lack of information as noticeably absent. And again, dad's reference to "the **doctor**" in line 2 is immediately followed with "She", and shortly thereafter, "her" (line 4). These are routine shortcuts for referring to a person both dad and son possess knowledge about, namely, mom's primary cancer specialist, who for a "couple days" has not been available.

Because dad was not able to talk to "any of the doctors", he remained uninformed about the purpose and findings of yet another bone scan (lines 6-8). But he is hopeful that he will soon "find out" and have new information to assess, to "learn some more" and reduce at least some of the surrounding uncertainty (lines 10-13). Importantly, his hope at this phase of the cancer journey is not raised (nor elaborated upon) in pursuit of false expectations for cure. Rather, dad is closely monitoring information and (as best possible) seeking to be educated about the evolution of mom's progressively failing health.

The upshot of dad's reporting is reiterated by son as he seeks, and receives, confirmation: "But other than that looks as though things are _relatively_ st_a_tus quo, huh" (lines 14-16). Although not discounting the potential importance of what the most recent bone scan might reveal, son treats dad as not possessing news that mom's condition had changed significantly (i.e., continued strong emphasis on pain management to manage, but not eliminate nor control her cancer). This is relatively good news, at least compared to many moments in the Malignancy corpus, when mom's diagnosis is bad and her condition is worsening. Dad's "st_a_tus quo" does not change mom's terminal prognosis, of course, but his reporting (and son's receptivity) exhibits ongoing monitoring and concern.

REFRAMING UNDERSTANDINGS OF REFERENCES TO NONPRESENT DOCTORS AND "THEY"

Doctors and medical staff are prominent figures for cancer patients and family members. By sheer frequency of references alone, it is clear that family members are constantly preoccupied with doctors' opinions, as well as actions that have or may be undertaken by anonymous and known medical staff. Whether reporting on routine matters, specific discussions with doctors, and/or treating doctors as resources for hope, it is clear that medical experts are treated by family members as critical when attempting to assess mom's condition, understand technical procedures, and navigate through an uncertain future and shifting prognosis.

Across diverse and routine circumstances, medical experts significantly impact what lay persons know and believe, and thus how they communicate about illness. To some extent, family members must rely on medical experts when forming their own technical understandings of illness circumstances. Talking with and about doctors (and medical staff) is a resource for obtaining information, and in turn, enacting their own authoritative positions by reporting what experts stated. Delicate balances are evident as family members talk about biomedical details they do not fully understand, display optimism and hope in the face of mom's failing health, and simultaneously manage who knows more about key events and circumstances comprising the family cancer journey. Several instances have been examined where specific interactional work is focused on who possesses more definitive knowledge about medical scheduling, results, and judgments. On many occasions, talk about matters such as prognosis for mom's dying also reveals that, and how, family members actively claim and defer to whomever knows more or less about particular topics. These discussions and reports make clear, however, that family members also live within an ongoing state of not knowing, even though they continually seek information from one another, and medical experts, that may not be readily available.

Family members subordinate themselves to such matters as medical experts' schedules, constantly waiting for some combination of news updates, biopsy results, and/or advice about advancing care. Though medical experts are at times doubtful and uncertain about treating and explaining cancer, despite their proficient skills, family members report what doctors said _objectively_ as authoritative resources whose attributed, hands-on familiarity uniquely qualifies them to be listened and attended to. In this important sense, medical experts become anchors for unsteady thoughts and feelings about a loved one's condition, professionals whose in-the-trenches investments of time and effort reveal their awareness of the impacts of living with and through cancer.

Through prosodically marked stretches of talk (i.e., intonation, pitch, rate), repeated instances have been provided in which the *voice* of reported authority is evident as serious, unemotional, and staccato reconstructions of what the doctor actually stated (or was attributed to have said). It is significant that speakers such as dad, son, mom, and aunt exhibited being more knowledgeable when reporting about doctors and medical staff, than when offering their own opinions about events surrounding mom's care. At root this makes perfect sense: As *lay* persons, family members do not typically have an authoritative basis — that is, a stock of knowledge at hand — for advancing complex, often technical claims about cancer treatments and care. However, as noted, they can and do act authoritatively on information they have received from experts and others. These reportings were shown to shift across doctors' and speakers' voices, including shifts across time domains (e.g., when son was reporting what dad had reported to him).

It is important to reiterate that whether reporting doctors' talk or actions, or offering their own opinions on biomedical issues, family members evidence their *lay* status in two primary ways. First, immediately prior to referencing such words and phrases as "needle biopsy results", "bone scan", or "morphine" numerous instances have been examined where speakers search (i.e., through stretching words and pauses), cut off, and/or initiate repair on their words. It is repeatedly evident that making references to such matters as treatment options is approached with hesitancy and dysfluency. Second, it was noted how speakers such as dad exhibited an inability and even disinterest when producing specific descriptions (e.g., "xra::y and scan or *whatever*", "the thyroid *stuff*", and "drip system >*whatever* the hell<"). In these ways both the limits of speakers' knowledge, and their exhibited stances toward procedures as matters they do not necessarily care to know more about, are also evident.

In the following chapter, analysis is extended to a series of moments involving how positive and negative assessments of doctors and medical care emerge within diverse interactional environments.

NOTES

1. This is not to say that medical experts and even cancer specialists never get diagnosed with cancer. But even on such occasions, it is possible but highly unlikely that these professionals will be adequately knowledgeable about complex and exacting details comprising a given cancer type. Nor are details about the most appropriate treatments, designed to promote healing, well understood.

2. Working with this collection of materials once again confirms how *a priori* conceptions of what might be studied become transformed as analysis continues. In the "shifting sands" of interactional understandings, research priorities simply change in the midst of generating and refining collections. What might initially be treated as important may not be the only, nor most prominent, set of phenomena to investigate. For example, we initiated this analysis with the goal of analyzing selected moments we had heard and attended to: How family members take on the "voice" of doctors when reporting what doctors had told them. We intended to focus on how enacted and "reported speech" (Beach, 2000b; Holt, 1996, 2000; Holt & Clift, 2006) is organized and how family members make sense of biomedical/technical matters. However, as this collection got built and more closely examined, these instances became subcollections in their own right. They are thus examined in this chapter, but not exclusively so. For example, it became apparent that medical staff were even more frequently referenced with "they" and "they're" references (i.e., deictic pronouns, Sacks, 1992). This expanded the size of the collection well beyond the focus on "doctors" and resulted in a corpus of varied instances.

   Although reported speech and actions are significant and clearly deserving of analysis on their own merits, working with a larger collection helped us to realize that even more encompassing activities occur throughout family cancer journeys. Priority has thus been given to analyzing social activities in order of their identified and apparent prominence, which the data selected for this chapter only begins to reveal.

3. Even when patients and family members provide written notification to medical staff about matters such as "no life support" or "do not resuscitate", decisions can continue to be made against such explicit wishes. By not being adequately informed, medical staff can and do make mistakes about patients' care.

4. In ordinary conversations, the practice of speakers' claiming insufficient knowledge (e.g., with "I don't know"), then routinely moving to immediately state what they do know and understand, is examined by Beach and Metzger (1997).

5. Immediately prior to this excerpt, son informed dad that he realized mom was home. Together they discussed that it was "tough" for everyone, circumstances that did not emerge by choice:

1) SDCL: Malignancy #39:4

Dad	They <u>dis</u>charged her.
Son:	<u>O:</u>h.
Dad:	They will not just w<u>a</u>rehouse her.
Son:	O::h okay.

Dad's references to "They" invokes decisions to "discharge" mom that were made not by a single individual in isolation, but an anonymous medical team. Exactly how this or related decisions get enacted remain evasive to nonmedical experts, but are no doubt altogether routine for professionals responsible for discerning when it is best to release a patient to care outside the hospital. These more general references to "They" proceed the following reference to "Doctor", presumably the person in control and assigned the responsibility of informing the family that, essentially, no bio-medical solutions existed for improving and healing mom's condition. In short, the colloquial expression is "there's nothing more we can do." In practice, such a phrase, or its equivalent, did not get reconstructed by dad in favor of the actual informing provided in Excerpt 21.

6. The term "elected" might be usefully contrasted with mom's earlier use of "verdict" (see Excerpt 2 in Chapter 4). Though here "elected" reflects a nomination or decision-making process, and thus some control by medical professionals, with "verdict" mom's cancer was depicted as not controlled by any party.

9

"she likes the doctor ... ↑ho:ly Christ come on"

Positive and Negative Assessments of Doctors and Medical Care

In the previous chapter a variety of social actions were identified as family members refer to, and report on, routine circumstances involving doctors, medical staff, and providing of care. One feature, addressed only in passing, involved how reportings may give rise to positive and negative assessments about both hospital and doctor care. Family members display support and frustration with the doctors and medical staff. This chapter examines the interactional features of family members' complaints about, frustrations with, and praises for doctors, medical staff, and care.

For example, as discussed in Excerpt 10 (Chapter 8), dad first praised one hospital then, in contrast, critiqued another:

1) SDCL: Malignancy #25:8-9

```
1   Dad:   ↑Yeah. And it's a (.) real nice little hospital? It's not a big
2          (1.2) mausoleum like (.) (name of hospital) is.

           ((17 lines deleted))

3   Dad:   °Yeah.° (name of hospital) was such a colossal (.) bitch the last
4          time she was in it because she couldn't get (.) people to take
5          care of [ ya   and ] =
6   Son:            [Uhm hm. ]
7   Dad:   = °a whole bunch of other stuff.°
```

The contrasts are evident: A "real nice little hospital" and "a big (1.2) mausoleum". The latter described as "such a colossal (.) bitch", because "she" (mom) couldn't get people to take care of "ya" (line 5). Dad's shift from "she→ya" (i.e, rather than "she→her") is one instance of what Sacks (1992) described as an *expansion* practice: "'you' can in fact be a way of talking about 'everybody'—and indeed, incidentally, of 'me'" (p. 349). By integrating dad's reformulation of mom's complaint with Sacks's original observation, "me" could be taken to mean "her". Further, dad's "ya" also places mom in a category of patients requiring (but not receiving) adequate care, where "'you' stands as a pronoun for the set of terms: 'everyone', 'someone', 'people,' etc." (p. 349). And as it was dad's assessment to report on mom's original complaint, with "Uhm hm" (line 6) son responds by aligning with an assessment about events he may identify with, but cannot report directly on (or at least chooses not to share similar experiences with poor hospital care).

Dad's negative critique, however, was followed by strong affirmation for mom's current doctor:

2) SDCL: Malignancy #25:9

```
1   Dad:   [     No::::   ] she likes the doctor the doctor does good
2              things for he:r that she can't.
3              (The hell with it [ya know.]) =
4   Son:                       [ Yeah.  ]
5   Dad:   = we'll drive so she can be comfortable.
6   Son:   °Okay.°
```

In contrast to prior experiences, their current doctor "does good things for he:r that she can't." (lines 1-2), one operational definition of providing quality care. The extent of support for the doctor is also laid bare: With emphasis ("hell", line 3), a longer drive is worth the effort for the sake of mom's comfort. In response to dad's reporting and stated conviction to drive, son aligns with dad's positions. It is dad who has directly observed and no doubt spoken with mom about the doctor's care. And in practice, any efforts to drive mom longer distances involve dad's efforts, not son's, further establishing dad's authoritative claims for making decisions.

Continued orientations to social epistemics—or claiming superior rights to assess, know, defend, take responsibility for, and act upon circumstances—have been repeatedly addressed in prior chapters. As evident in the above instance and below, what family members claim to know persists and is consequential for shaping agreements and disagreements, calibrating understandings and decisions about events, advancing and defending positions relative to their own knowledge and opinions about mom's health.

DISSECTING AN EXTENDED INSTANCE

The extended instance below, drawn from call #1, reveals a series of negative and positive assessments of doctors, staff, and care. These include dad's frustration with medical delay and treatment protocol (lines 4-17), son's sarcastic criticism (lines 25-26), and dad's reporting of a friend's recommendations for a doctor (lines 32-33). These moments are embedded within a variety of related social actions: (a) Multiple (19) references to "they/they're/they've", the majority of which refer to anonymous and/or unspecified medical experts; (b) Son's attempts to contribute to and assess dad's reporting, two of which are corrected as inaccurate by dad (lines 25-28, 53-54); (c) Repeated *lay* attempts by dad to depict medical procedures, including dysfluencies occurring immediately prior to technical descriptions (lines 9-10, 19, 22-24); and (d) Dad's invoking "hope" about future diagnostic and treatment procedures (lines 42-52). Each of these involvements will be examined in order of their occurrence.

Frustration, Support, and Disaffiliation

The excerpt begins as dad reports a prior conversation with mom about a "needle biopsy", specifically, whether mom knew what "they're" gonna do (line 2) and "are **they** gonna do bo:th?" (lines 2-3):

3) SDCL: Malignancy #1:5-6

```
 1    Dad:    It's >ya know< when I had (.) talked to her
 2            yesterday, I said .hhh ya know if they're gonna (.) do: a
 3            needle biopsy today, .hhh are they gonna do bo:th?=<
 4   →        And she said well she didn't think so.>=I said ↑ ho:ly Christ
 5            come o:n [ >ya know.< ]
 6    Son:             [ >Yeah it's like<] [>they got-<]
 7    Dad:                                 [ They:'ve ] already dragged
 8            this thing out e:ight days. I said why (.) .hhh if you're gonna
 9            go through a:ll the preparation an a:ll the rest of it, (0.7) two
10            ho:les isn't that much bigger deal than o:ne, [ once  ya ]=
11    Son:                                                 [ °Umhm.° ]
12    Dad:    = Get ta that part.
13            (0.7)
14    Dad:    Ya know if you gotta lay here another whole day and think
15            about goin' for the next one.
16    Son:    $Heh heh heh heh$ =
17    Dad:    = It might be tougher than doin' two at once. =
18    Son:    = Um hm.
19    Dad:    So they elected to do both. They did th- (0.2) the adrenal
20            gland first. That's why they got the results ba:ck on that one
21            quicker. .hhhh The other one'll take a little more time. .hh So
22            (.) then that'll be Monday before they have any answer: (.) as
23            I understand it on- what ki::nd and then once you know
24            what ki::nd then you can say okay.=
25  →  Son:   = Then they'll spend another week (0.3) deciding about what
26            color right?
27    Dad:    We::ll I don't (.) think so at that point. He has already said
28            that (.) .hhh uh he has co:ntacted .hhh you know who
29            Ma:ggie is, the friend of Katie's.
30    Son:    Ye::ah =
31    Dad:    = Okay well Maggie works for two cancer specialists. .hhh
32  →        A:nd (0.6) she recommended one. She said >you know< they
33  →        are both competent but this guy is more personable. .hhh  So
34            ((clears throat)) he was recommended to .hhh Lorraine and
35            Katie >ya know< by Katie. So .hhh uh: (Peters) tonight, (.)
36            he's going to be out of town for (.) tonight and tommorow
37            and then he'll be back Sunday. But =
38    Son:    = °Umhm.° =
39    Dad:    = .hhh He said he would have somebody else look in on her:.
40            =He also co:ntacted this cancer specialist so he will be in
41            Monday. (.) .hhh And they will do this bo:ne scan thing
42            tommorow. So .hhh n:o:: I would hope by Monday or
43            Tu:esday (0.5) pt they have <pin:ned do::wn> (0.7) the
44            particulars of what they're after. >Now they may not have<
45            the course of action all figured out, but [ .hhhh ] =
46    Son:                                              [°Umhm°]
47    Dad:    = they'll at least kno:w. (.) .hh  And maybe this is just
48            simplistically in my mind >but they'll know< .hhh what
49            ki:nd? they're dealing with. That way they should know
50            .hhh how quickly does it spread (.) what is- (0.5) what can
```

```
51              be done to: to stop it >you know< .hh radiation
52              [  or   chemotherapy   or      ] =
53  → Son:     [ Yeah where else has it gone. ]
54   Dad:      = Well that's part of the bo:ne scan.
55   Son:      Umhm.
```

In each instance, dad refers once again (see Chapter 8) to anonymous medical staff engaged in activities family members are neither skilled in, nor sure about (i.e., in terms of timing or occurrence). Here, as dad reports querying mom about if both procedures would be conducted at the same time or not, and that in response mom didn't think so, he vents his frustration with "↑ ho:ly Christ come o:n >ya know.<" (lines 4-5)[1] (see also Excerpt 7, below).

Returning to line 6, son immediately agrees with and even begins to contribute at the outset of dad's subsequent and elaborated complaint: "**They: 've** already dragged this thing out e:ight days." (lines 7-8), and "= It might be tougher than doin' two at <u>once</u>. =" (line 17). Although there may be legitimate medical reasons not to conduct two needle biopsies at the same time (e.g., different organ locations require different procedures, patients might tolerate one needle biopsy better than two, staff, location, and scheduling), it was either not apparent to dad or, if so, taken into consideration by him. As a husband and father, dad's lay priorities focused on minimizing mom's pain and discomfort as she undergoes preparation (line 9), as well as the anxiety emerging from waiting "another whole day" (line 14)— an extreme case formulation building his case against unnecessary delay (see Edwards, 2000; Pomerantz, 1984b).

His construction of concerns exhibits specific lay orientations to technical, medical procedures. For example, with "<u>a:ll</u> the preparation an <u>a:ll</u> the rest of it," (line 9), dad twice emphasizes "<u>a:ll</u>" as he legitimates (see Pomerantz, 1984b) what he envisions as inconvenient and discomforting procedures for mom to experience. His reference to "preparation" is overly general, just as "<u>a:ll</u> the rest of it" leaves unspecified (likely unknown) details involved in actually conducting "needle biopsies". And with "two <u>ho:</u>les isn't that much bigger deal than <u>o:ne</u>," (lines 9-10) dad summarizes medical procedures that, even though he does not fully understand them technically, nevertheless assumes their possibility and benefit for mom.

A Delicate Laughter

Son seems to be aligned with the positions articulated throughout dad's complaint. One particular moment, involving son's laughter (line 16), indicates that as recipient of dad's serious concerns he is not discounting, but even more strongly affiliating (but from his own perspective) with dad's serious concerns. In line 14 below, for example, dad does not display laughter or other humorous orientations to his own talk. Nor does he invite shared laughter from son in the next turn. Yet his actions provide an opportunity for son to laugh about mom's predicament. The basic question is, "Why that laughter here?":

4) SDCL: Malignancy #1:5-6

```
14   Dad:      Ya know if you gotta lay here another whole day and think
15              about goin' for the next one.
16  → Son:     $Heh heh heh heh$ =
17   Dad:      = It might be tougher than doin' two at once. =
18   Son:      = Um hm.
```

What is the orientation displayed by son, through laughter, as a recipient who previously monitored and appeared to affiliate with the full course of dad's prior complaint about mom's care? Is son simply "laughing off" dad's serious concerns? Or is he displaying some other orientation, uniquely rooted in his own experiences, as recipient of dad's stated problems?

Consider the first possibility: that son is "laughing off" dad's prior complaint. For example, as Glenn (2003, p. 64) has observed, following Sacks's (1992, pp. 10-12) comments about how others "laugh off" suicide threats they treated nonseriously, "The idiom 'laughing it off' captures this sense of laughing to show refusal to take seriously something by previous speaker" (see also Haakana, 2001). If son is heard and seen to be "laughing off" dad's complaint about mom's laying around, thinking about her next needle biopsy, it is an understandable reaction. Unlike dad, however, son has not directly observed and monitored (on a daily basis) the trials and tribulations mom is undergoing. Lacking this experience, he may not be able to identify fully with the breadth or depth of dad's concerns. After all, dad's voice of frustration is anchored in his unique immersion into the hospital setting, clinical observations and experiences that son has primarily heard about only as embedded in reportings during long distance telephone calls.

But the explanation of son "laughing off" dad does not seem well fitted to this set of moments. There is an alternative and viable possibility here, namely, that son's "$Heh heh heh heh$" (line 16) evidences his own delicate orientation to the troubles dad is describing. Son exhibits a nervous laughter indicating that he is, in his own manner and as informed by his residual stock of knowledge, *resistant* to what may be difficult news to hear about: the daily challenges involved in mom's activities as a patient, under the care (and to some extent, control) of at least several (if not numerous) medical experts. In this sense, son is not inviting dad to share laughter with him in the next turn, which dad does not do as he finalizes his elaboration by reference to what "might be tougher" (line 17). Instead, as recipient but now laugh-producer, son demonstrates that the very thought of waiting for yet another procedure is an unenviable position, one he identifies with but treats delicately. Son too is a consequential family member, impacted by the portrayals, complaints, and frustrations dad makes available as part of a routine update about mom's condition. Though son is not physically present as mom undergoes much of her cancer care, he is affected by her quandary.

Son's Sarcastic Comment and Two Disaffiliative Responses by Dad

Given the frustration dad has exhibited, it is not surprising that as dad moves forward with his summary and update, he states "So **they** elected to do both" (line 19). The term "elected" denotes a choice that "**they**" made, an enacted and deliberate decision among medical staff, but also actions taken without consultation with mom or dad (see also Excerpt #21 in Chapter 8). And the following dysfluency, "**They** did th- (0.2) the adrenal gland <u>first</u>." (lines 19-20), is akin to previously identified moments in which dad repairs, searches, and/or hesitates immediately prior to referencing technical procedures or terminology (and in this instance, a gland). His lay orientation to this round of procedures is further evident when dad summarizes anticipation of hearing results (i.e., when "they have any answer:") (lines 22-23):

5) SDCL: **Malignancy #1:5-6**

```
    22              .hh So (.) then that'll be Monday before they have any
    23              answer: (.) as I understand it on- on what ki::nd and then
    24              once you know what ki::nd then you can say okay.=
    25   → Son:    = Then they'll spend another week (0.3) deciding about what
    26              color right?
    27   → Dad:    We::ll I don't (.) think so at that point. He has already said
    28              that (.) .hhh uh he has co:ntacted .hhh you know who
```

29   <u>Ma</u>:ggie is, the friend of Katie's.
30   Son: Ye::ah =

With the preface "as I understand it", dad explicitly qualifies that his reporting is limited to his knowledge "on- on what <u>ki::nd</u> and then once you know what ki::nd then you can say okay.=" (lines 23-24). His cut off "on-" occurs prior to a generic description, a stretched "what ki::nd" repeated shortly thereafter, that fails to specify a particular type of cancer for a basic reason: As previously described, a lay person such as dad is not capable of articulating possible types, nor their implications for diagnosis and treatment.

However, he is on the verge of stating something about treatment with "then you can say okay =" (line 24). But before dad can continue, son next responds with "= Then **they'll** spend another week (0.3) deciding about what <u>co</u>lor right?" (lines 25-26). This sarcastic (i.e., nonliteral) offering by son actually aligns with dad's prior venting of frustration with the medical staff. However, it is not *what* son says, but the critical implication of his utterance that extends dad's complaints: that better care for mom might be made available. This is a form of humorous digging, without laughter, an action in pursuit of intimacy by inviting dad's own affiliation (see Jefferson, Sacks, & Schegloff, 1987). As consequential family members, and thereby collaborators in seeking quality care for mom, this utterance reveals how a son attempts to solicit his dad to join together in questioning, challenging, or otherwise constructing a negative stance toward the decisions and delays inherent in medical experts' actions. Yet, in response, dad's "We::ll I don't (.) think so at that point." (line 27) disaffiliates with son's effort. Dad offers a marked disagreement (see Pomerantz, 1984a) that not only rejects son's invitation, but also his offer to form such an alliance on how long medical experts' work takes and the detailed but trivial nature of their efforts (i.e., "deciding about what <u>co</u>lor right?", lines 25-26).

Dad's serious orientation to son's attempted sarcasm is similar to Drew's (1987) analysis of how some recipients, having been teased by prior speaker, offer a "po-faced" or serious response to the tease. Though son is not engaged in teasing per se, he does expand on dad's positions in a sarcastic and nonliteral manner. He achieves these actions by exploiting dad's prior actions, transforming dad's complaints into an opportunity for yet further excessive complaining. As evident in next turn, however, dad was not receptive to son's initiative. Anchored in dad's own first-hand observations and knowledge about mom's hospital care, he employs his disaffiliation as a resource for claiming the epistemic right to be critical. By so doing, he does not grant son the same right to be negative about matters (such as delay and scheduling). In this way, lacking dad's and other family member's updates, son is treated as essentially unaware of these matters: He possesses only second-hand knowledge that (apparently) does not qualify him as having the right to sarcastically and negatively assess others' medical care (see also discussion of lines 53-54, below).

As dad continues (lines 27-42), he describes that a family friend (Maggie) who "works for two cancer specialists" (line 31) recommended a competent, personal doctor who is out of town but will "have somebody else look in on her" (line 39). Because of these decisions, "they will do this <u>bo:ne</u> scan thing tomorrow.", and dad hopes that within a few days they will "have <<u>pin::ned</u> <u>do::wn</u>> (0.7) the particulars of <u>what</u> **they're** after." (line lines 41-44). He continues by qualifying his own possible and simplistic understanding that they will know about the kind of cancer involved, how quickly it spreads, and "what can be done to: to <u>stop</u> it":

6) SDCL: Malignancy #1:6

47   Dad: = **they'll** at least kno:w. (.) .hh And maybe this is just
48   simplistically in my mind >but **they'll** know< .hhh <u>what</u>
49   <u>ki:nd</u>? **they're** dealing with. That way **they** should know

```
50              .hhh how quickly does it spread (.) what is- (0.5) what can
51              be done to: to stop it >you know< .hh radiation
52              [ or    chemotherapy or-    ] =
53    →  Son:   [ Yeah where else has it gone. ]
54    →  Dad:   = Well that's part of the bo:ne scan.
55       Son:   Umhm.
```

In line 53, son's reformulates lines 49-51, agreeing with and summarizing dad's prior statement. But, once again, dad's "= Well that's part of the bo:ne scan." (line 54) offers an epistemic correction of son's version. Essentially, dad sets son straight with information dad does know about bone scans. Despite dad's self-proclaimed and simplistic understandings of the technical nature of many procedures, including bone scans, he invokes the knowledge he does possess to correct what son had offered as an agreement and summary.

One way to understand the background and narrative offered by dad is to recognize that his extended response was actually triggered by son's initial sarcastic critique (lines 25-26) of the delay, and even trivial nature, of the work done by medical staff. In a sense dad's lack of alignment with son's attempt to degrade professionals' efforts prefaced a defense of their efforts. This is due, in part, to the fact that it included input from both himself and mom (i.e., aunt's friend Maggie). Indeed, dad goes about evidencing that even though he was justifiably upset about needle biopsy procedures, son's attempt to comment about others' negative conduct (including his involvements with mom and largely unstated but implied interfacing with the medical staff) was not legitimate. Dad's own actions reveal that progress was being made in securing cancer specialists, moving as best and soon as possible toward bone scans, and basically figuring out the kind, nature, and treatment for mom's cancer.

It appears, then, that there were aftershocks from son's earlier attempt to join in on being critical. This resulted in dad's rejection and accounting for the inaccuracy of son's perspective. Even when son later (line 53) offered an otherwise benign comment about where else mom's cancer might have gone (i.e., spread), dad corrected son by recruiting a technical understanding about bone scans that dad otherwise knew very little about. Apparently, few degrees of freedom were made available to son, not necessarily because there were any outstanding conflicts between son and dad but, and perhaps more primally so, because dad simply spoke from a more authoritative position because he experienced mom's care more directly than son. Dad also, by observing and actually speaking with medical experts about mom's care, gradually became more educated about technical matters. One consequence is that dad defended his (and their/medical staffs') territory from a sarcastic comment by son. This is not to say that son knowingly or intentionally offered a comment that would elicit dad's defensive reaction. Rather, dad (for some unknown reason) was compelled to account for and legitimate that matters on his end were, in fact, being well managed.

MANAGING ADDITIONAL MOMENTS

From the instances above, involving son's comments and dad's responses, it becomes clear that reportings about doctors and medical staff reveal key insights about medical competence (or lack thereof). In the midst of these reportings, however, it is also apparent that and how family members' interactionally manage rights and privileges to assess the care of a loved one, claim knowledge about procedures, and ultimately establish (or defer) authority about the credibility of these types of reportings.

The excerpts below extend the single case analysis offered above. An attempt is made to begin to lay bare related yet diverse interactional environments within which doctors and medical staff are critiqued, put in their place, and even defended by family members.

Looking Toward (But Not Forward) to Christmas

Below are two excerpts (7 & 8), occurring within a 24-hour period and drawn from calls #10 (between son and aunt) and #12 (between son and dad). Looking ahead in anticipation of future events, both aunt and dad employ "Christmas" as a significant time frame for calibrating mom's remaining time.[2] Each addresses the basic issue of how long mom might have to live. In both excerpts, frustration is also exhibited regarding looming uncertainties and attempts by doctor and medical staff to treat mom's spreading cancer.

Following aunt's report that neither she nor dad assume that mom will live until "Chri:stmas" in line 1 (below), approximately one minute is deleted from this excerpt. Discussion focuses on how "mom's tough", an inherently uncertain future, and medication alternatives for treating mom during this phase of her illness. This is extended by aunt on line 3:

7) SDCL: Malignancy #10:11-12

```
1      Aunt:   but (.) ne:ither one of us believe that sh:e'll be here for
2              Chri:stmas.

              ((33 lines deleted))

3      Aunt:   Well ya know pt .hhh (.) I think that um::m (.) pt
4              if- if there's a po::sibility that this is so::mewhat
5              of a ma:tter of adjustments on medication in the past.
6              (.) Fa:irly re:cently =
7      Son:    = Ye:ah. =
8      Aunt:   = it has been that.
9      Son:    Yeah. =
10     Aunt:   = Which is what I'm also thinking.
11  →  Son:    But DA:MN! Come on. I mean it's li:ke a- they're
12             gonna adjust and then two days later it's a
13             cata:strophic adju:stme:nt. And two days la:ter it's
14             a cata:strophic adju:stment. An .hhh ya kno:w how-
15             how much can they keep clea:ning up after this me:ss.
16  →  Aunt:   O::h they can do a lo:t for a lo:ng ti:me. But I don't thi:nk
17             anybody he:re wants that.
18     Son:    No. You know ma- mom mentioned the no he:roic
19             me:asures. =
20     Aunt:   = O::h yeah. O::h yeah.
```

With considerable dysfluency (pauses, stretches, cut-off words), in lines 3-10 aunt attempts to describe for son how mom's medications have been adjusted in the past, more recently, and how these adjustments will likely continue. Son responds with an expletive and exclamation: "But DA:MN! Come on." (line 11) (see also dad's "↑ ho:ly Christ come o:n" in Excerpt #3, above). The source of his frustration rests with how often "they're gonna adjust" mom's medication in such "catastrophic" circumstances. The extremity of his concerns is further apparent as he exhibits irritation about their persistence: "how much can they keep clea:ning up after this me:ss." (line 15). Obviously, son constructs a troubled distinction between (a) medical staffs' attempts to make mom comfortable by adjusting medications and, if possible, prolong quality life, and (b) questioning just how long such "adjustments" should go on. His orientation represents a routine dialectic: Throughout often vague and ambiguous phases surrounding end of life care, family members frequent-ly struggle with stances toward medications, treatment decisions, and just what constitutes "quality of life".[3]

In response, aunt initially confirms and validates son by stating "<u>O</u>::h **they** can do a <u>lo:t</u> for a lo:ng ti:me." (line 16). Her attributions toward anonymous medical staff are replete with unstated implications. Aunt leaves hanging not only the ability of medical staff to unnecessarily prolong life, but their possible inclination toward such actions. Hers is a delicate and tenuous response to son's clearly emotional venting, simultaneously acknowl-edging the concerns he exudes—a "we" versus "they" orientation—while not explicitly holding "**them**" accountable for performing questionable actions. By hinting at but not directly accusing what "**they** can do", aunt at once aligns with son's obvious frustration, yet avoids taking an official position toward medical staff as *wrongdoers*: unnamed persons who would intentionally cause harm to mom or family.

As a resolution to this dilemma, in lines 16-17 aunt next makes clear that prolonging mom's passing is aligned with neither mom's nor family members' wishes. Her utterance serves as a reminder of earlier discussions with mom and others that instructions had been given for "no life support" (see Chapter 4). In turn, her assuaging action triggers son's dis-play of shared knowledge, providing him with an opportunity to utilize his own reporting of mom's stated "no he:roic me:asures" (lines 18-19). Almost ironically, son's reporting, aligned with aunt's prior position that the family will not allow unnecessary and prolonged adjustments, provides a resource for coping with (even reframing) his understandable frus-trations. He now displays recognition that the solution to his complaints (i.e., about repeat-ed "adjustments") rests solely with the family taking responsible action to ensure that mom's wishes are being met. And because he has a history of discussing such priorities with his mom, he can claim knowledge through his reporting of what mom had stated. And in response, aunt's repeated "O::h yeah. O::h yeah." (line 20) not only offers marked agree-ment, but claims her own epistemic authority as an informed family member well aware of mom's (and family members') preferences.

In these ways, together and authoritatively, aunt and son work through a primal frus-tration with medical staff's possible mishandling of mom's ongoing medication. They also collaborate in essentially detriggering son's displayed frustration and anxiety that, for a moment, became an outlet for expressing his annoyance with how medical staff are con-stantly making adjustments (i.e., "<u>c</u>leaning up after this me:ss.") (line 15). It is not as though son's venting overrode, or in any way took priority, over his memory of having spoken directly with mom about "no heroic measures". Rather, and understandably, part of the "me:ss" in the first instance is son's coping with the inevitable instability of mom's illness—conditions requiring ongoing adjustments by medical staff that are expected, at times even requested by family members, to best care for a dying mother about whom they are deeply concerned.

And therein lies yet another paradox of relying on talk in interaction to voice emotions and feelings about inherently uncertain cancer events that can not be fully controlled. The exact source of son's frustration—"**they're**" remedial actions—are the very behaviors attributed to medical staff as trained, competent, and caring professionals doing everything they can to comfort a terminally ill cancer patient (and her family).

The Evasive Doctor: "She's only got an educated crystal ball"

In a subsequent call, and with considerable uncertainty, dad offers an assessment that mom's death is at least a month away and could well occur during the Christmas holidays, most likely before "the end of the <u>year</u>" (line 3). Yet the difficulty of making such an assess-ment is evident in dad's "puhchuuuu" (line 4), an aspirated demonstration acknowledging the inherent difficulty of figuring out just how long mom might live:

8) SDCL: Malignancy #12:7

```
 1      Dad:   I- it may wind up bein' over the Christmas holidays or
 2             somethin'. I- >ya know< I don't know I- I- in my mind I can't
 3             (0.6) visualize this goin' past the end of the year, but lookin' at
 4             her to↑day I say puhchuuuu gotta be at least a month.
 5   → Son:   Hmkay. pt .hhhh Well yeah and I know Doctor (name) will
 6             never say anything in particular right. So- [hhhhh $huh ch$]
 7   → Dad:                                              [ We:::ll ya know]
 8             she doesn't have any- >ya know< she's only got an educated
 9             cr[ystal ball.] =
10      Son:     [ pt Sure. ]
11      Dad:   = She looks and she said >We:ll okay. So we got uh few more
12             tumors here we can radiate those that'll slow those down.
13             Then the next ones pop up ya know this is like-< .hhh trying to
14             squash mushrooms in a rainstorm. Eh ya know those suckers
15             just keep popping up eventually you're gonna lose but who
16             knows what eventually is. =
17      Son:   = Yeah pt .hhhh huh o:ka::y (.) Well (.) pt I will- hh .hh I will
18             unpack my ba:g: hhh [.hh and I'll keep] my lesson plans
19             current.
```

Following dad's attempt to "visualize" and (based on her appearance) estimate how long mom might live, son responds by offering a somewhat critical assessment: That the doctor "will never say anything in particular right" (lines 5-6). Similar to son's sarcastic utterance analyzed previously, "=Then **they'll** spend another week (0.3) deciding about what color right?" (Excerpt 3, line 25, above), son extends dad's reporting with a negative commentary on (in this case) a particular doctor's inability and/or unwillingness to offer a prognosis about how long mom might have to live. His critical orientation asserts knowledge akin to stereotypes that doctors (typically) are *evasive*: Speculating and predicting how long patients might live is withheld, in part to avoid wrong predictions, but also not to stifle hopeful approaches to healing and recovery.

It is not known whether, or how, son might have personally spoken with family members (or not) about this doctor's tendencies. But as son completes his utterance, he summarizes his critical assessment with "So- [hhhhh $huh ph$]". This exhalation (h's) is followed by laughter ($$) as he emphasizes his position. Son also invites dad's alignment through shared laughter, an attempt to garner dad's agreement with son's criticism of the doctor that is withholding prognosis. Yet in overlap (thus not responsive to son's aspirated laughter), and by stating the obvious, dad's response withholds the affiliation son is pursuing: "[We:::ll ya know] she's only got she doesn't have any- >ya know< an educated crystal ball" (lines 7-9; see also Excerpts 5 & 6 above, and Endnote 5 in Chapter 7). In lieu of joining with son in critiquing the doctor, dad actually supports the doctor's inability to predict how the future will unfold. Despite dad's knowledge about the doctor's expertise, he refuses to collaborate in unwarranted criticism and, further, to attribute any wrongful intentions. By supporting the doctor in this way, dad's actions counter son's negative portrayal. He once again, effectively and authoritatively, corrects son's own epistemic claim (as with Excerpt 24, above), an action that son's "pt Sure" (line 10) quickly acknowledges as relevant and appropriate.

Once again, dad's epistemic status is bolstered through a well-reasoned explanation, and more: a defense of actions taken by doctors and medical staff, rooted here in the fact that despite their education, even doctors cannot predict the future. As dad continues (lines 11-16), however, his reasoned explanation is further clarified. First, he reports doctor's biomedical orientation with "So we got uh few more tumors <u>here</u> we can radiate <u>those</u> that'll slow <u>those</u> down." (lines 11-12):

9) SDCL: Malignancy #12:7

11	Dad:	= She looks and she said ><u>We:ll</u> okay. So we got uh few more
12		tumors <u>here</u> we can radiate <u>those</u> that'll slow <u>those</u> down.
13		Then the <u>next</u> ones pop up ya know this is like-< .hhh trying to
14		squash <u>mush</u>rooms in a rainstorm. Eh ya know those <u>suckers</u>
15		just keep <u>popping</u> up <u>eve</u>ntually you're gonna <u>lose</u> but <u>who</u>
16		knows what <u>eve</u>ntually is. =
17	Son:	= Yeah pt .hhhh <u>huh</u> o:<u>ka</u>::y. (.) Well (.) pt I will- hh .hh I will
18		un<u>pack</u> my ba:g: hhh [.hh and I'll keep] my lesson plans
19		current.

Next (lines 13-16), dad shifts to a distinctive lay depiction that is one of the most metaphorical and visually alluring moments in the entire telephone corpus: Tumors are characterized as "popping up" and likened to "trying to squash <u>mush</u>rooms in a rainstorm."—"<u>suckers</u>" that cannot be controlled, that "you're gonna <u>lose</u>" to, even though you are uncertain about just when that might be. Cancer, in this comparative sense, is likened to "nature running amok": a frenzied, uncontrollable state of affairs symptomatic of events such as the case here—a rich natural environment for growth (e.g., dark, wet, and warm)—or even natural disasters such as floods, hurricanes, or, avalanches.

Marked with agreement and a sigh acknowledging dad's depiction ("= Yeah pt .hhhh <u>huh</u> o:<u>ka</u>::y", line 17), it is the inevitability and inherent uncertainty of mom's progressive illness that son is responding to. And with repeated dysfluency, indicating a troubled orientation to the circumstances they are faced with, son invokes a figurative expression about unpacking his bags yet remaining vigilant by stating "keep my lesson plans current" (see Excerpt 10, Chapter 7).

Protecting Mom from "the good ol' doctor"

The topic of mom's receiving radiation is addressed four calls later, as aunt (mom's sister) further speculates that the doctor may (or may not) offer "answers" about how long she think mom might have to live. Unlike Excerpt 8 (above), however, son does not provide a negative comment about doctor's unwillingness to offer a prognosis. Rather, he acknowledges (line 7), with some uncertainty, aunt's lay conclusion that a doctor's decision to radiate demonstrates a belief that mom has "↑ more <u>ti::me</u>." (lines 5-6):

10) SDCL: Malignancy #16:7-8

1		Aunt:	And maybe by today we'll have some <u>kind</u> of answers from
2	→		<u>Doctor</u> (name), as to (.) ↑ jus' <u>how</u> long ↓ she thinks she's go:t.
3			I don't know.
4		Son:	.hh[hhh]
5		Aunt:	[If s]he's gonna ↑<u>rad</u>iate then, she thinks there's ↑ more
6			<u>ti::me</u>.
7		Son:	↑ Yeah ap<u>par</u>ently. .hh
8		Aunt:	Either tha:t or she's going to <u>deci:de</u> there- or she's jus- (.)
9	→		ya know <u>play</u>ing the (.) .hhh the <u>good</u> ol' <u>doctor</u> let's keep 'er
10			goin' as long as we <u>ca:n</u> at which point I will <u>see</u> to it that she
11			has a change of mind. =

```
12    Son:    = Mm: hm. hh (.) .hh[h]
13    Aunt:                      [I] ca:n't sta:n:d to watch your mom
14            suffer.
15    Son:    ↓ N:o hh .h[hh] Well.
16    Aunt:              [e i]
17    Aunt:   It ain't- it ain't in me.
18    Son:    If there's- if there's any (0.6) significant change in
19            information.
20            (0.2)
21    Aunt:   Honey,=
22    Son:    = Let me know. [hhh]
23    Aunt:                  [you] will be the >f:ir:st (.) person< (.) I call.
24    Son:    ↑ O:kay.
25    Aunt:   O↑ka:y:?
```

By linking together a treatment procedure with a doctor's belief, it is evident that aunt is attempting to figure out what doctor is thinking from actions taken to radiate mom's tumors. Left unspecified are just what "↑ more ti::me." consists of, and the often complex relationships between radiating to prolong life vs. provide comfort to mom as her cancer progresses (i.e., by shrinking particular tumors, thus easing pain). As aunt continues (lines 8-11), an alternative line of action is attributed to the doctor: That she will play "the good ol' doctor"—in this instance, a stereotype of a doctor whose voiced position is "let's keep 'er goin' as long as we ca:n". This typecasted, categorical depiction is not offered by aunt as actual reported speech of the doctor. Rather, aunt provides a critique of reasoning and decision-making associated with prolonging life for no good lay reason, positions that may stand in start contrast to what is constructed as traditional biomedical decision making.

By no means complimentary, aunt formulates an oppositional stance as a staunch defender of mom's rights and stated preferences: "at which point I will see to it that she has a change of mind. =" (lines 10-11). Unequivocally, aunt announces her commitment to confront the doctor—to put her in her place—if and when the "the good ol' doctor" attempts to use her medical authority to keep mom alive beyond whatever mom and family might consider appropriate. The exact point at which appropriate or inappropriate medical care is imposed is also left unspecified. But as son affiliates with aunt's defensive stance, a critical issue is made apparent: "[I] ca:n't sta:n:d to watch your mom suffer." (lines 13-14), which son next and again aligns with as aunt further states "It ain't- it ain't in me." (line 17). This bottom-line concern and personal disclosure that she simply cannot tolerate unnecessary suffering assumes ownership of the epistemic right and need to be not just her sister's advocate, but a faithful protector. The adversary, in this instance, is a known doctor whose actions may be contrary to mom and family members' wishes. The consequence is unwise and possibly incompetent medical care, the very kind of care that negative depictions of "good ol' doctor(s)" may seek to provide. Certainly, references to "good ol' doctor(s)" may also be quite positive (e.g., as when describing the personal care offered by doctors in an endearing fashion). But the case built here by aunt is one anchored in protecting her sister from a doctor that might keep mom alive beyond her (and family members') wishes.

Aunt's personalized claim to protect her sister is basically not addressed by son. As noted, his "↓ N:o" (line 15) aligns with avoiding mom's suffering. But son then immediately shifts away from further discussion about aunt's concerns to requesting that he be updated should "any (0.6) significant change in information" (lines 18-19) occur. This topical shift does not disregard aunt's stance in opposition to the doctor. Nor does it provide stronger confirmation of aunt's epistemic claim for authority, for example, by more actively affirming aunt's concerns or extending discussion by disclosing his own concerns about prolonging mom's life.

In response, it is with an endearing "Honey,=" (line 21) that aunt reassures son that he will be the first person she will call. As son has just shifted away from aunt's fervent position-taking against the doctor, this is one way for aunt to address, even compensate for, son's lack of uptake. She ensures son's importance, yet by so doing also retains her epistemic access to updated news. These actions further establish her claimed role of centrality to the primary business of monitoring and managing mom's care, which son acknowledges but does not fully confirm. Such contrasting orientations reveal how the negotiation of family roles, and the authority claimed to establish primary responsibilities, are often subtle but delicate matters when working together to cope with ongoing illness.

Attributing Knowledge to Doctors

Just as doctors' authority may be challenged on a number of grounds by family members, so too may doctors be treated by family members as more knowledgeable than patients they are caring for. Below, dad appears to be contrasting what prior doctors have said about mom's release from the hospital (lines 1-4), with opinions of two additional doctors—one of whom, dad reported, "↓ said °she was in no shape° to come home." (line 6):

11) **SDCL: Malignancy #25:3-4**

```
 1     Dad:   But you know they're keepin her as comfortable as they can.
 2            But (.) there's no way she's comin' home right now that I can
 3  →         see, cause the doctors have said you know maybe she'd come
 4  →         home Friday. But (1.0) both of the doctors (.) hers Doctor
 5            (name 1) and (name 2) was the one I talked to Wednesday
 6            ↓ said °she was in no shape° to come home.
 7     Son:   Mm hm:::.
 8     Dad:   So. =
 9     Son:   = Okay well. =
10     Dad:   = Today I'll pop in and she'll go I'm ready.
11     Son:   Shhh:.
12     Dad:   Um (0.4)I don't th[in:k  so.]
13  → Son:                     [ Believe] the doctors $before you believe
14            her.$ =
15     Dad:   = Oh yeah yeah.
16     Son:   If you'd believe her she would've been dead already huh.
17     Dad:   Well yep. (0.8) A couple of times I figured that was pretty
18            close. =
19     Son:   = Mm hm:::.
20     Dad:   °It hasn't worked out that way so far.° So: okay fine, we'll take
21            it.
22     Son:   Okay.
```

Dad's initial "**they're/they**" (line 1) occur as plural references made to a medical team, persons coordinating their actions to ensure mom's comfort. It is not known whether dad can identify particular team members nor the specific tasks they perform. However, dad's shift to the "**doctors** have said" (line 3) occurs in unison with his ability to report what doctors have stated. Similarly, dad's following "**doctors/Doctor**" (line 4) are deployed in the context of referring to specific individuals, "both...one I talked to" (lines 4-5). From these few instances, then, it is clear that "**Doctor/doctors**" are used in reference to known others who dad has heard speak and/or spoken directly with.

Dad then proceeds to contrast doctor's professional judgment with mom's own evaluation: "= Today I'll pop in and she'll go I'm ready." (line 10). This reporting of yet another routine hospital visit by dad is offered as though mom is acting independently from doctors' evaluations. As son's initial "Shhh:." response (line 11) indicates and previews, both dad and son (lines 12-15) cast doubt on mom's ability to adequately assess her own condition for release. Explicitly formulated by son with "[Believe] the **doctors** $before you believe her.$ =", he initiates shared laughter which dad does not provide. Dad's "= Oh yeah yeah." does, however, strongly agree with son's assessment while also reasserting his first-hand, epistemic knowledge (see Heritage, 2002): A position that mom's "I'm ready." was, indeed, not to be believed. And just as dad and son had collaborated in formulating doctors' opinions as more believable than mom's, so too does son next provide further evidence of mom's faulty reasoning. He proceeds to make reference to statements mom had made in the past, namely, that she would soon die. As alluded to by son, if what mom stated in the past were true she'd be "dead already" (line 16)—an outcome that, of course, had not yet occurred.

As this excerpt comes to a close, a delicate and potentially despairing moment is addressed and managed. With "A couple of times I figured that was pretty close" (lines 17-18), dad slightly disaffiliates with son by clarifying that mom's assessment (that she would soon die) had not been totally awry. On the cusp of addressing mom's dying, dad's softly spoken "°It hasn't worked out that way so far.°" leaves unstated, but hints at, mom's condition as tenuous, evolving, yet nevertheless terminal. Immediately balanced with "So: okay fine, we'll take it", dad offers a resigned and even thankful recognition that whatever time remaining with mom is appreciated.

In these touching moments the dialectics of despair and hope are once again intertwined. But in this instance, the shift toward hope is modified by resignation—an acceptance that mom's death is imminent, making the value of time together something to "take" whenever and however provided. As is evident, simply believing doctors' rather than mom's opinion, that she is ready to leave the hospital and come home, in no way dismisses the intimate and familial bonds with a mother and wife.

Offering Advice about "that dipshit doctor"

Prior to the final excerpt for this chapter, son had been discussing with his ex-wife and her brother (Mike) the recent cancer diagnosis of their dad. Relying on his experience with the uncertainty associated with mom's cancer journey, son acknowledges the "big question mark" everybody must be experiencing (lines 2-3). He then produces a revealing utterance (lines 3-5), comprised of three interrelated features: (a) a bottom-line assessment of "what this really means"; (b) an "I hope to hell" reference,[4] previewing son's wish that the subsequent and upcoming trouble he is wary of is being avoided; and (c) "that dipshit **doctor** that's .hh [they always go to.]":

12) **SDCL: Malignancy #39: 6-7**

```
1    Son:   pt .hh I don't know (.) hh at this point what else to think 'cuz
2           there's .hh ya know .hh everything is kind of a big question
3           mark at this point I'm sure fer everybody. .hh As to what
4           this really means I hope to hell he's not going to that dipshit
5    →      doctor that's .hh [they always go to.]
6    Mike:                    [Well  mom said s]omething about suing
7           him.
8    Son:   .hhh  hh Yeah well see part of my concern is that if he's been
9    →      goin' to that dipshit doctor an' he's had this for a year like
```

```
10 →              my mother did .hh heh an' ya know the doctor hasn't
11                figured it out then that could be a problem.
12    Mike:       They said it's as big as a walnut.
13    Son:        Oh okay .hh well.
14                (0.7)
15    Mike:       Anyways.
16    Son:        Yeah. I mean they can .h they can do ch- chemo. They can
17                do radiation with so[mething like that they might do surgery.
18    Mike:                           [(                                      )
19                Well they said the first option is to remove the lung.
20    Son:        Mm hm.
21    Mike:       If the other one can (.) live on it's own.
22    Son:        Well ya know John Wayne had that done.
23    Mike:       Mm hm.
```

In lines 1-5, son's utterance treats the very possibility of a bad doctor, the one "they always go to" (line 5), as a fundamental and critical issue to be steered away from. Son treats the importance of avoiding this doctor as even more significant than the uncertainty son had just referred to. His negative critique triggers Mike's report that his mom "said something about suing him." (lines 6-7). As son's "dipshit doctor" triggered Mike's reference to "suing", it can be seen that a derogatory characterization of a medical expert can also function as a lay criterion for malpractice claims. In addition to technical incompetence and medical errors, poor relationship skills and the inability to foster empathic, trusting relationships have been determined to be primary predictors for malpractice claims (e.g., see Suchman, Markakis, Beckman, & Frankel, 1997).

Just what son means is clarified as his elaboration next confirms Mike's reporting, repeats "dipshit doctor", and likens their dad's treatment during the past year to his mom's, where "the doctor hasn't figured it out" (lines 9-11). With Mike's "They said it's as big as a walnut." (line 12), he demonstrates son's prior concern with a failure to provide early detection for cancer. Treated as news by son in line 13 (but not overly surprising information), he immediately relies on his background understandings about mom's illness—provided by dad in call #1, but now utilized by son as a basis for his own epistemic authority to speak on the topic—to list medical experts' treatment options as chemo, radiation, or surgery. And when Mike reports that they "said the first option is to remove the lung" (line 19), son turns to another dimension of his stock of knowledge, namely, "Well ya know John Wayne had that done." (line 22).

PREOCCUPATIONS WITH DOCTORS,
MEDICAL STAFF, AND EPISTEMIC AUTHORITY

It is not surprising that family members routinely offer positive and negative assessments of medical experts, their procedures, as well as the bureaucracies and institutions they work within. A series of relevant instances have been examined in this chapter, including moments where medical professionals are put in their place and family members have exhibited being frustrated with:

- A large, impersonal hospital as grounds for rationalizing a longer drive to ensure mom's comfort from a particular doctor;
- The imposition and inconvenience of needle biopsies, as well as an implied lack of consultation with the family about those procedures;

- The length of time, delay, and focusing on trivial matters;
- Looming uncertainties about the constant adjustments made by medical staff to prolong mom's life, actions that may well go against the expressed wishes of mom and family;
- A doctor's (stereotyped) unwillingness to offer a specific prognosis and/or avoid prolonging mom's life unnecessarily;
- A "dipshit" and apparently incompetent doctor, involved in diagnosing and treating son's ex-wife's dad for cancer, who couldn't figure out what the "problem" might be.

Also examined were a smaller but no less important collection of moments when family members offer praise and support for doctors and medical staff who:

- Are worth a longer drive to ensure mom's comfort, especially when mom likes the doctor, who cares for her in ways mom (and family) cannot;
- Are competent and personable, organized and capable of enacting specific and appropriate treatment plans;
- Do the best they can predicting uncertain futures, because they do not have "an educated crystal ball";
- Keep mom as comfortable as possible and should be believed (more than mom) about mom's condition and ability to be released to her home;
- Are a source of hope when seeking additional information and assurance.

Marbled throughout these family members' discussions, of what they like and dislike about medical care, are repeated moments when efforts are made by speakers to invoke knowledge as a basis for their actions. These *social epistemics* represent a series of often delicate moments comprised of actions such as claiming, restricting, granting, correcting, and bolstering the right to act authoritatively on matters relevant to mom's cancer care. The following Chapter 10 extends the attention drawn to epistemics since the first data excerpt in Chapter 3 (i.e., between dad and son). Additional key moments are analyzed involving the use of few words, in the midst of achieving the interactional work of sharing commiserative space.

NOTES

1. Dad's "↑ ho:ly Christ" offers yet another example of invoking the deity, and clearly in a troubling circumstance, over which there is little control, and in need of an alternative and more comforting remedy. His intoned and emphasized "↑ ho:ly" adds further impetus to his frustration—a sacred plea for intervention against procedures unduly imposing pain or discomfort upon mom. As a caregiver, dad's position is forwarded as both protective and, as he continues, justifiable.
2. The assessments reported by aunt and dad are reasonably accurate—mom died in November, prior to Thanksgiving:

   SDCL: Malignancy #10: 11

Son:	= I- I keep wo:ndering (.) if we can even (.)
	re:alistically think about <u>Thanksgiving</u>.
	[.hhh ahhh]
Aunt:	[I don't kn:ow.]
Son:	And right now >it sure doesn't sound that way <u>does</u> it?< =
Aunt:	= <u>No</u> it doesn't sound that [way.] =
Son:	[No.]

> Aunt: But the:n (0.4) .hhh ya kn:ow (.) your mom's tough.
> Son: Um hm.

3. Numerous and complex relationships among stability and ambiguity and the inherent flux of cancer journeys are addressed in Chapter 6. Son's frustrations and confusions are altogether common and perhaps most apparent in debates and controversies surrounding "right to life" and "euthanasia". Though not addressed here in any detail, the communicative dimensions of these societal dialogues are addressed by Hyde (2001).

4. Son's "I hope to hell", a colloquial expression, offers an interesting twist on more typical invocations of hope (see Chapters 12 & 13). Though certainly unconsciously produced, son displays a wish that by sending a negative possibility to "hell", it may not impact what might otherwise be a more positive outcome (i.e., working with a better doctor).

V

ENDURING AND ENDEARING
MOMENTS ACROSS CALLS

10

"SH:I:T...YEAH $I KNOW.$"

Sharing Commiserative Space and Claiming Epistemic Authority

Reporting about difficult moments, speakers often state some version of"I just didn't know what to say." Family members in the Malignancy corpus repeatedly display that very few words are available for expressing thoughts and feelings about cancer circumstances. At particular moments, there is little else to say about the events they are entangled within. Mom (as cancer patient) and impacted family members (e.g., dad, son, aunt/mom's sister, Gina/ex-wife), exhibit difficulty putting into words just how trying and perplexing it is to be confronted with and manage the realization that they are in the very midst of experiencing the angst of cancer. Marked by social actions such as response cries (e.g., "Shit", "Oh boy", "Phew", "This sucks", "Yuck"), extended silences, and abbreviated responses (e.g., "Yeah", "I know", "Yeah I know", "You're right, it's yuck"), speakers demonstrate the cumulative impact and trouble cancer has created (and is creating) in their lives.

Though minimal in length, analysis of these brief verbal exchanges reveal complex and significant social actions comprised of two primary features: (a) *Sharing commiserative space* involves providing empathic and aligning responses, designed to exhibit understanding and appreciation for what each other is experiencing. Though few words are all that are available, family members demonstrate being in and affected by the realities they are facing together; and (b) In moments of otherwise joint commiseration, family members also *claim epistemic authority* by staking out territory:

- Who knows and experiences what, and more, about cancer circumstances?
- Who is in a primary position to report on and care for mom and other family members?

There is an inherent dialectical tension, therefore, as speakers simultaneously orient toward being with one another yet independently capable of experiencing, knowing, and thus assessing (or not) different events associated with mom's cancer (see Beach, 2003c; Heritage, 2002; Heritage & Raymond, 2005; Pomerantz, 1984a; Raymond & Heritage, 2006; Stivers, 2005). These contrasting orientations occasion the ongoing management of "territorial preserves" (Heritage & Raymond, 2005):

> By examining how such rights to knowledge and action are shared by speakers, or how they are distributed among them, or how they might be violated, and how they are used

to establish agreement, or how they might be used to foster conflict, we can begin to identify how identities are produced and reproduced in specific episodes of interaction. (p. 47)

Consider a basic instance, occurring during son's phone call with mom, when he first spoke with her about being diagnosed with cancer (see Chapter 4). Mom is in the hospital and is not only diagnosed with a serious cancer but, though son is unaware, already beginning to undergo treatment for cancer. The following exchange occurs approximately two minutes into the phone call:

1) SDCL: Malignancy #2:3

```
1      Son:    .hh hhh (.) Whadda you do: with this kind of thing. I mean-
2              (.)
3      Mom:    >Radiation chemotherapy.<
4  →          (1.4)
5  →   Son:    Oh bo:y?
6  →   Mom:    Yeah.
```

With extended silence followed with "Oh bo:y?" in line 4, son treats mom's initial response to his query (line 3) with hesitation, surprise, and a realization that he is in a position to recognize the serious nature of mom's condition. There is something remarkable about mom's response and dilemma that has triggered son's response cry. As previously discussed in Chapter 4, that mom does not respond to son's prior query by discussing personal coping, but rather biomedical treatment solutions, may well contribute to son's delayed and affective response. In line 5, his "Oh bo:y?" response cry (Goffman, 1981; Good & Beach, 2005; Goodwin & Goodwin, 2000; Wilkinson & Kitzinger, 2006) addresses the dilemma mom is confronting, including the basic fact that she is now faced with experiencing treatments, that is, regimens commonly known to be employed to reduce, slow down, and possibly eliminate tumor and cancer growth that are not without side-effects. In this way, son's "Oh bo:y?" not only exhibits his own recognition, but offers alignment by orienting to mom's predicament as remarkable and troubling. Though his "Oh"-preface displays a "change of state" in his orientation and some independent ability to assess mom's predicament (Heritage, 2002), son is not in a position to know exactly what mom is experiencing.

In response, mom's "Yeah." (line 6) achieves more than agreement with the actions achieved through son's "Oh bo:y?". In second position, she also asserts her ability (as cancer patient) to more fully realize the impacts of diagnosis and treatment. Although son can and did offer surprise and even dreaded comprehension of the seriousness of mom's illness, mom claims the superiority of her right to know. As the person whose ill body and experiences are intertwined, her "Yeah." simply (and elegantly) stakes out a territory of knowledge that son cannot bring into play.

There are, then, repeated moments when family members come together to commiserate about their shared problems, but also mark out distinct territories unique to their lifeworlds. In the ways speakers organize these moments interactionally, sharing commiserative space should not be understood as devoid of the routine affairs inherent to managing roles, status, authority, and territories of knowledge comprising family relationships. Ironically, it is in the very midst of what appears as "commiserating together" that inherently delicate and (at times) even conflicting orientations are displayed by interactants:

As family members routinely enact their identities, it becomes evident that how these parties deploy resources for managing epistemic primacy and subordination reflects what appears to be a basic dilemma of self-other relations. . . . This dilemma appears to be a direct product of participants' management of their intersubjective grasp of the world, the relationship they build with one another based on that intersubjective grasp, and their simultaneous insistence on the independence of their access to the events under discussion . . . what we might term the "distance-involvement" dilemma in constructing intimate self-other relations generally. In acts of affiliation, persons must manage the twin risks of appearing disengaged from the affairs of the other, or over-involved and even appropriating of them. (Raymond & Heritage, 2006, pp. 47-48)

Excerpt 1 (above) and others, examined in more detail throughout this chapter, reveal how inherent difficulties exist when being caught up within unfortunate and uncertain matters regarding illness. Such events and possibilities, though not easily controlled, must nevertheless be interactionally managed as resources for coping with the moment-by-moment contingencies of cancer (and certainly other illness) journeys. Family member make available to one another that, as a consequence of gradually assimilating and absorbing bad cancer news, there exists a fundamental inability to say much, or talk further then and there, about dealing with additional bad news. As noted, few words are all that get utilized in such difficult moments. Yet these moments are dense with key social actions speaking directly to the "distance-involvement" dilemma described above. It is within these brief and passing moments that the shared, yet distinct life worlds of speakers are evident and consequential for shaping both the dynamics of family life and the inevitable unfolding of a progressive cancer journey.

This chapter will first focus on three extended discussions from calls #1 (between dad and son), #2 (between mom and son), and #10 (between son and aunt/mom's sister). From these longer involvements, a collection of shorter excerpts (such as Excerpt 1, above) will be extracted and analyzed in detail, as will moments from an assortment of other calls throughout the Malignancy corpus. These moments further exemplify patterns that emerge whenever speakers share commiserative space yet simultaneously claim epistemic authority. This collection of moments will be employed as resources for addressing the following questions:

- What are the constituent features of moments where very few words are spoken?
- How does "Who is being affected more by the cancer journey?" get played out interactionally?
- Stated somewhat differently, how do family members assert and claim the rights to more direct experiences and consequences of bad cancer news?
- How do speakers (particularly the son) rely on response cries as resources for affectively responding to prior (triggering) depictions of cancer circumstances?
- How do recipients of response cries claim primary knowledge about the events being managed, and further account for the relevance of events as remarkable?
- What relationships exist between commiseration and epistemic claims of cancer impact?
- Why and how do these types of interactions occur during topical transitions from bad to good news?

LOCATING A SEQUENTIAL ENVIRONMENT
FOR 'SHARING COMMISERATIVE AND EPISTEMIC SPACE

The next instance to be analyzed (Excerpt 2, below) occurs during phone call #1, several minutes following dad's informing son (in Excerpt 1, above) that "It is: malignant." (see Chapter 3). The delivery and receipt of news is routinely followed with further elaboration about the events and circumstances constituting the news (typically, mom's and thus the family's condition). It is at or near the termination of what Maynard (1997, 2003) described as Post-Assessment Elaborations (PAE's) that these moments, comprised of relatively few words, normally occur (see Figure 10.1).

Speakers orient to sequence and topical closings, at or near transitional attempts to shift from bad to good news, in a number of related ways: (a) Displaying that few words are sufficient, indeed all that may be available, to express shared concerns, experiences, and knowledge about the cancer journey; (b) Owning the impacts of cancer; and (c) Claiming epistemic authority and superiority about the events being assessed. Together, speakers demonstrate being involved in and impacted by the news. They also claim being differentially, and at times more impacted by the news, than other speaker/family member.

The following instance provides an example of the overall sequential environment within which speakers work together to assess and shift from bad to good topics. Following dad's initial delivery and son's receipt of mom's cancer news (NDS/Chapter 3), dad proceeds to elaborate (PAE) on mom's condition and treatment options for approximately three minutes. This elaboration was replete with technical details and a cumulative sketch of an unknown, but potentially dreaded, future. In lines 1-7 (below), dad addresses yet further uncertainties about whether mom's cancer may have spread and the possibility that the family must await results from the "bo:ne scan":

2) SDCL: Malignancy #1:7-8

1	Dad:	[But] ya know it's a very <u>slo::</u>w growing thing. So if it is sti:ll
2		in <u>tha:t</u> fa:mily of (.) of cancer then ya say >well okay.< It's
3		<u>un</u>likely it's anyplace <u>else</u>. = They can just treat these two bu-
4		pt .hh (0.3) .hhh But °that we won't know° ah- at least 'til
5		tomorrow and may not have the results of the bo:ne scan
6		back til Monday. = >I don'(t) know how long it takes ta get
7		that back.<
8 →	Son:	°Hm:.° pt .hhh Oh <u>bo:y</u>.
9 →	Dad:	A::hh ye:ah: hhhhh (.) <u>But</u> she seemed to be doing (.) as I said
10		pt .hh at this point it was mostly (0.2) <u>co:n</u>firmation and
11		resignation.
12	Son:	[Mmhmm:.]
13	Dad:	['Cause she] said, .hhh I just hurt too <u>b:ad</u> to be anything else
14		(.) >ya know.< It <u>ha::d</u> to be som- (0.4) <u>some</u>thing drastic.
15 →	Son:	Mmhm.
16	Dad:	And she was really having some problems with pa:in today.
17		She had .hh one and a half (0.2) ><u>perco</u>dans< in her and it
18		wasn't hardly slowin' it down.
19 →	Son:	°Mmm wow.°
20 →	Dad:	**.hhh <u>But</u> (0.2) she did have two nice things ha:ppen today.**
21		She was on her way <u>do:wn</u> and .hhh and was ↑kinda <u>de</u>pressed
22		or con<u>cer:</u>ned I guess with having >to go down< for these needle
23		biopsies and ↑<u>Bi</u>ll showed up.

It is in response to further delays that son reflectively considers, then responds with "Oh <u>bo:y</u>." (line 8). Goodwin (1996, p. 394) describes how response cries emerge in particular interactional environments:

[Triggering Event] + [Response Cry] + [Elaborating Sentence]

News Delivery Sequence (NDS) → Post-Assessment Elaboration (PAE) →
Sharing Commiserative Space → Claiming Epistemic Authority →
Topic Termination and Transitions

TIE: Topic Initial Elicitor (e.g., How's things?)
INI: Itemized News Inquiry (e.g., Is something up?)
↓
1. Announcement
2. Response
3. Elaboration
4. Assessment
↓
Post-assessment Elaboration (PAE)
↓

Sharing Commiserative Space and Claiming Epistemic Authority:
Resources for doing the work of expressing and closing down difficult topics.
Speakers' methods for displaying that there is much to say, but few words
are needed or available to express shared and individual experiences.

↓
Topic Transition & Termination
↓
Hope/Bright Side Sequences

Figure 10.1. Overall Sequential Environment: Situating the Co-Occurrence of "Sharing Commiserative Space" and "Claiming Epistemic Authority"

Although this basic pattern can vary depending on the participation frameworks being examined,[1] some triggering event prompts a speaker's next response cry, followed by post-cry elaboration that further accounts, justifies, and/or explains that the prior triggering event merits such a "response cry" reaction. As Goodwin (1996) has observed, "The occurrence of the response cry thus locates (or at least notes the existence of) some other event and formulates it in a particular way, i.e. as something that has the power to elicit strong reaction visible in the cry" (p. 394).

As noted, the triggering event above—the spreading of cancer and further delay of bone scan results—gives rise to son's response cry. In turn, dad does not immediately elaborate but responds with "A::hh ye:ah: hhhhh" (line 9). As with Excerpt 1 (above), dad agrees and aligns with son's "Oh bo:y." assessment. But his response is comprised of three notable features: (a) He also offers his own and extended reflection ("A::hh"), (b) a stretched "ye:ah:", and (c) an emphasized aspiration ("hhhhh"), hearable in two related ways: (a) as frustration and/or impatience with the ambiguities and uncertainties emerging from mom's cancer; and (b) as dad's having not only already considered the circumstances triggering son's response cry, but managed the on-site details of mom's diagnosis, testing, and (at present) unspecified prognosis. It is these experiences, and the hands-on knowledge generated by being with mom in the home and hospital settings, that dad expresses through his immediate response to son's response cry. In these ways, dad personalizes and enacts ownership of more direct access to events being depicted—events that he (and not son) can report directly on—and thus claims the rights to more fully and authoritatively speak from his unique lived experience.

With "Oh bo:y." son offers a "relevant display of emotion with minimal lexical resources. . . . The very simple lexical and syntactic structure of Response Cries masks a more elaborate grammar of practice" (Goodwin & Goodwin, 2000, p. 18). So too is this the case with dad's next "A::hh ye:ah: hhhhh", an abbreviated but revealing response. Together, these paired actions exemplify an efficient, even elegant packaging of emotional impact. At the root of both son's response cry and dad's tailored response is the ability to claim experiences legitimating the stance of each speaker whose life has been negatively influenced by mom's diagnosis and treatment (i.e., a consequential family member):

> Central to the organization of Response Cries is a particular kind of experience that requires appropriate access to the event being responded to . . . the party producing the Response Cry is making an embodied assessment of something they know in a relevant way [requiring] appropriate access before producing a response that agrees with an assessment just made by his co-participant [requiring] specific kinds of experience and forms of access to the entities being assessed. (Goodwin & Goodwin, 2000, pp. 16-19)

In lines 9-14 (Excerpt 2, above), immediately following dad's "A::hh ye:ah: hhhhh", further evidence is provided that the attention being given to events surrounding mom's care are indeed justified. Dad continues by describing mom's general orientations as "mostly (0.2) co:nfirmation and resignation" (lines 10-11). He then moves to directly report on what mom said: "I just hurt too b:ad to be anything else (.) >ya know< It ha:d to be som- (0.4) something drastic." (lines 13-14). Incrementally, dad recruits mom's own voice as a resource for speaking about pain and a "drastic" discernment—epistemic knowledge dad himself did not have access to, except as a hearer, who now invokes mom's depiction to further validate and account for the reasonableness of son and dad's present actions.

Both son and dad, then, rely on their own specific experiences to assess what they know to be troubling (frustrating, ambiguous, uncertain) about the testing mom is undergoing, including the dreaded possibilities of what such testing might reveal (see Peräkylä, 1993, 1995). In mom's absence, her voice is personified by dad to characterize her sense, as a wounded storyteller (see Chapter 4), that something "drastic" was wrong with her health and well-being. In these ways, whoever knows more (and more directly) about what is actually occurring, in mom's life as well as his/her own, establishes a family hierarchy regarding the cancer journey: Mom to dad to son.[2] With this lens in mind, it is more clearly understood that son's response cry was fully justified in its own right. So too is dad's next assertion equally warranted, conveying yet more authority to speak on these matters. Even as a conduit for reporting what he had heard mom say, dad is able to relay information not otherwise available to a concerned son—a person who simply did not have access to events (and thus experiences and knowledge) possessed by dad and mom. In practice, speakers in ordinary and extraordinary circumstances work out what is accessible, and thus reportable, moment by moment.

Returning to Excerpt 2 (above), it is important to notice that following dad's report of mom sensing "somethin drastic", with "Mmhm" (line 15) son continues to monitor and facilitate dad's ongoing telling. But as dad further elaborates mom's "pa:in today"—so bad that a strong dose of medications "wasn't hardly slowin' it down."—son responds with a quiet "°Mmm wow.°":

3) SDCL: Malignancy #1:8

   19 → Son: °Mmm wow.°
   20 → Dad: **But** (0.2) she did have two nice things ha:ppen today.

Son's response cry, though quietly offered, is no less potent as an expression of impact. Rather, it appears that further details about mom's suffering overwhelmed son's ability to more fully respond or comment. Unfolding information has now become, since the opening News Delivery Sequence of call #1 several minutes earlier, a progressive portent of bad news (Maynard, 1997, 2003). Yet there is additional and more convincing evidence that son's suppressed voice made clear that he had reached a *tolerance threshold* for more bad news. In next turn, dad responds to son by immediately shifting away from further bad news and toward what Holt (1993) has described as bright side sequences: noticeable shifts from bad to good news. In this way, dad treats son's "°Mmm wow.°" as being impacted, but also having made available an inability (and/or unwillingness) to hear yet more details about mom's condition. As recipient, dad thus designed his next turn to avoid further elaboration about mom's pain. He pursues an explicit focus on "two nice things" that happened today in her life, a bright and hopeful set of events that begins to counter the prior (and residual) consideration of inherently bad news.

Small and otherwise unrecognized utterances, such as son's "°Mmm wow.°", can and do have significant impacts on how next speaker might change topics and direction in conversation.[3] In the instances above, and as the pendulum of joint attention swings, this shift might be roughly characterized as momentarily moving from despair to hope (see Chapters 12 and 13). The occurrence and predominance of bad news events does not entirely preclude drawing attention to other, more positively valenced, happenings in everyday life.

MOVING IN AND OUT OF COMMISERATIVE AND EPISTEMIC SPACE

The second and extended instance (below, 2:42 in length) is included in its entirety for several reasons. First, readers will gain a fuller appreciation of these remarkable, delicate, and reveling moments between mom and son. Second, the overall sequential organization and location of moments involving sharing commiserative space and claiming epistemic authority (bold face, below) can be better understood as situated in ongoing dialogue. Third, from this longer spate of conversation, selected moments will subsequently be drawn out and examined in more detail. So doing allows for better descriptions and explanations of contrasts between mom and son's orientations.

Portions of Excerpt 4 (below) have been analyzed earlier in this chapter (i.e., lines 31-36) as a preview for working with a larger set of instances involving moments when few words (but complex and important social actions) are deployed by speakers. Attention is drawn to these dense and rich involvements in other chapters as well (see Chapters 4, 11, & 12). For example, Chapter 4 examined such matters as how mom begins (lines 1-7) by depicting the extremity of her worst-case scenario, some of the inherent difficulties faced by son when responding to mom's blunt and extreme characterizations of her illness (e.g., lines 11-19), the dialectics of hope and despair (e.g., lines 20-51), mom and son's revealing apologies (lines 49-50), and a preview of the complex relationships between response cries, claiming epistemic knowledge, and *hope* (marked with *→ below and addressed in more detail in following Chapters 12 and 13).

Among the many distinct moments in this excerpt are those when speakers respond to some prior, triggering event as remarkable, even overwhelming, to the point that the ability to say much about those topics is impeded. Five such moments are examined below. These recur in the midst of mom and son being engaged in the work of closing down troubling, and transitioning to related (particularly "hopeful"), topics. Yet in each instance, mom's preoccupation with the serious nature of her illness draws attention back to difficult, tenuous matters:

4) SDCL: Malignancy #2: 2-5

1	Mom:	There's an adenoma type that is uh- °worse°. = But this is
2		<u>very</u> fast very <u>rapid</u>.
3	Son:	Mm hm.
4	Mom:	.hh Ah very difficult to <u>tre</u>:at. = There's a very <u>sma</u>:ll
5		percentage of people that would- that do: uh re:<u>spond</u>?
6		(0.8)
7	Mom:	<u>A</u>:nd we're talkin' uh (0.6) at that maybe five years.
8		(1.5)
9	Son:	H:mm:.
10		(0.6)
11	Mom:	So:, (0.4) it's °<u>r(h)e::al b(h)a:d</u>°. ((voice breaks))
12		(0.8)
13	Mom:	[[((coughs))
14	Son:	[[pt .hhhh I guess.
15		(0.4)
16	Mom:	**And uh: >I don't know what else to ↑tell you.<**
17		(1.0)
18	Son:	.hh hhh Yeah. (0.2) um- ((hhhh)). Yeah, I don't know what
19		to say <u>either</u>.
20 *→	Mom:	**No there's nothing to say.>You just-< .hh I'll wait to**
21		**talk to Dr. Leedon today = he's the cancer man and =**
22	Son:	= Um hmm.
23 *→	Mom:	See what he has to say, and (0.4) just keep goin'forward.
24		I mean- (.) I might be real <u>lucky</u> in five years. It might just
25		be six months.
26		(0.4)
27	Son:	**Yeah.**
28	Mom:	°Who knows.°
29	Son:	pt .hhh Phew::.
30	Mom:	↑Yeah.
31	Son:	.hh hhh (.) Whadda you <u>do</u>: with this kind of thing.
32		I mean- (.)
33	Mom:	>Radiation <u>chem</u>otherapy.<
34		(1.4)
35	Son:	**Oh <u>bo</u>:y?**
36	Mom:	**Yeah.**
37		(0.5)
38 *→	Mom:	My only <u>ho</u>pe- I mean? (.) my only <u>choice</u>.
39	Son:	Yeah.
40 *→	Mom:	It's either that or just lay here and let it <u>kill</u> me.
41		(0.1)
42 *→	Mom:	And that's not the human con<u>dition</u>.
43	Son:	No. (1.0) I guess [not.]
44	Mom:	[No.] (.) So that's all I can tell you
45		(°sweetie.°)
46		(0.8)
47	Son:	.hhh HHHUM.
46		(0.8)
49	Mom:	°Yeah I'm <u>sorry</u>.°
50	Son:	$We<u>ll</u>::$ I should think <u>yeah</u> um- (0.2) Me too.

51	Mom:	°Yeah°.
52	Son:	I guess maybe it's good I didn't know yesterda:y. (1.5)
53		But uh- (0.2) here I was thinkin' (.) gee this medication's sure
54		makin' you depressed.
55		(0.2)
56	Mom:	°Yeah.°
57	Son:	I mean I understood that you would be depressed. But I just
58		thought (.) wo:w. (0.6) .hh This is really- (.) really hittin' you hard
59		this medication. And I got all do:ne and then dad told me.
60		= And I thought (.) well (0.4) .hh The hell with th' medication huh?
61		tsh .hhh =
62	Mom:	= °Yeah.°=
63	Son:	= It's ahh- (.)
64	Mom:	= Yeah. See it's already metastisized. It's already gone
65		°someplace else even?°
66	Son:	Mm hm.
67	Mom:	That's what makes it? >that's partially what makes it< so: (.)
68		ve:ry serious.
69	Son:	Mm hm.
70		(1.4)
71	Son:	.hhh hh
72		(1.2)
73	Son:	pt Sh:i:t. hh
74	Mom:	Yeah $I know.$
75	Son:	$Heh heh.$
76	Mom:	I kno:w.
77 *→	Son:	Well where's our magic wand mom.
78 *→	Mom:	$It- he$ (.) .hh °beats the hell out of me.°
79		(2.2)
80 *→	Mom:	I guess the o:nly thing: (.) I: can do: is (.) after I'm done
81		ree:ling from this,=
82	Son:	Mmhm.
83 *→	Mom:	=.hh is find a reason ot keep fighting and (.) to keep being
84		hopeful. (0.5) You know that- that's about all you can do.
85		>↑That's all a person can do.<
86	Son:	How can you do: that. (0.2) That's [gotta] =
87	Mom:	[We::ll.]
88	Son:	= Be tough. >I mean?< I don't mean to sa:y that sounding like
89		a-
90	Mom:	Here comes your Papa::?
91	Son:	A:hhh.

"it's °r(h)e::al b(h)a:d°...pt .hhhh I guess"

Beginning with line 11, mom provides a bottom-line assessment of her prior description of a very serious diagnosis (see Chapter 4):

5) SDCL: Malignancy #2: 3

11 →	Mom:	So:, (0.4) it's °r(h)e::al b(h)a:d°. ((voice breaks))
12		(0.8)
13	Mom:	[[((coughs))

```
14 →   Son:    [[pt .hhh I guess.
15             (0.4)
16 →   Mom:    And uh:>I don't know what else to ↑tell you.<
17             (1.0)
18 →   Son:    .hh hhh Yeah. (0.2) um- ((hhh)). Yeah, I don't know what
19             to say either.
20 *→  Mom:    No there's nothing to say. ((continues))
```

Mom's "°r(h)e::al b(h)a:d°" offers an apt portrayal of her condition. But her summary, in addition to an incremental pursuit of response from son (see Chapter 4), also reveals an orientation to considerably more emotions. She moves away from describing cancer types, tendencies, and possible prognosis. On the cusp of crying (see Hepburn, 2004), mom progressively personalizes her dilemma by displaying difficulty accepting such bad news. Though it is hard to describe, there is an amalgam of fear, anxiety, and sadness in her voice. In her own, unique way she articulates what she is experiencing in the very course of facing the dire possibilities depicted only moments before. In practice, mom's "°r(h)e::al b(h)a:d°" is similar to providing her own *response cry* to a prior, personalized and dreaded, future. Her utterance is akin to "a natural overflowing, a flooding up of previously contained feeling, a bursting of normal restraints [from being] unable to shape the world the way we want to" (Goffman, 1981, pp. 99,100).

The descriptions mom has offered about cancer, and her voiced realization of just how bad it is, leave son in a precarious position. Here (and in the prior call #1), he exhibits having minimal technical background about cancer, nor personal ability to fully know what mom must be experiencing. His "pt .hhhh I guess." response (see also line 43), following a marked (0.8) pause, reflects his basic inability to offer more than a speculation regarding mom's rather blunt descriptions (see Chapter 4). He is, literally, enacting the stance of only a partially knowing recipient, a family member not in a position to comment more fully on the content, impacts, or implications of mom's prior "°r(h)e::al b(h)a:d°". Beyond what he might "guess", son does not elaborate further about any conjectures he might have. He thus defers to having the ability to assess what mom has presented. This is the case even though son demonstrates being caught up in the emotions mom has exhibited. His voice is audibly shaky, more restrained and less likely to cry than mom, but nevertheless influenced by the affect she made available with "°r(h)e::al b(h)a:d°".

Together, mom and son have reached a juncture where there is apparently little more that can be said. Though mom has provided an extreme case to son, actively pursuing his response through blunt and then personalized characterizations, son has withheld commenting beyond "pt .hh I guess." (line 14). Not surprisingly, then, mom states ">I don't know what else to ↑tell you.<" (line 16). Following (1.0), with son's own aspirated voice near breaking and an attempt to respond that initially fails, he repeats mom's sentiment but from his perspective: "Yeah, I don't know what to say, either." (lines 18-19). In agreement, mom states "No there's nothing to say." (line 20) before moving to talk about her doctor (see Chapter 11).

"pt .hhh Phew::...↑Yeah"

Despite explicitly stating there is nothing more to tell or say, mom only briefly elaborates about the doctor before shifting back to a prior topic: "five years" (line 7). But now she translates a more generic metric (line 7) into "I might be real lucky in five years. It might be just six months." (lines 24-25).[4] Faced with mom's living for five years if she is "lucky", and the indexical "It" referring to dying in "just six months", son pauses (0.4) and simply states "Yeah." (line 27). This is *not* a claim of his own epistemic authority to assess the accuracy of mom's statement. Rather, son acknowledges her ability to reasonably lay out the scope of prognostic possibilities. However, as evident (line 28) with her next "°Who knows.°", produced quietly and reflectively, even mom is uncertain about what the future holds:

6) SDCL: Malignancy #2: 3

```
27   Son:    Yeah.
28   Mom:    °Who knows.°
29   Son:    pt .hhh Phew::.
30   Mom:    ↑Yeah.
```

Triggered by a glimpse into an unknown yet dreaded future, where mom projects six months to five years (at the outset) as the approximate and likely time she has before death, son's "pt .hhh Phew::." (line 29) is a response cry that is quasi-syntactic. Instead of a fully formed and grammatical word, son utters an aspirated "Phew::"—a meaningful and strong reaction to recognizing, with mom but in his own way, what has just emerged as a basic and lingering fact: Mom's diagnosis is not only serious, but fraught with an inevitably vague future. And with "↑Yeah." (line 30), mom makes known that the immediate and ongoing impact *for her* is even greater than what son's "Phew::" has conveyed. It is mom's body that has been invaded with cancer, and her projected (though ambiguous) lifespan that is being discussed. Through a simple shift of intonation (↑), mom's "Yeah" thus offers considerably more than acknowledgment or agreement with son's assessment. More consequentially, she asserts her undisputed right to know and speak about what other family members are caught up in and impacted by, yet cannot experience directly: being a cancer patient whose life is being threatened.

As their conversation continues, lines 31-36 were examined in Excerpt 1 (above). Given the preceding analysis, however, it can now be seen that son's "Oh bo:y?" response cry (line 35) occurs only seconds following his prior "Phew::." (line 29). That two response cries would occur in such close proximity, by the same speaker, even more fully discloses the intensity of the interactional environment mom and son are producing together. His proclivity toward having little to say (as with "I guess" in line 14, and stating he does not know what to say in lines 18-19) is evident. But even when he utters response cries, his strong and emotional orientations are seen as cumulatively impactful. Just as mom evidences a tendency to move back into difficult topics, such as a bad prognosis and how serious her condition really is, so is son progressively triggered to speak minimally, but in very revealing ways, about his experiencing the turmoil that mom has yet deeper access to.

"So that's all I can tell you (°sweetie.°)...(0.8) .hhh HHHUM"

And as with lines 20-23, in lines 38-42 mom again (*→) refers to "hopeful" possibilities (i.e., about radiation and chemotherapy). The pattern discussed previously (see Figure 10.1, p. 215)—of raising and responding to difficult topics → referencing hopeful possibilities → sharing commiserative space and claiming epistemic authority → topic shift—is reified in this environment as well. For example, consider lines 42-52:

7) SDCL: Malignancy #2: 4

```
42 *→  Mom:   And that's not the human condition.
43     Son:   No. (1.0) I guess [not.]
44     Mom:                      [No.] (.) So that's all I can tell you
45            (°sweetie.°)
46            (0.8)
```

```
47      Son:    .hhh HHHUM.
48              (0.8)
49      Mom:    °Yeah I'm sorry.°
50      Son:    $We::ll::$ I should think yeah um- (0.2) Me too.
51      Mom:    °Yeah°.
```

As with line 14 (Excerpt 5, above), in line 43 son can only guess about the position mom has taken regarding the "human condition". Mom's choices about receiving treatments (or not) are treated by son as hers alone, matters she is not seeking advice about but pronouncing as her "only choice." (line 38). Next, mom treats son's inability to comment as sufficient to state, "So that's all I can tell you (°sweetie.°)" (line 44; similar to line 16). Her endearing "(°sweetie.°)" makes clear that she is affectionate toward, and concerned about, the impact of this information on her son. She is capable of tailoring her talk to son as a loved recipient, despite being understandably preoccupied with her own choices and decisions.

Once again, son appears at a loss for words. Following yet another marked (0.8) pause, he offers a loud emotional sigh (but nothing more) in consideration of mom's endearing effort (line 47). As discussed in more detail in Chapter 4, mom's next apology, and son's response, are revealing and paradoxical moments in managing these delicate moments (see also Excerpt 17, below).

"**pt Sh:i:t**. hh... Yeah $I know.$"

In lines 52-61 (Excerpt 4, above) son initiates and elaborates his recollections from "yesterday", a topical shift that redirects attention to mom's medications. In response, mom again (line 64) provides additional bad news about her condition. She does not focus on medication, however, but on the cancer spreading (i.e., "it's already metastasized", line 64):

8) SDCL: Malignancy #2: 5

```
64      Mom:    = Yeah. See it's already metastasized. It's already gone
65              °someplace else even?°
66      Son:    Mm hm.
67      Mom:    That's what makes it? >that's partially what makes it< so: (.)
68              ve:ry serious.
69      Son:    Mm hm.
70              (1.4)
71      Son:    .hhh hh
72              (1.2)
73      Son:    pt Sh:i:t. hh
74      Mom:    Yeah $I know.$
75      Son:    $Heh heh.$
76      Mom:    I kn:ow.
```

Although she adds new information to their conversation, mom's tendency, reenacted here, is to continue to extend a general topic (bad cancer news) both speakers have displayed difficulties talking about. Just as mom and son have repeatedly run out of things to say about such intimidating and perplexing matters, so too does slipping back into (almost closed) topics emerge as a primary preoccupation by mom. These "no close closings" (see Button, 1987, 1990; Sacks, 1992) demonstrate the compelling and complex nature of the diagnosis mom has received from medical experts. Though delicate and difficult to address, these topics are sufficiently critical, and layered with issues, that mom continues to pursue their consideration regardless of their tenuous nature.

The result is one form of an *interactional do-loop* (∞): Speakers cycle in and out of similar topics, entrapped in matters not easily remedied nor terminated, visibly enacting a tendency to discuss again—but with added information or emphasis—what they are interested in, concerned and/or preoccupied with (e.g., see an analysis of "second stories" in Chapter 11). In turn, and predictably, the interaction in lines 69-72 is marked by extended pauses and son's minimally acknowledging, but otherwise saying, nothing. It is in response to mom's further elaborating bad cancer news that son's silence is ended with a poignant response cry: "pt Sh:i:t. hh" (line 73). Voiced with emphasis and audible exasperation, son's expletive bears the brunt of yet additional information that the cancer is spreading (see also Excerpt 15 in Chapter 13).

Though abbreviated, son's "pt Sh:i:t. hh" is not a minor expression of fear or frustration. If the already identified tumors were static, mom and the family could face a serious illness requiring immediate and focused treatment. But the very nature of "metastasis" does not allow for a static or motionless conception of health problems. With the possibility of spreading cancer cells comes the progressive realization, evident in son's response cry, that the mere identification of tumors is only half the battle: Where else has the cancer migrated and colonized? Can such spreading be detected, and halted? When can it be known, *for sure*, that other areas of the body have been invaded (or not)? Is certainty even a possibility when confronting a potentially progressive illness such as cancer? These types of potent questions are, of course, drawn from a much larger set of possible, recurring queries by patients, family members, and medical experts alike.

Son's "pt Sh:i:t. hh" offers more than a recognition that metastasis increases dangers beyond the already serious identification and treatment of tumors. This expletive simultaneously curses the bad news *and* acknowledges a lack of control over such a rogue illness. Just as these orientations are readily available to son as a concerned family member, even more so is mom in a position to move beyond agreeing with son to an explicit claiming of personal impact. With "Yeah $I know.$" (line 74), mom "owns" the problem by upgrading son's already overt position that metastasis amounts to further bad news. Yet by laughing through $I know.$, mom also exhibits her ability to manage these troubles and thus be resistant to the daunting task of dealing with a spreading cancer (Glenn, 2003; Jefferson, 1980a, 1984a,1984b). At this moment she does not discard the capability of facing these challenges. But with laughter, mom invites son to share her troubled yet persistent orientation toward dealing with whatever news emerges. In line 75 son's $Heh heh.$ aligns with mom. He displays hearing and being receptive to mom's invocation of the authority as a claim of personal knowledge, which she next reasserts with "I kno:w." (line 76). As with prior instances (e.g., lines 20-23, 38-42), it is at or near these junctures that mom has shifted to matters related to "hope". Here, son takes the initiative via reference to a "magic wand" (see Chapters 12 & 13), which mom transforms into the task of remaining "hopeful" (line 84).

A REAL RUSSIAN ROULETTE

A series of instances have been examined where speakers deploy few (but potent) words to accomplish primary social actions in family life. Particular events trigger a response cry (or related utterance, such as "°r(h)e::al b(h)a:d°"), actions assessing prior issues as surprising, remarkable, and/or troubling. Agreement and alignment follows from the next speaker, and commiserative space is momentarily shared. Yet it has been shown that a claim of knowledge, revealing authority to speak even more directly about that being assessed, may follow. While these claims are seemingly independent of having just shared commiserative space, they are triggered by such sharing. Or, as with son's "I guess", a speaker may also defer, because he was unable to know just what mom was experiencing. Next, elaborations or accounts emerge, justifying the positions taken as legitimate. These actions, en route to attempts at topical closure, can also give rise to invocations of hope as a transition is made from bad to (comparably) good topics.

In Excerpt 9 (below), this overall sequential structure is once again evident as son and aunt have been discussing his plans for traveling home (see Chapters 5 & 6). With <u>geez</u> <u>w</u>ait." (line 1) and "S:h<u>it</u>." (line 2), son realizes there is a scheduling problem that he has forgotten (see Goodwin, 1987). Son's problem, of arranging for someone to take his class-es, is left hanging in favor of informing aunt that he will call "you guys" (aunt, and/or like-ly dad) to update them of his plans (lines 7-8). In turn, aunt next informs son (lines 9-10) that she and dad will likely be at the hospital (so that he knows where and how to contact them). It is these trials and tribulations of traveling—involving forgotten details, rearrang-ing plans, and staying in contact with one another—that son addresses in line 11:

9) SDCL: Malignancy #10: 7

```
 1    Son:     A̲ctually (.) g̲eez w̲ait.  ] (.) Hang o̲n. (.) .hhh umm
 2             (.) .hhh Couldya- couldya make it- .hhh S:h̲it. See the t̲hing
 3             is (.) .hhh I t̲each at noon, (.) .hhh um-kay (.) .hhh so if
 4             s̲ome̲body is gonna t̲ake my classes tomorrow I gotta get to um
 5             before then.
 6    Aunt:    Okay-
 7    Son:     uhhm .hhh (.) pt-pt .hhh W̲ell ↑ why don't I c̲all (.) you
 8             guys.
 9    Aunt:    And we'll probab- one of us if not b̲oth of us will be at
10             the hospital.
11    Son:     O̲:kay. .hhhhh W̲(h)e̲:ll hh (0.7) J̲e̲:sus this's (.) y̲u̲:cky isn't it.
12    Aunt:    ↑Yeah it is.
13    Son:     U̲:m hhhhhhhh
14             (0.2)
15    Aunt:    And it's a r̲eal R̲uss̲ian r̲oulette.
16    Son:     Yeah. It s̲ure is.
17    Aunt:    Ahhhh
18    Son:     We̲:ll .hhh
19    Aunt:    You could (.) m-well (.) you could c̲all. (0.3) (I was
20             gonna say)you could call the h̲o̲:spital, but then I don't
21             know if that's (.) necessarily wise either.
22    Son:     N̲O. .hhh (.) [ummm]
```

Prefaced as an aspirated sigh, with ".hhhhh W̲(h)e̲:ll hh (0.7)" son momentarily draws his attention away from traveling and reflectively takes stock of the circumstances they are embroiled within. The upshot of his contemplation, "J̲e̲:sus this's (.) y̲u̲:cky isn't it.", neg-atively assesses experiences both aunt and son have access to. Once again, a deity ("J̲e̲:sus") is invoked in the midst of trouble, where events are not fully controlled (and, though spec-ulative, in a situation where some comfort and/or remedy from unsolicited circumstances would clearly be preferred by participants). Previewed by his original "g̲eez" (line 1), both references explicitly mark the unfolding interaction as troubling.

As son states "this's (.) y̲u̲:cky isn't it.", his assessment treats aunt as fully knowing and aware of what he is talking about: "this's" does not articulate details of the challenges they face, nor does the slang "y̲u̲:cky" elaborate on the disgust (or revulsion) inherent in deal-ing with mom's cancer (including traveling under ambiguous circumstances). In response to son inviting aunt's confirmation with "isn't it.", her "↑Yeah it is." aligns but provides more than agreement. With upward intonation and emphasis, she also claims "y̲u̲:cky" as her own. Though son offers little in response (line 13), his next "U:m hhhhhhhh" begins to search for what to say next. However, this action is momentarily abandoned in favor of an extended outbreath, acknowledging the frustration of recognizing—together in shared commiserative space, yet also independently—that the travel, coordination, and overall task of dealing with mom's cancer is a wearisome burden.

Indeed, following a brief pause, aunt extends and further accounts for their shared commiseration by stating "And it's a real Russian roulette." (line 15). Readers familiar with this "game", often depicted during tense movie scenes, will recall that a single bullet is place in the cartridge of a pistol, spun, and placed at the head of an involuntary (and scared to death!) participant. The trigger is pulled, resulting in an empty chamber or an unlucky (and dead) person. If the person is fortunate enough to survive the odds (typically, one in six), successive spins add further suspense to an already tense situation. And so the "game" continues.

In Excerpt 9 (above), both son and aunt have offered assessments ("yu:cky" and "real Russian roulette") that are inclusive of one another yet each, in turn, claims personal knowledge anchored in his/her own experiences and rights as consequential, impacted family members. Son literally includes himself as a family participant in the "roulette" when, as with aunt's earlier "↑Yeah it is.", son replies with his own "Yeah. It sure is." (line 16). Fittingly, aunt's following "Ahhhh" (line 17) offers a final, exasperated utterance summarizing their prior moments together before son ("We:ll .hhh") begins to transition back to the topic of making a phone call, which aunt continues (lines 19-21).

Having already acknowledged how "yu:cky" it is, alternative focus is subsequently given to the inherent uncertainty, anxiety, and potentially lethal outcome of their present lifeworlds. Approximately two minutes later, having just discussed with son whether they believe mom will live until Christmas or even Thanksgiving, aunt again invokes "Russian roulette":

10) **SDCL: Malignancy #10: 11**

```
1  Aunt:  A:nd if it is an- an ya know these are re:al- (.) it's like
2         Russian roulette. =
3  Son:   = Yeah. =
4  Aunt:  =all thi:s guess work.=
```

It is with considerable difficulty (and dysfluency) that mom attempts to describe an uncertain future with "re:al-" consequences, an effort she abandons with "it's like Russian roulette. =" (lines 1-2). Son quickly agrees, and aunt further clarifies that her prior reference amounts to "= All thi:s guess work. =" (line 4). A sharp distinction is thus drawn between "guessing" and "knowing", and it is clear that predicting the death of a loved one is fraught with ambiguity (e.g., see Chapters 4-7).

"It's de:vastating... IT SUCKS!"

Moments before Excerpt 10 (above), following aunt informing son that she would do her best to work with his dad to manage affairs at home (see Excerpt 8, Chapter 11), she reports that "we're do:ing okay." (line 2). This reporting, and offering of assurance to son, is almost immediately contrasted with "= It's de:vastating." (line 4):

11) **SDCL: Malignancy #10: 10**

```
1  Aunt:  [A n d] a- on the way home your dad and I ya know there was a
2         little joking back and forth. (.) We're do:ing- we're do:ing okay.
```

```
 3   Son:     Aright. =
 4   Aunt:    = It's de:vastating. I mean no matter how [you cut it.] =
 5   Son:                                              [ $Ye:ah$. ]
 6   Aunt:    = It's de:vastating. =
 7   Son:     = Yeah.
 8   Aunt:    Ah:- umm (.) We talked about (.) ya know (.) wh- what we
 9            re:ally think about this. And um:: (.) both of us a- agree that
10            tha:t a::h =
11   Son:     = IT SUCKS! [$ heh heh heh heh heh heh heh$]
12   Aunt:                [    (We:ll)        ye::ah,      ] and that's a
13            real sweet way of putting it. =
14   Son:     =Yeah I know.
```

That dad and aunt are able to joke, and "do:ing okay" (line 2), does not alleviate the difficulties of facing cancer as a family. With "I mean no matter how [you cut it.]",[5] aunt self-repairs (see Schegloff, 1992; Schegloff, Jefferson, & Sacks, 1977) by explaining that they are overwhelmed despite reporting doing well. Son's "$Ye:ah$." (line 5) offers agreement but, with laughter, also displays that he is being impacted by these disturbing circumstances. With a repeat of "It's de:vastating." in line 6, aunt emphasizes her assessment and, once again, son's next "Yeah." lays claim to also being distressed.

Son makes clear that the devastation aunt reports experiencing is not hers alone, but his as well. Though it is aunt who next begins to elaborate by reporting what she (and dad/we) "re:ally think about this" (lines 8-9), it is son who interjects by exclaiming "= IT SUCKS! [$ heh heh heh heh heh heh heh heh$]" (line 11). His utterance initiates one form of a *collaborative turn sequence* (see Lerner, 1987, 1989), "a syntactically fitted continuation of the current speaker's utterance-in-progress" (1989, p. 173). Occurring in the very midst of aunt's turn construction, son interrupts at precisely the moment where aunt herself appears to be searching for how to state what aunt and dad agree on ("a::h ="). It is clear that aunt has *not* reached a possible completion point with her utterance, but is on the very cusp of launching into further details about her and dad's perspectives. This is quite a reasonable place for son to interrupt, yet do so in a manner avoiding overlapping and simultaneous talk. What he has secured is a turn-space for offering a frank revelation of *his* unique perspective. With "= IT SUCKS!", son seamlessly exhibits that he is well qualified to finish aunt's thought and thereby lay claim to a slightly delayed, but no less affective, demonstration as a son who is not only devastated but hearably upset. In very lay and practical terms, son translates and upgrades aunt's two prior "It's devastating." references by even more explicitly venting frustration about what it is like to experience and deal with mom's serious cancer. His prior "Yeah." responses (lines 5 & 7) to aunt's assessments were previews of a subsequent and less concealed orientation to being directly affected. And with his following extended laughter (line 11), he at the same time exhibits an ability to be resistant to, and thus manage, the troubles both son and aunt are addressing.

Immediately following "= IT SUCKS!", and in overlap with son's laughter, aunt responds to son's preemptive completion and extends a collaborative turn sequence: "This action is the acceptance or rejection of the preemptive completion as a proper continuation and completion of the pre-empted turn-constructional unit" (Lerner, 1989, p. 173). With "(We:ll) ye::ah that's a real sweet way of putting it.=" (lines 12 & 13), aunt equivocates on acceptance and rejection. Her "(We:ll)" prefaces a disagreement (Pomerantz, 1984a), not with "= IT SUCKS!", but with son's assertion as being stated too "sweetly". In this way, aunt escalates son's own escalation: She stakes out a position that son's interruptive completion was inadequate (i.e., too mild), that the dire circumstances could be depicted even more forcefully (though perhaps less politely), and that *her* experiences allow for such discernment. With "Yeah I know." (line 14), however, son treats aunt's assessment as not being new news. He declares his own recognition that "= IT SUCKS!" is not sufficiently harsh to truly capture the daily challenges of being a family member of a loved one diagnosed with a (terminal) cancer.[6]

SIMILAR PATTERNS, DIFFERENT SPEAKERS

While commiserating about shared difficulties, it appears inevitable that aunt and son also invoke their authority to claim territories of knowledge and experience—routine matters when negotiating roles and identities in family life. In subsequent phone calls, and indeed throughout the Malignancy phone call corpus, specific troubling events trigger varied forms of response cries and/or related affective displays, providing next speakers the opportunity to claim shared (if not more authoritative) knowledge. These matters were framed in previous chapters as interactions exhibiting which speakers are not only more knowledgeable, but experiencing greater impact and thus consequences of being family members (and, as below in Excerpt 14, a cancer patient). For example in Chapter 6 a series of interactions were analyzed between son and Gina (his soon-to-be and eventual ex-wife) as son repeatedly provided updates about mom's condition and his travel plans. These News Delivery Sequences (NDS's) contrasted tenuous relationships between the *stability and ambiguity* associated with mom's illness. In the following two instances, son's descriptions about how mom is doing, are assessed by Gina with similar "Oh my God" response cries:

12) **SDCL: Malignancy #11:1**

```
1    Son:    =↑Not pulling throu::gh but at least s:ta:bilized=an:d
2            of course I can only be gone so: lo:ng.= So .hhh if it
3            looks like she's gonna (.) hang in for another (0.2)
4            couple of wee:ks, then I'll wanna wait a couple of
5            weeks but,=
6    Gina:   =Oh my $G(h)o[::d.$
7    Son:    [Ye:ah ri:ght, .hh uhm, hh So
8            that's in fact< that's what I thought this pho:ne call
9            was,= I'm- I'm waiting, (.) to hear from,=
```

13) **SDCL: Malignancy #18:2**

```
1    Gina:   sta:bilized 'er again.=A:nd ba:sically
2    Son:    We:ll (.) the:y've sta:bilized 'er again.=A:nd ba:sically
3            what they said i:s .hhh keep you're le:sson pla:ns
4            current:, a:n don't unpa:ck your ba:g comple:tely.=But-
5            (.) I don't need ta sho:w up: quite ↑(ch)yet.=So:=
6    Gina:   =< O:h my G(h)o::d. >
7            (0.3)
8    Gina:   You poor thi::ng. hhh
9            (0.4)
10   Son:    pt So tha:t's:=↑really all I can tell ya.
```

In Excerpt 12, son responds with "Ye:ah ri:ght,", claiming personal knowledge as the family member able to report about and experience more directly what mom is going through. He then shifts topics toward whom he is waiting to hear from, further revealing his being caught up with ongoing and (somewhat) urgent matters. Similarly, in Excerpt 13 it is son's initial lack of response to Gina's "= < O:h my G(h)o::d. > ", and her pursuit of response with "You poor thi::ng. hhh", that demonstrates (without explicitly stating) his being in a troubled position not requiring an immediate response. Gina relies on and uses her knowledge that despite all son's efforts to ready himself for travel, these plans are now put on hold, and that this amounts to a very difficult situation. When son does speak, his "pt So tha:t's:=↑really all I can tell ya." (line 10) closely resembles mom's previously analyzed "And uh: >I don't know what else to ↑tell you.<", and "So that's all I can tell you (°sweet-ie°)." (Excerpt 4, lines 16 and 44-45), moments where topical closure is sought by the speaker most frustrated by difficult circumstances.

"Yuck huh...You're right, it's yuck"

Who is in a better position to directly claim personal knowledge about cancer than mom herself? Though each family member experiences the cancer journey in a unique and legitimate matter, only mom is actually dealing with being diagnosed with life-threatening cancer. When contrasting how different family members assert primary knowledge and experience (e.g., when dad informs son of what the doctor told him, son and aunt discuss shared but different experiences about talking with mom, or son informs Gina of mom's changing condition and his travel plans), it is clear that speakers having more direct access to personal experiences are in a position to more authoritatively claim epistemic authority.

In a phone call between son and mom (below), as son queries "What's happening with you?" (lines 3-4), mom replies "Not a <u>stinkin</u> thing that I can think of. They really <u>don't</u> <u>know</u> what's wrong." (lines 5-6):

14) SDCL: Malignancy #28: 1-2

```
 1   Son:   At the marketplace ah and although its kinda drizzly so I'm
 2          afraid it might not- might not be a very good day for it. But
 3          other than that yeah same ol' same ol' here. (.) What's
 4                 happening with you?
 5   Mom:   Not a stinkin thing that I can think of. They really don't know
 6                 what's wrong.
 7                 (2.0)
 8   Mom:   All I know is that it hurts like hell whatever it is.
 9   Son:   $Ha ha ha.$ Yeah, [  d    a    d       s-    ] =
10   Mom:                     [They just don't know.]
11   Son:   =dad said they found some stuff in your spine?
12   Mom:   Well they did.
13   Son:   That's not very fun.
14   Mom:   No. But what we don't know is ya know what is causing this major
15                 pain.
16   Son:   Hmph.
17   Mom:   And ah sometimes it's there and sometimes its gone.  (1.0) I woke
18                 up this morning and it was there. I mean it definitely was there.
19   Son:   Hm mmm.
20   Mom:   And-
21                 ((Tape cuts off))
22   Mom:   Today's gonna be a rough day. And I fall back to sleep >and I
23                 wake up again and it's gone.<
24   Son:   Hmm. (0.7) So it just comes and goes and there's no rhyme nor
25                 reason to it huh.
26   Mom:   Right right.
27   Son:   How bizarre huh. That must be awfully frustrating.
```

28	Mom:	**It's very painful.**
29	Son:	Yeah um well. (0.6) And to not be able to predict it. >I mean if you
30		could if you could just know that it was gonna hit you every
31		morning and you could get up and the first thing you do is take a
32		pill< that might be a little easier but- **Yuck huh.**
33	Mom:	**You're right, it's yuck.**
34	Son:	Dad said though there's a p:ossibility you might get to go home
35		maybe early next week huh.
36	Mom:	Yeah.

When speakers utter "I don't know", claiming insufficient knowledge (see Beach & Metzger, 1997), they often proceed by stating what they do know. Similarly, when mom replies "Not a <u>stinkin</u> thing that I can think of.", she next nominates what "They" (i.e., medical experts) are unable to figure out "what's wrong"—an important concern and topic elaborated throughout Excerpt 14 (above). In this sense her "<u>stinkin</u>" previews negative experiences: frustrations occurring because "All I know is that it hurts like hell whatever it is." (line 8), "they found some stuff in your <u>spine</u>" (line 11), "That's not very fun." (line 13), and confusion about what is "<u>causing</u> this major pain" (lines 14-15). Yet, in following moments, mom also claims unequivocal rights to know and experience that pain, even though such pain cannot be adequately explained.

Throughout this excerpt, son's initial actions reveal that he is able to report what dad told him about mom's spine (lines 9 & 11), then identify and commiserate with the fact that it is not "fun" (line 13). And his careful monitoring of mom's descriptions continues. Later, he summarizes and reformulates mom's prior description of pain (lines 24-25), and again identifies and commiserates with her frustration (line 27):

14) SDCL: Malignancy #28: 1

22		Mom:	Today's gonna be a rough day. And I fall back to sleep>and I
23			wake up again and it's gone.<
24	→	Son:	Hmm. (0.7) So it just comes and goes and there's no rhyme nor
25			reason to it huh.
26	→	Mom:	Right right.
27	→	Son:	How bizarre huh. That must be awfully frustrating.
28	→	Mom:	It's very painful.

It is mom, however, who is in the position to knowingly claim "Right right." (line 26). She confirms that son's prior paraphrase offered a reasonable version of her confusing experience with pain and sleep. And although son can observe that it is "bizarre" and attribute how for mom "That must be awfully frustrating" (line 27), it is mom who definitively states "It is very painful." (line 28). The shift from "bizarre and frustrating to painful" is, in part, a matter of access to direct experience: Only mom can report on how it is the pain that draws her primary attention, bizarre and frustrating as the experience might be.

Son continues by elaborating that if the pain could be predicted, such pain might be eased by taking a pill (lines 29-32). He then concludes as follows:

15) SDCL: Malignancy #28: 2

32	Son:	Yuck, huh.
33	Mom:	You're right, it's yuck.

Mom aligns with son's "Yuck" assessment, validating his ability to know that this is not a pleasant experience for her. And with "it's yuck", mom does not undermine son's prior assertion, but by repeating his word (see Stivers, 2005) does claim primary rights to speak about and know "yuck" as practically experienced. Not having direct access to what mom has claimed as her own, son next shifts to reporting what dad informed him about mom leaving the hospital (lines 34-35).

Few Words and Revealing News Delivery Sequences (NDS's)

This chapter is brought to a close by briefly considering how it is possible that important news, and speakers' orientations toward delivering and receiving such news, can be achieved with such brevity and efficiency. In contrast, for example, Chapter 3 focused on an extended excerpt in which dad informed son that mom's tumor was diagnosed as "malignant". This and other NDS's—again, comprised of initiating, announcing (1→), responding to (2→), elaborating (3→), and assessing (4→) the valence of the news (e.g., as good or bad)—was revealed as a rather elaborate and complicated set of critically important moments. Later, in Chapter 6, a contiguous series of other NDS's were closely examined as son updated his (soon to be) ex-wife about mom's changing condition and thus travel plans. These NDS's (see also Excerpts 12 & 13, above) were more condensed, yet sufficient to accomplish a host of actions necessary for news to get updated.

Analysis of prior excerpts in this chapter has revealed how delicate social actions can be achieved through very few words. Similarly, the two excerpts below (16 & 17) evidence how entire News Delivery Sequences (NDS) can be compressed into short but meaningful exchanges between family members and friends. In the following excerpt, son's itemized news inquiry (INI) receives a brief response from dad (line 2) that confirms mom's being home but does not add further information:

16) **SDCL: Malignancy#39: 4-5**

```
 1 INI→Son:    Yes:. .hh (0.5) I understand mother is home?
 2 1→   Dad:    Yes she is.
 3 2→   Son:    A:nd how is that going.
 4 3→   Dad:    A:::hhh (.) tough.
 5 2→   Son:    pt On everybody on her on you o:n who.
 6 3→   Dad:    All of the above.
 7 4→   Son:    Oka:y.
```

When son next queries "how is that going" (line 3), dad only states "A:::hhh (.) tough." (line 4). His searching yields "tough", about which more could obviously be said but is withheld by dad. Son again clarifies (line 5) by providing dad with a listing of possibilities. And, again, dad's "All of the above." (line 6) inclusively confirms but does not volunteer additional information. It is in response to dad's repeated confirmations, yet withholdings, that son simply acknowledges dad's news with an "Oka:y." offering less of an assessment of the minimal news dad has provided and more of a recognition that at this moment dad is unable and/or unwilling to delve into just how and why it is "tough", and who exactly is involved.

Though it is not possible to know for sure, I initially wondered whether mom (now at home) is capable of hearing dad's comments, and if so, if dad is building his talk to accommodate her potential eavesdropping. In mom's presence, dad would understandably avoid informing son how "tough" it is to have mom home. Of course, even if mom's overhearing is what prompts dad's withholdings, it remains for son to figure out why and how dad deploys so few words—neither volunteering additional information on his own, nor in response to son twice seeking clarification (lines 3 & 5). But an inspection of the ensuing conversation between dad and son reveals otherwise:[7] Dad does, eventually, provide details not likely to be disclosed in mom's hearing. This promotes speculation about whether mom was ever a factor in dad's initial and displayed hesitancy to more fully respond to son's queries. Or, was dad (for his own reasons and in his own ways) simply reticent to divulge information known only to him?

In the final instance, a friend (Shannon) calls son at his home and asks "What're you doin'.", a topic initial elicitor (TIE) that is not designed to address or pursue particular topics (which INI's, as in Excerpt 16, above, are):

17) SDCL: Malignancy #52:1

1	Son:	Hello. Doug here.
2	Shannon:	Hi: the:re.
3	Son:	Hi.
4 TIE→	Shannon:	What're you doin'.
5 1→	Son:	Packing.
6 2→	Shannon:	Packing?
7 3→	Son:	Uh huh.
8 4→	**Shannon:**	**O:h no::.**
9	**Son:**	**Yup.**
10	**Shannon:**	**O::h Doug I'm sorry:.**
11	**Son:**	**Yeah me too. .hhh hh**

Though Shannon's opening query (line 4) was not designed to raise a particular topic or agenda, it becomes evident that son's one word response—"Packing." (line 5)—names an activity known to Shannon as troubling. By withholding further explanation, leaving unspecified *why* he is packing, he attributes knowledge to Shannon as capable of providing her own meaningful and relevant solution. With her next "Packing?" (line 6), repeating what son had said but with upward intonation, Shannon offers surprised recognition, but does not yet specify the significance of son's utterance. Acknowledged with "Uh huh.", son again does not elaborate, but leaves it for Shannon to make explicit her understanding of his circumstances. In this way, son acts as if she knows what he is referring to, and proceeds accordingly.

With "O:h no::." (line 8), a triggered and surprised response cry, Shannon confirms that son's attributions were correct. On her own volition, this oh-prefaced utterance displays realization that son is "Packing." because his mom is finally dying. Though she does not lay out the details of her assumption, son's "Yup." confirms both what and how she stated "O:h no::.". What remains unspoken by both speakers nevertheless reveals intersubjective agreement. This is further evident as Shannon next offers "O::h Doug I'm sorry:." (line 10). Her oh-prefaced condolence demonstrates sincere concern for what son must be experiencing, for the difficult trip he must now take, for the loss and grief he is facing—though it cannot be known with certainty what the motivations prompting her sympathy might have been. It is evident, however, that the primary action achieved through Shannon's "O::h Doug I'm sorry:." is *not* apologizing for having offended son (see Chapter 4; Robinson, 2004). Rather, she is expressing compassion for son's circumstances.

In turn, it cannot be unequivocally determined what son's response, "Yeah me too. .hhh hh" (line 11), is specifically addressing. But it is clear that he is claiming the obvious right to be sorry as well, either for his mom and/or himself, thus aligning with Shannon but owning the circumstances as a burden he must bear. His sigh, ".hhh hh", only partially reveals the emotions he is experiencing—frustration, sadness, fear?—though these too remain undisclosed, part of his life-world that language neither reveals nor adequately captures. Whether few words or many are spoken, it is an understatement to observe that a chasm often exists between speakers' internal emotions, the words they deploy, and the actions achieved through their utterances.

NOTES

1. Goffman's (1981) original descriptions of "response cries" more fully described individual's psychological states than their socially organized status within talk in interaction. Goodwin and Goodwin (2000) have extended Goffman's notions by focusing on an

> embodied display that that the party producing it has been so moved by a triggering event that they temporarily "flood out" with a brief emotional expression. This is followed a moment later by a fully formed syntactic phrase which accounts for, and explicates, the speaker's reaction by describing something that is remarkable in the event being responded to. . . . The event is so powerful that an actor spontaneously "floods out" on encountering it and emits an involuntary, emotionally charged Response Cry. (p. 16)

For example, in an examination of how young girls and family members organize gift openings at a birthday party, Good and Beach (2005) discovered a slight alteration of Goodwin's (1996) response cry sequence. The following structure emerged as enacted within particular contingencies of a birthday party:

> *[Triggering Event (opening of gift)] + [Enthusiastic Response Cry] +*
> *[Positive Assessment] + [Elaboration Sequence/Thanks].*

So too do the matters addressed between family members, on the phone, yield basically the same but slightly different structures—such as the person responding to a response cry being the speaker, who further elaborates just why the event being discussed is remarkable.

2. There are some exceptions to this hierarchy, such as when dad is told something from doctors (or other medical staff) that mom was not privy to. For example, when mom later becomes unable to speak and is generally incoherent, it is dad who receives more direct medical information than mom.

3. This moment might be usefully contrasted, for example, with Jefferson's (1981, 1993) analysis of "Yeah" as speakers move to close down others' talk and shift toward fuller speakership. Similarly, "Okay" has been shown to be an additional resource for acknowledging yet seeking closure on prior speaker's turn at talk in order to facilitate movement toward other matters (see Beach, 1990a, 1993b, 1995b, 1996, 2002b).

4. Regarding "six months → five years", readers are once again reminded that mom died 13 months following diagnosis (see Timeline in Chapter 2). Phone call #2 occurred on the second day, following diagnosis, so the scenario mom portrays—relying no doubt, at least in part, on what doctors have informed her—is a mixture of good and bad news: She lives seven months longer than the worst-case six-month projection, yet dies considerably earlier that the five years she would be "lucky" to experience.

5. Might aunt's "I mean no matter how [you cut it.]" possibly be understood as an *unintended pun* (see Beach, 1993a, 1996; Jefferson, 1996; Sacks, 1992)? With "cut it", is a (subconscious) reference made to mom's cancer, or tumors, as well as a preoccupation with different modes of treatment? Though surgery was not considered as a viable option for mom's condition, "cut" could also imply "reduce or minimize". Or perhaps not. As I have discussed elsewhere (1996, Chapter 5), these kinds of matters—in which speakers' language is tailored to, indeed parallels, the very circumstances they are caught up within—were repeatedly addressed by Harvey Sacks in his early lectures (e.g., see Winter 1969 & 1971, 1992 in lectures), and later by Gail Jefferson in subsequent positions on "poetics" (1977, 1996). As stated earlier, Sacks (1992) observed: "Well, who knows? Noticing it, you get the possibility of investigating it. Laughing it off in the first instance, or not even allowing yourself to notice it, of course it becomes impossible to find out whether there is anything to it" (p. 292). Or as Jefferson (1977) wryly noted, and despite evidence to the contrary,

analysts may well come off as "screwy" for raising such possibilities. Perhaps this is best cap-sulized in a written note she received from Sacks concerning poetic talk: "Not for circulation; they'll think we're both batty."

6. Minutes later, for example, son is more harsh as he more directly discloses his feelings. He further relies on response cries (1→, 2→) to vent his frustration, and anger, about mom's being "tough" and working to live as long as possible:

SDCL: Malignancy #10: 12

Son: =It seems like a hell of a lot of work fo- for no<u>thing</u> (.) <u>t</u>o <u>me</u>.

Aunt: Ye:ah. =

Son:1→= At this poin<u>t</u>. (.) I mean **O::h BOY**. So she can lay in the bed for another three days. **SO:: WHAT**.

Aunt: Um hm.

Son: .hhh <u>B</u>ut uh-

Aunt: Well ya know pt .hhh (.) I think that um::m (.) pt if- if <u>t</u>here's a <u>po::s</u>ibility that this is <u>so::mewhat</u> of a ma:tter of adj<u>ust</u>ments on medication in the past. (.) Fa:irly <u>re</u>:cently =

Son: = Ye:ah. =

Aunt: = it has been that.

Son: Yeah. =

Aunt: = Which is what I'm also thi<u>nk</u>ing.

Son:2→But **DA:MN**! <u>Come</u> on. I mean it's li:ke a- they're gonna adjust and then two days later it's a <u>cata</u>:strophic adju:stme:nt. And two days la:ter it's a <u>cata:strophic</u> adju:stment. An .hhh ya kno:w how- how much can they keep <u>c</u>lea:ning up after this me:ss.

Aunt:3→<u>O</u>::h they can do a <u>lo:t</u> for a lo:ng ti:me. But I <u>d</u>on't thi:nk anybody he:re wants that.

Son:4→No. You know ma- mom <u>men</u>tioned the no he:roic me:sures. =

Aunt:5→= O::h yeah. O::h yeah.

Son:6→A::h hhh.

Aunt:7→We've alr:eady dis<u>c</u>ussed that. When I ta:lked to the doctor this morning (.) a::h Doctor Wylie wa:sn't in and an associate of hers ca:lled and he <u>a:sked</u> me th:at, <u>because</u> (.) of what <u>I</u> was <u>telling</u> him what was <u>g</u>oing on. And (.) an ya know it- it cha:nges i:n (.) two three hours. =

Son: =Um hm.

Aunt: And he said- w:ell he said u::m (.) ya know do I ne:ed (.) ya know what does she -ya know about li:fe support do we need aah to:- to wor:ry about things. >And I said <u>no</u>.<

Son: Um hm.

Aunt: I said there <u>won't</u> be any hero<u>ic</u> mea:sures.

Son: Umkay.

Aunt: And I said so you make absolutely cl:<u>ear</u> in your he:ad that that's <u>exact</u>ly where we're all at. (1.0) A::nd a she's <u>not</u> on li:fe support systems.

In (2→) it is apparent that son focuses his criticisms on "they're/they", anonymous medical staff (see Chapters 8 & 9) who keep adjusting to mom's emergent condition, "<u>c</u>lea:ning up after this me:ss.". In successive turns, aunt establishes her authority to address son's concerns by report-ing experiences son (living out of town) has not been involved in. With aunt's "<u>O</u>::h"-prefaced response (3→) she first claims specific knowledge that although mom's life can be prolonged for a "lo:ng ti:me.", such actions are not aligned with family wishes. Son responds by reporting what he knows (4→); referring (without stating so) to his phone call #3 with mom about life support, where "mom <u>men</u>tioned the no he:roic me:sures. =". By repeating "= O::h yeah. O::h yeah." (5→), however, aunt displays being fully aware of mom's statements and position. Followed by a sigh from son (6→), aunt's "We've alr:eady dis<u>c</u>ussed that." makes reference to a conversation son was apparently not a part of. Aunt proceeds to report on a phone discussion with the doc-tor (7→) that very morning, in which the doctor specifically asked about "li:fe support". In no uncertain terms, aunt reports not only that there should be no life support (i.e., no "hero<u>ic</u> mea:sures") but that "And I said so you make absolutely cl:<u>ear</u> in your he:ad that that's <u>exactly</u> where we're all at."

Being in a primary position to report more recent and direct experiences than son, aunt thus asserts her right to enact the role of defending mom and family member's wishes. In her own words, she is a staunch advocate of no life support, a spokesperson able and willing to direct medical care "locally" and to insure there are no misunderstandings about the critical issue of unnecessarily prolonging mom's life.

7. The extended excerpt appears below:

SDCL: Malignancy #39: 4-5

Son:	yes:. .hh(0.5) I understand mother is home?
Dad:	Yes she is.
Son:	A:nd how is that going.
Dad:	A:::hhh (.) tough.
Son:	pt On everybody on her on you o:n who.
Dad:	All of the above.
Son:	Oka:y.
Dad:	Uhm. =
Son:	→= Is it w- i- this sounds terrible t'say is it worth it.
Dad:	( ) It's not a choice.
Son:	Okay.
Dad:	They <u>dis</u>charged her.
Son:	<u>O:</u>h.
Dad:	They will not just w<u>a</u>rehouse her.
Son:	O::h okay.
Dad:	Doctor said you know take her home (.) handle her with hospice and she can be ther:e and know she probably like the surroundings better etcetra and she wasn't overly thrilled but .hh you know.
Son:	Hmm.
Dad:	But I brought her home (0.8) Friuda:y. Let's see we left I dunno ten eleven o'clock I guess. .hh And they have elected to do radiation on both the <u>upper</u> and lower s<u>pine</u> to try and reduce the tumors in there and see if they can (.) make it any less painful for her.
Son:	Mmm.

Following the NDS, son queries whether it is "worth it" (→). Dad then progressively offers additional details that would most likely not have been discussed had mom been present (as initially speculated). That said, it is of course possible that dad simply walked into another room with the phone, and/or that mom was the one who walked out of the hearing of dad's phone call, thus allowing dad to be less constrained when offering information to son. These *scenic*, ethnographic details are typically not discernable when working with phone call interactions—compared, for example, with what video recordings of face-to-face encounters can (but may not) reveal.

11

STORIES-IN-A-SERIES

Tellings and Retellings About Cigarettes, Devastation, and Hair

Family members tell and retell many stories during the Malignancy phone calls. This chapter examines a series of such stories, conversations reflecting enduring and endearing qualities: three discussions about cigarettes across three separate calls in a 24-hour period and one later cigarette story; two "devastation" stories, told by aunt to son, across two different calls; and two stories about "hair," during two different calls, between dad and son.

Analysis of these interactions allows for stories in a series (e.g. see Jefferson, 1978; Norrick, 1997, 1998, 2000; Ryave, 1978; Schegloff, 2004) to be understood as practical, centrally important achievements for family members. Though in the midst of a cancer journey, family members remain in close contact and work through whatever delicate moments may arise. One prominent feature of these stories is how relationships get managed through a wide array of social activities: claiming entitlement as a story teller, animating own and others' voices, avoiding conflict about family alliances, venting frustration, assessing another's demeanor, pursuing and withholding affiliation, soliciting responses, organizing play and humor. Taken together, the sampling of actions comprising these stories provides rich insight into how family members communicate about the trials and tribulations of everyday life.

THREE STORIES ABOUT "CIGARETTES"

Analysis begins with three stories about cigarettes, occurring across three phone calls within a period of one day. As mom was diagnosed with lung cancer, the relationship between her smoking behaviors and illness do not go unnoticed by dad and son. When talking with son, dad offers the initial and revealing story in call #12. In two subsequent calls (#16 & #18), son provides reconstructed versions of dad's story to aunt and Gina. Approximately one week later, dad initiates a fourth story involving cigarettes to son. It will be shown that these stories, each unique and interesting on its own merits, are also intertwined through curious and subtle practices for organizing continuity in everyday affairs.

Dad's Initial Reporting: ">Jesus Christ ya forgot my cigarettes.<"

Prior to Excerpt 1 (below) dad had just informed son that because mom's medical condition had stabilized, he should not travel to visit mom and the family (see Chapter 6, Excerpt 2). However, dad urges son to remain in a state of readiness (see Chapter 7), as a call to travel in the near future is likely to occur. As evident in line 1, marked by laughter, son receives this news with troubled disbelief. He then states "<u>This</u> is- this is <u>weird</u>. hhh":

1) Malignancy #12:3

```
 1      Son:    =$.hhh huh huh hh hh .hhh$ This is- this is weird. hhh =
 2      Dad:    = Yeah  [(        )] >I mean ya know< ya go =
 3      Son:         [O:yvey:]
 4      Dad:    = home at night and (.) ya cry yourself to sleep thinkin'
 5              w::ell this is the end of it.° Ya come back the next day and
 6  →           she says- ((mimicking wife's voice )) >Jesus Christ ya forgot
 7  →           my cigarettes.<
 8      Son:    $Humphhhh .hh$ =
 9      Dad:    = O:::h gimme a break. =
10      Son:    Yeah. hhh .hhh heah .hh So what'd the doctor have to say
11              specifically anything. =
12      Dad:    =We:ll. (0.2) Th- the thyroid is too high, the pa:in: is
13              tremendous and it will just slowly keep accumulating.
14              They will leave her o:n (0.8) u::h the morphine stuff.
15              (0.4)
16      Dad:    But it will be pill form instead of this drip system and they
17              will just keep the pain under control.
18              (0.8)
19      Son:    Okay. [ .hh hhh hhhh hhh hh  ]
```

With "<u>weird</u>" son depicts the bizarre nature of having his considerable efforts to arrange travel plans put on hold (see Chapters 5 & 6), followed with "O:y vey:.". As summarized in *Wikipedia*:

> Oy vey! (*Yiddish*: __ __) is an exclamation of dismay or exasperation meaning "woe is me" or "oh, no". This exclamation was borrowed from *Yiddish*. A related exclamation is "vey iz mir" (__'_ __)—"woe is me" or "oy very iz mir" (*Yiddish*: __ __'_ ___). (http://en.wikipedia.org/wiki/Oy-vey)

With "O:y vey:.", son encapsulates his experience of being caught up in the inherent problems of managing unpredictable, and uncertain trajectories, of mom's changing condition. His utterances gives "expression to feelings of shock or sorrow . . . Different cultures have formulated a variety of quasi-verbal ways of instinctively reacting to distressing situations" (http://www.ucalgary.ca/~elsegal/Shokel/920302_Oy_Vay.html).

He also confronts the inherent problems of managing the unpredictable and uncertain trajectory of mom's changing condition. This sequential environment reveals one version of a normalized interactional practice: "at first I thought, but then I realized" (see Halkowski, 2006; Jefferson, 2004b; Sacks, 1992). In these moments, son's "<u>This</u> is- this is <u>weird</u>." contrasts his thoughts and feelings about what was going to happen (i.e., traveling home for mom's dying) with the strange realization that he must deal (indeed is now dealing) with the consequences of an unexpected event (i.e., mom's stabilization). The improvement of her health is not treated as good or bad news. Nevertheless, son orients to hearing the news as an odd rupture of his expectations (Maynard, 1996). In a very short period of time mom's looming death has been postponed, and thus so too have son's plans to travel home.

In response, as a concerned and loving husband, dad extends son's prior "<u>weird</u>" with his own story. He provides a "my-world" or "my-side telling" of similar troubling events (see Heritage, 1984a, 1998, 2002; Pomerantz, 1980, 1984a).[1] As he is entitled, dad speaks directly about stark and troubling contrasts anchored in his own life experiences. Beginning with line 2, dad's "Yeah" first acknowledges the bewilderment evident in son's "<u>weird</u>." reaction. He then moves to offer a basis for knowing and claiming that the kinds of dilemmas son has depicted are equally evident, yet manifest differently, in his daily life (see Chapter 10). Employing the generic "ya" three times (lines 2, 4, & 5), dad is inclusive of son but also situates his experience as unique to him. As noted previously, Sacks (1992) observed how "The openness of 'you' means that 'you' can in fact be a way of talking about 'everybody'—and indeed, incidentally, of 'me'" (p. 349).

Dad describes a scenario where he arrives home (presumably, from visiting mom at the hospital). With his "ya cry yourself to sleep" (line 4), it is not possible to know whether dad actually "cried himself to sleep" or invoked a colloquial, figurative expression to portray the depth of sadness he was experiencing. Either way, he reports the emotional turmoil of facing his wife's apparent and imminent death (°w::ell this is the end of it.°, line 5). By shifting to the next day (again, presumably, when he returns to the hospital), with "she says-" dad directly reports what mom said by mimicking her voice (see Buttny, 1997; Holt, 1996, 1999, 2000; Holt & Clift, 2006): ">Jesus <u>Christ</u> ya forgot my cigarettes.<" (lines 6-7). Here, and in son's subsequent retellings (Excerpts 2 & 3, below), speakers' voices are *prosodic achievements*—interactional resources for demonstrating, through intoned and animated constructions of particular utterances, the affective significance of specific social actions (e.g., see Beach, 2000b; Couper-Kuhlen & Selting, 1996; Freese & Maynard, 1998; M. Goodwin, 1990). Produced at a fast pace and with emphasis, dad invokes the deity "<u>Jesus Christ</u>". He begins to animate mom's demeanor as demanding and upset, prosodically making available to son that he treated her unsolicited behavior as not just unexpected, but uncalled for and even insensitive. Mom's blunt criticism was enacted by dad as unmerited, especially (as framed in his story) when contrasted with the compassion and grief he had experienced just the night before (i.e., when trying to get to sleep at home). But he does not explicitly reveal these or related feelings. Rather, he leaves it to son (as recipient) to specify the upshot of the event he has experienced, and now makes available, for son's reply.

It is likely that mom had no access to dad's trying (and perhaps crying) moments the prior evening. And as a hospitalized cancer patient, she may well have been enduring her own private (e.g., irritating, anxious, fearful, lonely) experiences since dad last visited. A specific request may even have been made for dad not to forget her cigarettes, which dad simply forgot. But who knows? These possible events do not dismiss her sharp action, if and when it occurred as dad reported it. Whatever the background exigencies giving rise to mom's reported utterance and demeanor, that is what dad provided to son. And that reporting is what son must next be responsive to.

With "\$Humphhhh .hh\$" (line 8), son aligns himself as receptive to dad's own quandary, but does not further comment on it. It is in the absence of any further elaboration by son that dad next summarizes his reaction with a marked "Oh-prefaced", and incongruous, "= <u>O</u>:::h <u>gi</u>mme a <u>break</u>. =" (line 9; see Beach, 1996; Heritage, 2002). Treating mom's action as absurd, and in the absence of a more specific upshot provided by son, dad makes his own case that he is deserving of special understanding: As a husband undergoing uncertain and grievous circumstances, he deserves a "break" (see Endnote 2). Though son has the opportunity in next response, he again passes on making dad out to be blameless in this delicate situation and/or to hold mom accountable for her actions. Son withholds further commentary with "Yeah. hhh .hhh heah .hh So what'd the <u>doctor</u> have to say specifically anything. =" (lines 10-11). His brief acknowledgment token "Yeah.", subse-quent laugh particle "heah", and shift away from dad's story about mom — that is, to solic-iting news about what the doctor reported (see Chapters 8 and 9) — fail to treat dad's call for a "break" as having invited more specific agreement or alignment from son. Instead, son draws attention back to biomedical updating, information only the doctor could provide to dad, which dad is capable of overviewing (lines 12-17).

The preceding analysis makes clear that son repeatedly *withheld* further commentary on dad's troubling story (i.e., lines 8 & 10-11). Son does not fully acknowledge or elabo-rate on dad's reported wrongdoing by mom, appeals for commiseration, and even possible collaboration in critiquing mom. In essence, son carves out a neutral stance (see Wu, 2004) No pursuit is made of potentially complex relationships between mom's smoking, her can-cer, and how the family has dealt with her ongoing addiction to cigarettes. These obvious-ly connected and consequential matters remain unaddressed by son. Son's withholdings, however, do not necessarily provide evidence that he failed to hear what dad had stated, nor that the significance of dad's story about mom was misunderstood. It may well be that the upshot of dad's reporting was ambiguous for son, placing him in a conflicting situation of aligning with dad about his dying mother's (alleged) behavior yet simultaneously avoiding criticism of her actions.

But who knows what son was experiencing? His acknowledging yet shifting response, when questioning dad about news from the doctor, could be recruited as evidence of son's ambiguity. But what can unequivocally be seen is that son does not pursue, but redirects attention away from further complaints about mom and toward news about her condition.

Son's First Retelling: "given 'em hell"

Consider a call with his aunt (mom's sister) later that same day, as son tells her about dad's original "cigarette" story:

2) Malignancy #17:2

```
 1    Aunt:  [What'd-] did Dr. Wylie ↑say to him (.) >do ya know?<
 2           (0.8)
 3    Son:   No not <really.> hh u:m hhh (.) Ya know that they were gonna
 4           radiate these tumors in her le:g and that- they were gonna
 5           put 'er on ↑pill form morphine (.) .hhh after a while n:: .hhh
 6           u::h
 7           (0.4)
 8    Son:   An'that was about it. An' that there no >there wasn't quite
 9           the immediate danger they thought there was last ni:ght an'
10           that's basically,< .hhhh a:ll::.
11           (1.0)
12    Son:   ↓Ya know dad said °ya know° last night (.) .hhh <it was one
13  →        way an'> this morning she's m- .hh given 'em hell for
14  →        forgettin' her cigarettes (.) ya know. pt hh An' so $hhh hhh
15           hh .hhh$ =
16    Aunt:  = Okay. So she was much better this m[orning.]
17    Son:                                        [ Ye: ah.] Much better
18           apparently.
19    Aunt:  ↑I'll take every day I c'n get without your mother suffering. =
20    Son    := ↑Ye:ah.
21           (0.6)
22    Son:   hh .hh ↓Yeah. I- I agree.
```

In lines 1-10 son responds to aunts' query, requesting an update (via dad) from the doctor. Son responds by summarizing what dad had informed him: that the doctor reported about radiation, morphine, and mom being in less danger than last night (thus son was canceling his travel plans). When he then continues by initiating a version of dad's "cigarette" story, several noticeable contrasts or "transformations" (Ryave, 1978, p. 131) can be observed between dad's first telling and son's retelling. Offered as direct reported speech ("dad said"), in lines 12-13 son references "last night (.) <it was one way", but does *not* describe dad's reported emotional turmoil ("ya cry yourself to sleep" in Excerpt 1, line 4, above) about facing mom's death. Rather, in his own terms, he portrays dad's version of mom's action this morning (i.e., ">Jesus Christ ya forgot my cigarettes.<", lines 6-7 In Excerpt 1, above): Mom was "given 'em hell for forgettin' her cigarettes" (lines 13-14, above). Though left unarticulated in dad's original story and son's response to it, son's "given' 'em hell" constructs dad as recipient of a hard-line action by mom. In this moment, son also specifies the upshot of mom's action by stating what she was doing through her utterance. He does not prosodically voice her action, but leaves it for aunt to determine the orientation mom was taking in her talk in interaction (as dad did for son in Excerpt 1, above).

As with dad's initial story, also left unstated is any reference to the ironic nature of these circumstances: a soon-to-be-dying mother, diagnosed with lung cancer precipitated (at least in part, see Chapter 15) by excessive smoking, holding her husband accountable for forgetting to bring her cigarettes—and to the hospital, of all places. Making these connections explicit, as well as any more specific hint of ridicule, was *not* evident in son's retelling. Such linkages are intersubjectively known and understood by son and aunt, yet remain unspoken. Indirectly, then, son concludes his brief retelling with "An' so $hhh hhh hh .hhh$ (lines 14-15). He stops short of providing a particular point, outcome, or moral to the story—an action that would commit son to a particular, and possible derisive stance (see Wu, 2004), that he is taking toward mom. In its place son offers aspirated laughter, displaying his recognition that what he has just provided is indeed a delicate matter, but not inviting aunt to laugh with him (see Haakana, 2001).

After all, aunt is mom's sister. By reporting the "cigarette" incident, and hinting yet remaining noncommittal as to mom's blameworthiness, son leaves it for her to provide the conclusions that son had left unarticulated. And not unlike son's second response to dad in Excerpt 1 (above), aunt's "= Okay. So she was much better this m[orning.]" (line 16) briefly acknowledges son's retelling, but next immediately shifts attention away from son's retelling and toward mom's current state of health. Her pivotal use of "= Okay." pays only minimal attention to what son had reported, en route to a next-positioned matter she treated as more significant (see Beach, 1993, 1995a, 1995b): not mom's potentially moody or inappropriate behavior, but how her current health had stabilized so quickly from a near-death experience. In addition, following son's acknowledgement that mom was apparently better (lines 17-18), aunt further clarifies the basis of her priorities by reporting "↑I'll take every day I can get without your mother suffering. =" (line 19). In this way, aunt does not explicitly reject the opportunity to collaborate with son about the inappropriateness of mom's actions. Rather, as Drew (1984) observed:

> From what is reported the inviters/proposers are enabled to see for themselves that their invitation is being declined. Thus through just reporting, recipients not only manage to avoid outrightly or directly doing a rejection; particularly, they also have speakers (coparticipants) collaborate in seeing that, objectively or reasonably, an acceptance is not possible. (p. 146)

Indeed, as evident in son's repeated agreement (lines 20-22), aunt had successfully made it clear that even though mom may be engaging in some questionable actions, for aunt (mom's sister) emphasis needs to be given to minimizing mom's suffering. In the way aunt designed her talk, no attempt was made to gang up on mom in her absence, especially when her health was so fragile. And for son, now faced with pursuing collaboration from aunt in making mom out to have conducted herself in a questionable manner, or aligning with aunt's priorities about mom's health and suffering, it is clear that his actions reveal that he chose the latter. As noted previously, son thereby steered clear of any possible conflict about family alliances. Specifically, he avoids pursuit of wanting to criticize his mom (aunt's sister) in the very midst of her cancer struggles. Son's responsive actions, then, are a very objective and reasonable way of dealing with aunt, who displayed an inability to accept son's invitation to possibly collaborate in blaming mom.

Son's Second Retelling: "≠>Where are my cigarettes $anyw(h)ay .hh hhh$"

Son's second attempt to reconstruct the original telling, about what dad had said about mom's "cigarettes", occurred in the next call that same day. Analysis provided earlier (see Excerpt 3, Chapter 6) focused on how son, prior to Excerpt 3 (below), informed Gina that mom had stabilized. Although he should "keep his lesson plans current and not unpack his bag", he was postponing his travel plans. He also informs Gina that mom remains in the hospital, could live for a few more weeks, and is "incoherent." The following excerpt occurs next:

3) Malignancy #18:2

```
     1   Son:    But they think that they're gonna >get her ba:ck< to where
     2           she's- hhhh she floats in an' o:ut.
     3           (0.2)
     4   Gina:   °Mm hm.° =
     5   Son:    = U:hm (0.2) and I guess she- .hhhh sh- at one point $dad
     6           said$ that (ch')a:ll of a sudden she said (0.8) (( mimicking
     7 →         mother's voice )) ↑>Where are my cigarettes $anyw(h)ay
     8 →         .hh hhh$ >.hh An' he said< sounds like she's back to normal
     9           again for a little bit there. =So .hhh S[he-
    10   Gina:                                          [>Who'd ya talk- who'd
    11           ya talk to toda:y.<
    12   Son:    pt .hh U:h (0.8) Just da::d this morning.
```

As with dad's original telling and son's first reconstruction about "cigarettes" to aunt, his second reporting of dad and mom's talk occurs in an environment where mom's health condition and treatment regimen are being discussed. In lines 5–9, son transitions away from describing mom's prognosis and coherence by initiating a second retelling. The beginning of his utterance (line 5) is marked with dysfluency. He first reflects on what he is going to say, and with "I guess she-" abruptly cuts-off the perspective (and distance) he was going to report the story from. Followed by "hhhh sh-", a noticeable inbreath and another cut-off thought, son then states "at one point $dad said$" (lines 5–6). These actions reveal how son was moving away from what he *guessed* mom had done, and toward what he'd heard dad (as recipient) *report* about her behavior. This shift, from son's speculation to a reconstruction of what dad had told him, allows for a more authoritative telling-to-come.

Two preliminary and distinct differences can be observed, however, and each reveals how son progressively assumes authorship to improvise the story as teller. First, in this second version, son continues to reduce emphasis given to the temporal unfolding of the event. In Excerpt 1 (above), dad's original description included his emotional turmoil of being "home at night." In Excerpt 2 (above) these details were glossed, becoming "last night (.) it was one way" in son's retelling to aunt. For Gina, son simply states "at one point $dad said$ that (ch')a:ll of a sudden she said." Thus, from one retelling to the next, the particular sequential events leading up to mom's ">Jesus Christ ya forgot my cigarettes.<", and dad's surprised reaction, became diminished (see Schegloff, 2004).

Second, with "$dad said$", the retelling to Gina also provided son the opportunity to frame the event as presently laughable. Though this is different from how dad originally reported mom's utterance, and dad's reaction to it, son now emphasizes the event as humorous. But why that now?

Framing his retelling as laughable could simply have emerged naturally, even over a short amount of time (i.e., less than one day), as a resource for taking perspective of the event by making light of it. Despite dad's original depiction of his emotions about mom's dying at home and mom's bothersome utterance the next morning at the hospital, son is in a position to reframe the event in a less serious and emotional manner.

Yet a more plausible and interactionally grounded explanation can be advanced: Son is designing this retelling specifically for Gina's hearing. As son's ex-wife, not mom's sister, his "$dad said$" offers an enticement for soliciting Gina's hearing and attention as story recipient. And as a second retelling, not a first (i.e., for aunt), son can rely on his prior experiences and adjust his story accordingly. In Excerpt 2, it was shown how aunt's "=Okay. So she was much better this m[orning.]" (line 16) acknowledged but decidedly shifted away from any sense of collusion *against* mom. This reaction by aunt did not explicitly reject, but neither did it overtly affirm or further encourage son's story. One upshot of aunt's response is son's subsequent adaptation for a second retelling (to Gina). As noted in Chapter 5, when son talked with different airline representatives, stories may become increasingly streamlined and tailored across repeated retellings (see Beach, 2000b; Norrick, 1997; Sacks, 1992; Schegloff, 2004). With airline agents, son adjusted his story formats to enhance the likelihood that he would be more likely to receive discounted airfares. So too may son have shaped this retelling, as laughable, to boost Gina's acceptance of a not-yet-delivered story (see Jefferson, 1979).

Returning to Excerpt 3 (above), it can be seen that son shifts intonation and prosodically mimic's mom's voice by stating "↑>Where are my cigarettes $anyw(h)ay. hh hhh$" (lines 7-8). This reconstruction retains mom's harsh demeanor, but (as with Excerpt 2, above) alters what mom actually said to dad. Son's own humorous stance on mom's utterance is evident, in part, as he laughably states "$anyw(h)ay .hh hhh$". He then reports dad as stating "An' he said< sounds like she's back to normal again for a little bit there"—an embellishment also revealing son's own interpretation of events that dad did not actually convey. Yet regardless of son's laughable framing of the story, and added features, Gina responds with ">Who'd ya talk- who'd ya talk to toda:y.<" (lines 10-11). Like aunt, Gina next and also draws attention away from son's story about mom's "cigarettes." But here she offers no acknowledgment of the point son was trying to make, nor of the relevance of son's story to mom's health. Instead, Gina seeks additional information about who son had been in touch with.

Contrasting Three Proximal Cigarette Stories

Dad's original telling to son, and two subsequent retellings by son (to aunt and Gina) yielded the following actions: only minimal acknowledgment from recipients, no belittling collaboration, and marked shifts away from the initial focal point of the stories—Mom's ">Jesus Christ ya forgot my cigarettes.<." In the original telling, son's laughter showed appreciation for dad's predicament, but provided only brief acknowledgement to dad's "=

O:::h gimme a break. =" before asking what the doctor had to say. Similarly, aunt and Gina's responses to both son's retellings about mom's suffering and condition, were treated as more important than pursuing either what dad had said or how mom's actions were inappropriate. As evident in Excerpts 1-3 (above), recipients dealing with mom's dying—son, aunt, and Gina alike—displayed little interest in criticizing mom in the final few weeks of her life.[2] In particular, son's own responses to dad's original telling did not vary in any significant way from aunt and Gina's reactions to son's retellings.

For son, then, the dual roles of first being a story recipient and subsequently (twice) a story teller were thus enacted differently. Although he displayed an unwillingness to draw attention to mom's actions when responding to dad's original story, he twice raised these same actions (as teller) when speaking with aunt and Gina. It is curious how once information is received, it then becomes available as a resource for informing others about one's own (and others') experiences via story telling. In this set of instances, retelling about mom's "cigarettes" utterance became son's entitlement. This is not a result of son hearing mom speak originally, as it was dad who reported to son what he had heard. Rather, by initiating his stories as retellings he treated aunt and Gina as potentially interested recipients who could not only identify with the incidence, but perhaps be collaborators as well—just as dad had initially done with son.

Son also associated dad's reporting about mom as something mom might normally do. In Excerpt 3, he reports to Gina how dad stated that "sounds like she's back to normal again for a little bit there.". Even though dad did not utter this statement, son relied on his own understanding to assess the situation in this manner. And if it is true (which we do not necessarily know), at least by implication son is also taking a position toward the kinds of interactional patterns mom and dad routinely enact together. This is information that both aunt and Gina would possess knowledge about; that is, as knowing recipients with shared and thus intersubjective information that could be relied upon by son to design his story, and to solicit their hearing and response.

The previously observed tendency for retellings to become condensed and/or recontextualized versions of earlier reportings (e.g., see Arminen, 2004; Holt & Clift, 2006; Norrick, 1997; Ryave, 1978; Schegloff, 2004), can be verified by closely reexamining Excerpts 1-3. What is deleted and added by a storyteller also shapes progressively new and different versions of what actually occurred. Just as son altered dad's original telling, might it also be assumed that dad's initial report glossed specific and relevant details about his visit to see mom in the hospital? This inevitably occurs in stories, more or less, because it is impossible (in the absence of actual recordings of interaction) to recapture the detailed and sequential organization of conversational participation. In ordinary conversations and institutional interactions alike (e.g., see Atkinson & Drew, 1979; Bergmann, 1992, 1993; Drew & Heritage, 1992), there are subtle distinctions between actual and reported events (see Chapter 1 & 2). Real time and reconstructed realities offer inevitably different versions of same events (see Beach & Dixson, 2001). For example, in son's retelling to aunt he did not prosodically voice mom's demeanor, but stated "given 'em hell." In the next retelling to Gina, he animates what mom said and then provides his commentary (though he attributed it to dad) in order to normalize mom's actions. These retellings have also been shown to deviate in key ways from dad's original reporting.

One common feature across all three stories is that, as Bergmann (1993) has observed regard gossiping, there is a "morally contaminated character" (p. 99) inherent in talk about absent others' personal and private lives (see also Bergmann & Linnell, 1998). It can be difficult to manage a "high degree of intimacy" (p. 153) when trying to calibrate just how much to say about another to different recipients (see also Beach, 2000b). And in response, if recipients treat what prior speakers' have nominated as issues to be further commented on, how do speakers pursue topics and collaboration about absent others? What if initial speakers' actions are taken as lacking discretion, as having gone too far? In these moments, as in each of the three excerpts above, avoidance of possible derogatory talk about others can and does occur.

Simply because the focus of talk is about intimate others—even beloved family members facing terminal cancer—does not mean that problems inherent in managing possible indiscretions will magically go away. These three excerpts about "cigarettes" make clear that delicate issues and potential conflicts are omnipresent, and thus omnirelevant features of everyday life for family members. Universally, family interactions are political encounters. In the Malignancy phone call corpus, a dying mom remains uniquely her own person, long-developed patterns in relationships continue to be enacted, and there is little time out from managing which issues and topics to pursue and those best left alone. And although the obvious connection between cigarettes and mom's cancer remains unstated, it is still known by each speaker. Yet it remains an empirical question to determine just how this shared knowledge is handled throughout interactions.

As storytellers, dad and son discreetly raised the possibility for recipient collaboration about mom's smoking, her illness, and overall demeanor. But these were overlooked in favor of emphasizing mom's health and well-being, a priority that all family members' actions treated as sacred: on such hallowed ground, at least for the moment, others' faults can be (and are) readily accepted and forgiven.

A FOURTH AND FINAL "CIGARETTE" STORY

As Kubler-Ross (1969b, 1974) described years ago, as did Groopman (2004) more recently, *accepting* and *forgiving* troubles caused by illness are practical achievements requiring ongoing and considerable efforts. Approximately one week following Excerpts 1-3 (above; see also Timeline in Chapter 2), a discussion between dad and son focuses on dad's experience following mom's release from the hospital, as not just her husband, but as primary caregiver who needs to closely monitor her daily actions. This excerpt, slightly longer than two minutes, involves complex social activities that could be examined in considerably more detail than possible within the space available here. Preliminary attention will be drawn, however, to how a fourth story about mom's cigarettes and smoking arises (lines 1-43). Discussion then shifts to a related concern about mom's state of mind and overall demeanor (lines 44-73):

4) **Malignancy #41: 8-9**

1	Dad:	So:: you gotta <u>help</u> her up an' then you gotta <u>walk</u> with her
2		'cuz she f<u>e</u>ll yesterday mo<u>rn</u>ing here in the kitchen.
3	Son:	O<u>:h</u> you're <u>kid</u>ding.=
4	Dad:	= °Yeah.° (0.2) Came around the co<u>r</u>ner I said >Okay wait a
5		minute.=I h<u>a</u>ve to go to the bathroom. But I went the other
6		wa:y, and she was gonna walk around here and get a
7 →		<u>cigarette</u>.< =
8	Son:	=<u>U</u>h huh.=
9	Dad:	= H- half way across the kitchen <u>floor</u> between the two
10		<u>coun</u>ters it- her leg gave out, an' down she <u>went</u>.=
11 →	Son:	O:hh <u>J</u>(h)e:su:s. .hh $Heh heh she's still **smo::king**.$=
12	Dad:	=Huh?=
13 →	Son:	=I said and she's <u>still</u> **smo:king**.
14 →	Dad:	°(She's still **smoking**.)°
15	Son:	<u>G(hh)o::d</u> (hh) .hh
16	Dad:	(Yeah, it's my life's <u>fight</u>.)=

17	Son:	=<u>Yea</u>hh I guess.=
18	Dad:	(.)
19	Son:	It's kinda a <u>mo:r</u>bid way of l<u>oo</u>king at it. But ↑ye:ah you
20		kno:w, what the hell huh.
21	Dad:	Yeah. ↑Probably when- when the funeral directors do the
22 →		crem<u>a</u>tion and I give 'em a **carton a <u>cig</u>arettes** an' say lay 'em
23		on <u>top</u>.
24	Son:	Mm hm.=
25	Dad:	=They're gonna bitch.[Heh heh.
26	Son:	[Heh heh heh [<u>hh</u>
27	Dad:	[Well I will (.) <u>ser</u>iously
28		think of that every time I'm thin- = u::m na:::h ↓I won't do
29		that. But ↑<u>I'm</u> gonna think about i[t °heh heh.° =
30	Son:	[<u>Ye:</u>ah.
31	Dad:	= Ya'know, °God damn.° An' you gotta <u>watch</u> because eh
32 →		shit >you know when she fell she had a **cig<u>a</u>rette** in her
33		↑<u>ha:nd</u>.< =
34	Son:	=Mm [hm.
35	Dad:	[(Heh heh.)=
36	Son:	=Well and the way she falls as<u>le:ep</u> you gotta watch that too
37		huh.
38	Dad:	Ya'know she's gotta do it (.) standing up out here at the
39		<u>coun</u>ter. I won't give it to her in <u>there</u> unless I'm sitting right
40		there l<u>oo</u>king at her 'cuz (.) go to sleep burn her <u>ha:nd</u>
41		[(or somethin'.)
42	Son:	[Mm hm.=
43	Dad	=(Fire) do somethin' so.=
44	Son:	=.hh So she's <u>not</u> <u>thin</u>kin' real straight.
45	Dad:	Not even <u>c</u>lose. (.) And <u>not</u> <u>too</u> <u>sweet</u>ly either.
46	Son:	<u>O:hh</u> .hh hey ↑that's gotta be <u>tough</u> on you <u>too</u>.
47		I know you were sayin' that she was- she was getting
48		<u>snar</u>kier amd <u>sna:r</u>kier jus'-
49	Dad:	(°Yep.°) ↑<u>We::ll</u> she's <u>frustra:</u>ted. =
50	Son:	= <u>S(h)ure</u>.
51	Dad:	Ya know, pt doesn't- (.) <u>if</u> she understands on the <u>in</u>side
52		she sure doesn't v<u>e</u>rbally. >Ya'know,= it's gonna be like aunt
53		<u>Es</u>ter< you don't know <u>how</u> much is sh- is truly going on
54		<u>ac</u>curately in her ↑<u>mi:nd</u> but-
55	Son:	Mm hm.=
56	Dad:	=You listen to what comes out her <u>mo:uth</u>, ya'know that-
57		tha:t gets con<u>fu</u>sed.
58		(1.1)
59	Dad:	You know she'll be standing here saying well (.) o<u>ka:</u>y get
60		some flour and sugar (.) a::nd I'm gonna make breakfast.
61	Son:	$Heh he(h)[h. hh
62	Dad:	[O::↑<u>ka:y</u>. (.) Thursday morning she came out
63		poured herself a cup o' coffee put <u>or</u>ange juice in it and
64		started drinkin.=Said <u>boy</u> you make lousy
65		co[$ffee$. °Hah hah hah.°]
66	Son:	[Hhhh heh heh heh.]
67		I guess I shouldn't <u>la:</u>ugh, but that <u>is</u> kinda funny.
68	Dad:	(°Mm ye:ah.°)=

69	Son:	=But that's like aunt Esther puttin' the plastic=
70	Dad	:=M:m ↑h:m.=
71	Son:	=Pe- pot on the stove and tryin' to cook it huh?
72	Dad:	Sa::me=thing?
73	Son:	How are you gonna be able tuh- g:o to work. hhh

In lines 1-43, six references to cigarettes and smoking occur. Dad begins by addressing the need to help mom walk (line 1), an extension of previously mentioned problems associated with mom's sleeping, eating, and requiring aid getting to the bathroom. He then announces that mom had fallen yesterday in the kitchen (line 2), which son marks with surprise (line 3). This incident occurred because as mom was trying to get a "cigarette." (line 7), her "leg gave out" (line 10). Although son's "=O:hh J(h)e:su:s." (line 11) displays more concern than previously (line 3), his next ."hh $Heh heh she's still smo::king.$=" does not address mom's well-being (or other related topics). Rather, he treats her continued smoking as the remarkable news, which subsequently gets clarified for dad prior to his quiet confirmation (lines 12-14). More than affirming mom's smoking, however, dad's utterance "(°She's still smoking.°)" (line 14) is replete with resignation: a quite acceptance, but *not* a condonment, of behaviors he is unable to change. Like son's prior "=O:hh J(h)e:su:s." (line 11), his next and aspirated "G(hh)o::d (hh) .hh" (line 15) invokes a deity that, once again, occurs in a troubling circumstance that cannot be controlled as evident, for example, through his display of disbelief and even revulsion.

Mom's recent fall in the kitchen, now associated with actions related to smoking addiction, is placed into a larger context and temporal framework as dad states "(Yeah, it's my life's fight." (line 16). Although dad's resistance is not treated as news by son—that is, as a known battle, fought but not won—son next reframes the fight as tied to the past. Focusing on the present, son continues with "It's kinda a mo:rbid way of looking at it. But ↑ye:ah you kno:w, what the hell huh." (lines 19-20). At this point in mom's illness, what further harm is mom's smoking going to do? What difference does it make? Though son prefaces his utterance as "mo:rbid", it is not as gloomy as it might appear. For example, hospice workers often report that if a person is dying, yet continues to be reliant on cigarettes, why not afford them that familiar comfort? Trying to "change the leopard's spots" at this juncture is highly unlikely to succeed. Attempting to alter long-engrained behaviors can often promote further and unnecessary turmoil within the family. Further, just how much shorter will a person's life be if their smoking continues? Late in terminal illness phases, it is generally agreed that it is at least equally important to enhance quality of life rather than only lengthen the days/weeks before death. And if so, in these circumstances smoking should not only be "allowed" but facilitated—if and when patients and family members are in an environment (such as home, rather than a hospital or care facility) where smoking will not adversely affect others (i.e., through second-hand smoke).

Thinking About Cremating Mom
with a Carton of Cigarettes

Son's "what the hell" position, however, is not what dad addresses next. Dad does not pursue the possibility that mom's continued smoking would not do considerable harm. Instead, he plays off son's "mo:rbid" theme by describing how "funeral directors" will "bitch" when he asks them to lay a "carton of cigarettes" on top of mom during her cremation (lines 21-25). Dad shifts attention not away from mom's smoking, but in favor of *venting his frustration about mom and cigarettes* with a future-oriented, hypothetical set of events (see M. Goodwin, 1990; Holt & Clift, 2006). As dangerous objects, cigarettes are known and considered as contributing to mom's cancer and imminent death. Her use of cigarettes (likely in the face of his ongoing resistance) has been the source of dad's concerted efforts for change over a long period of time (i.e., "life's fight."). This frustration is encapsulated through a somewhat grisly yet humorous depiction of a cremation involving a carton of mom's cigarettes on top of mom's body. Dad symbolically and sarcastically portrays a scene equivalent to burying a loved one with the most important possessions of a lifetime.

Having deployed and received dry wit and dark sarcasm, dad and son simultaneously treat this as laughable (lines 25-26). Dad then continues by making explicit that he will think about it, but after "I'm thin- = u::m na:::h", he reconsiders out loud and admits that "I won't do that." (lines 27-29). Though dad displays his emotions (e.g., frustration, anger, resentment) as justifiable, he also makes apparent that turning these particular thoughts into actions is not just easier said than done, but that such actions would be inappropriate. Once again it is evident that unspoken limits for pursuing mom's indiscretions and alleged wrongdoing (see Beach, 1991, 1996) are at work as dad organizes his talk. Boundaries for civility are not externally imposed rules mandating speakers' alignment (e.g., see Heritage, 1984b, Chapter 5). Rather, as with this instance, dad's envisioning of an action based on resentment is closely followed by going on record that he will *not* actually carry it out. Though he may "seriously think" (lines 27-28) about giving funeral directors a carton of cigarettes to lay on mom's body to be cremated with her, he also states "↓I won't do that. But ↑I'm gonna think about it °heh heh.°." (lines 28-29). Marked by dad's quiet laughter at the completion of his utterance, the delicate and often tenuous relationship between doing and thinking exemplifies a dialectical tension exceedingly common as speakers manage everyday social life.

Legitimate Concerns About Smoking and Fire

What dad does do, however, is launch a new reporting about the inherent dangers of mom's smoking (lines 31-43). These are legitimate concerns prompting watchful actions from caregivers. With the expletives "°God damn.°" and "shit", dad emphasizes that mom had a cigarette in her hand when she fell in the kitchen. And in response, son draws attention to the fact that mom may well fall asleep smoking (lines 36-37). In each instance, the possibility of mom getting burned and creating a fire do not go unnoticed (lines 40-43).

ASSESSING MOM'S DEMEANOR AND ACTIONS

One way for son to explain mom's actions is that "she's not thinkin' real straight." (line 44), an assessment upgraded by dad's "Not even close." (line 45). But dad has been impacted by more than mom being "confused" (line 57), which dad states later and, as will become clear as analysis proceeds, is meaningful for unfolding interaction. It is not just mom's thinking, but the demeanor of her actions that dad addresses next with "And not too sweetly either." (line 45):

5) Malignancy #41:9

44	Son:	=.hh So she's not thinkin' real straight.
45	Dad:	Not even close. (.) And not too sweetly either.
46	Son:	O:hh .hh hey ↑that's gotta be tough on you too.
47		I know you were sayin' that she was- she was getting
48		snarkier amd sna:rkier jus'-
49	Dad:	(°Yep.°) ↑We::ll she's frustra:ted. =
50	Son:	= S(h)ure.

51	Dad:	Ya know, pt doesn't- (.) <u>if</u> she understands on the <u>in</u>side
52		she sure doesn't v<u>e</u>rbally. >Ya'know,= it's gonna be like aunt
53		<u>E</u>sther< you don't know <u>how</u> much is sh- is truly going on
54		<u>acc</u>urately in her ↑<u>mi:nd</u> but-
55	Son:	Mm hm.=
56	Dad:	=You listen to what comes out her <u>mo:uth</u>, ya'know that-
57		<u>tha:t</u> gets con<u>fu</u>sed.

With "<u>O:hh</u> .hh hey ↑that's gotta be <u>tough</u> on you <u>too</u>." (line 46), son even more fully recognizes how difficult it must be for dad as husband and caregiver. Son draws attention away from mom's behaviors and toward the offering of commiseration and support for his dad. He connects dad's "And <u>not too sweet</u>ly either." by reporting that dad had earlier stated that mom "was getting <u>snar</u>kier amd <u>sna:r</u>kier" (lines 47-48). It should be carefully noted that "snarkier" appears nowhere on any of the family phone calls in the Malignancy corpus. It is possible, of course, that son had spoken with dad during a nonrecorded call (e.g., from his office), and that during that discussion dad had actually employed "snarkier." It is equally plausible, however, that what son is referring to is dad's original ">Jesus Christ ya forgot my cigarettes.<" (Excerpt 1, lines 6-7 above)—the focal utterance previously analyzed in some detail, not only as uttered by dad, but also as reconstructed by son to aunt and Gina (Excerpts 2-3). If so, what son is producing is a here-and-now version of the gist or general essence of dad's earlier portrayal: unsolicited and biting behaviors now translated by son as "snarkier." Might the derivative of son's improvised slang be "snarling"?—growling, sneering, and scornful actions displaying disrespect for dad? Whether "snarling" is the actual derivative or not, alone or in combination with other terms (e.g., "shark"), son's "snarkier" is minimally designed to extend dad's prior "<u>not too</u> <u>sweet</u>ly." And he does so by taking a stance against any treatment that is unmerited and insensitive.

With son's "<u>snar</u>kier amd <u>sna:r</u>kier", dad is now provided with a ripe opportunity to elaborate further on mom's untenable behavior. But this opening is also passed by as dad quietly confirms, but then accounts for the reasonableness of mom's actions: "(°Yep.°) ↑<u>We::ll</u> she's <u>frustra:</u>ted. =" (line 49). Again, mom's culpability is not pursued. The option of critiquing mom is replaced with a compassionate grasp of mom's lifeworld experience. Her frustration is a normal and understandable reaction, as affirmed with emphasis by son's aspirated "<u>S(h)</u>ure." (line 50).

Three Embedded and Humorous Stories

It is with that shared understanding in place that dad returns to mom's inability to display that she comprehends what is going on (lines 51-57). Mom is compared to elderly aunt Esther who, across the calls, has been repeatedly invoked as lacking understanding and doing weird things. With this comparison as a background dad launches into two embedded stories (1→ & 2→, below), followed by one initiated by son (3→, below), each exemplifying humorous aspects of mom's (apparently increasing) confusion. The first example dad provides (1→, lines 59-62) involves mom announcing that she plans on making breakfast out of sugar and flour:

6) Malignancy #41:9

59 1→	Dad:	You know she'll be standing her saying well (.) <u>oka:</u>y get
60		some flour and sugar (.) a::nd I'm gonna make breakfast.
61	Son:	$Heh he(h)[h. hh
62 2→	Dad:	[):: ↑<u>ka:y</u>. (.) Thursday morning she came out

```
63              poured herself a cup o' coffee put orange juice in it and
64              started drinkin.=Said boy you make lousy
65              co[$ffee$. °Hah hah hah.° ]
66    Son:         [ Hhhh heh heh heh. ]
67              I guess I shouldn't la:ugh, but that is kinda funny.
68    Dad:    (°Mm ye:ah.°)=
69 3→ Son:    =But that's like aunt Esther puttin' the plastic=
70    Dad:    =M:m ↑h:m.=
71    Son:    =pe- pot on the stove and tryin' to cook it huh?
72    Dad:    Sa::me=thing?
73    Son:    How are you gonna be able tuh- g:o to work. hhh
```

Son responds by laughing, and in overlap, dad produces what I have described as an *incon-gruous* "O::↑ka:y." (Beach, 2002c): a display that something is "*not* okay"—that is, that some prior actions are heard and understood to be somehow at odds or out of place with "okay producers'" position toward those actions. Dad displays recognition that despite mom's good intentions, she is presently unable to prepare a breakfast the way she no doubt used to. His "O::↑ka:y." makes this position available to son in an abbreviated, yet highly efficient, manner.

A second embedded story (2→, lines 62-68) is tied to the first, but shifts to "Thursday morning." Mom is described as pouring orange juice into her coffee, then stating to dad "boy you make lousy co$ffee$." (lines 64-65). This is a classic instance of dad doing noth-ing wrong and getting the blame for it! Dad and son begin laughing at precisely the same moment. Each responds to how a false accusation can be laughed off because of mom's innocent, inherently funny, yet revealing action of pouring juice into her coffee.

Son's laughter does not go unnoticed by dad, as he states "I guess I shouldn't la:ugh, but that is kinda funny." (line 67). While he was laughing *with* dad they were also laughing together *at* mom (see Glenn, 1995). Son's utterance is designed to ward off the appearance of being mean-spirited and in other ways deprecating his ill mother. She is, after all, not simply a person doing funny things in the kitchen: Her mental acuity is diminished from pain medications and the toll of a protracted cancer journey.

However, mom's actions do remind son of aunt Esther: "=But that's like aunt Esther puttin' the plastic pe- pot on the stove and tryin' to cook it huh?." With "Sa::me=thing?" (3→, lines 69-72), dad agrees with (line 70) and confirms son's assessment. This is the third and final triggered story, the theme being funny cooking stories involving mom and aunt Esther. Each story—mom's proposing to make breakfast with flour and sugar, pouring orange juice in her coffee, and Aunt Esther's cooking with a plastic pot—makes clear the importance of humor as a collaborative and interactional resource for reframing otherwise troubling circumstances. These humorous moments are short-lived, however, as son next shifts back to more serious concerns about caregiving, namely, how dad is going to go to work *and* care for mom (line 73).

Retrospective: "bill payin' time"

Approximately four minutes later in the same call, a discussion ensues about dad's work/home schedule and updates from the doctor about mom's deteriorating condition. Son has just asked dad if he is "doin alright?", and dad reports "Most of the time." he is, that he can't dwell on it because it will drive him crazy, and he will "do what I have to do" by keeping mom comfortable, fed, and warm. Dad then offers a revealing summary, inte-grating and providing insight into key moments across Excerpts 1-4 (above). The excerpt below begins as dad informs son that "°this is killing me° you kno::w" (line 1):

7) Malignancy #41:13

```
1    Dad:   I you know I:- °this is killing me you kno::w ([        ).=
2    Son:                                            [Heh .hh hh
3    Dad:   = Hell of a lot of life isn't a choi:ce = yikno:w, and you do this
4           ↑for the ones you love. An' so it's yiknow (.) bill payin'
5           time.=
6    Son:   Ye:ah. hhh .hhhh whe::w.
7    Dad:   And yes it gets tough on times yiknow, 'cuz you're tryin' to
8           be nice an' you're tryin' and you get- (.) he:ll: because you
9           ho:ver: or you get hell because you're not doin' what she
10          wants or you know- (0.5) Bu:t (.) yiknow >she asks for
11          somethin' and then ↑o:kay I'll go do that. And by the time
12          you get back< that's not what she wanted an' =
13   Son:   = Mm hm. =
14   Dad:   = Whatever you °kn[ow)°-
15   Son:                     [Ye:ah.
16          (0.3)
17   Dad:   ↑A:nd it's not ra:tional behavior so you- yiknow you gotta
18          stop and think wa::it a minute (              ) stay
19          pleasant overall an' don't get all bent out of sha:pe over it.
20   Son:   Right.
21   Dad:   And I don't always do that ↑too gracefully.=
22   Son:   =Heh heh [   heh.   ]
23   Dad:            [Heh heh.]=
24   Son:   =That's right this is gonna teach ya tolerance like nothing
25          else in the wo:rld huh.
26   Dad:   °Oh yeah°. (.) Yeah I guess (.) (       ).
```

As dad continues, his role as a caregiver and husband is framed in a larger context, a philosophy of living and coping (lines 3-19) that allows him to fulfill his responsibilities and move forward. In lines 3-5 he emphasizes that "life isn't a choi:ce" when caring for those you love, invoking the cliché "bill payin' time." to characterize the inevitable costs of living—in this case, being a family member caring for a dying wife. Although son can agree and identify with these costs, he cannot claim first-hand knowledge as a primary caregiver. Thus, his responsive "Ye:ah. hhh .hhhh whe::w." (line 6) aligns with dad's description and shares commiserative space (see the previous Chapter 10), offering appreciation for what dad is going through. But as son can only partially know what dad's hands-on experiences consist of, he does not act as though it is part of his *territorial preserve* (see Raymond & Heritage, 2006): Son simply lacks authority to speak directly about such caregiving responsibilities.

TWO "DEVASTATING" STORIES

In the previous chapter, focusing on the *epistemics* of family relationships in the midst of a cancer journey, a set of moments were examined in which aunt twice states "It's devastating." (see Excerpt 11, Chapter 10; lines 33-47 in Excerpt 8, below). As aunt expressed being overwhelmed by disturbing cancer circumstances, so also did son display his turmoil with "IT SUCKS." Each speaker demonstrated being negatively impacted by mom's cancer, actions reflecting their unique yet shared experiences of daily living.

In Excerpt 8 (below) these utterances are placed in a larger context: Aunt is telling a story to son about discussions she'd had with dad. Several calls later, in Excerpt 9 (below), aunt again reports her devastation to son, as a topic raised in yet another discussion with dad. Her tellings, and son's responses, provide a useful backdrop and lens for understanding prior excerpts (1-7, above) about dad's caregiving experiences. Analysis of these excerpts also provides additional insight into how family members simultaneously manage caring for mom and one another.

As aunt begins to describe her talk with dad, son makes clear that he wants to support dad as much as mom (lines 3-7). She then transforms son's concern—that is, being there for dad and mom—by reporting that she and dad had a "real nice lo:ng talk" about "th:at kind of <u>stuff</u>" (lines 8-9):

8) Malignancy 10: 9-11

1	Aunt:	Yeah well the <u>two</u> of us just kinda <u>sat</u> (.) and lo:o<u>k</u>ed.
2	Son:	Um hm.
3	Aunt:	Ya know (.) and you kn[ow]
4	Son:	[I want] to be there as <u>m</u>:uch for dad
5		(.) [as-] as =
6	Aunt:	[Ye::ah.]
7	Son:	= mom at this point too.
8	Aunt:	Um hm. Well I- your <u>d</u>ad and <u>I</u> had a real nice lo:ng talk <u>this</u>
9		afternoon about th:at kind of <u>stuff</u>.
10	Son:	Um hm.
11	Aunt:	I- I- we- we got some (.) re:al good ideas as to the dire:ctions
12		that we:'re go:ing in >because as I said to him< (.) it's going
13		to be <u>he</u> and <u>I</u>.
14	Son:	Ye:ah.
15	Aunt:	And (.) <u>I</u> <u>c</u>an't do it alone (.) a:nd <<u>neither</u> can <u>he</u>.>
16		(1.0)
17	Son:	Nor should either of you have to re:ally.
18	Aunt:	<u>Nope</u>. Not if we've got each oth:er to do this (.) and I said
19		he's gonna have to be (.) le:<u>ss</u> stoic
20		[(.) <u>more</u>] open because <u>I</u>: will =
21	Son:	[$Heh.$]
22 →	Aunt:	= be (.) ju:st as **de:vastated**.
23	Son:	Um hm.
24	Aunt:	A:nd <u>c</u>an't- and won't have the abi:lity ta kinda:a to- to
25		ana:lyz:e (.) ya know it's called you just gotta put it out. =
26	Son:	= Ye::ah.
27	Aunt:	Be<u>c</u>ause I <u>c</u>an't- I won't be able to do:: (.) the <u>typ</u>ical let's try
28		to analyze this.
29	Son:	Ye::ah. <u>I</u> know what ya mean.
30	Aunt:	And so (.) <u>I</u> think we've got ourselves pretty we:ll squar:ed
31		away.
32	Son:	[Umkay.]
33	Aunt:	[A n d] a- on the way home your <u>dad</u> and <u>I</u> ya know there
34		was a little <u>joking</u> back and forth. (.) We're <u>do</u>:ing- we're
35		<u>do</u>:ing <u>okay</u>.
36	Son:	Aright. =
37 →	Aunt:	= It's **de:vastating**. I mean <u>no</u> <u>matter</u> <u>how</u> [you cut it.] =
38	Son:	[$Ye:ah.$]

```
39  →   Aunt:    It's de:vastating. =
40      Son:     = Yeah.
41      Aunt:    Ah:- umm (.) We talked about (.) ya know (.) wh- what we
42               re:ally think about this. And um:: (.) Both of us a- agree that
43               tha:t a::h =
44      Son:     = IT SUCKS! [$ heh heh heh heh heh heh heh$]
45      Aunt:              [         (We:ll)        ye::ah,    ] and that's a
46               real sweet way of putting it. =
47      Son:     = Yeah I know.
```

With "th:at kind of stuff" (line 9), aunt makes indirect reference to the general topic of "being there" for one another. On lines 11-15, she then transitions by reporting what she had stated to dad—that, essentially, they must rely on one another as co-primary care-givers: "as I said to him< (.) it's going to be he and I." (lines 12-13). Though it remains unstated, son's "Ye:ah." (line 17) next recognizes and agrees with aunt's description that she and dad (living near and with mom) will share the on-site, hands-on responsibility of car-ing for mom—tasks that both aunt and son agree can't and shouldn't be done alone (lines 15-18).

In order to rely on dad, however, aunt reports informing dad that he must "be (.) le:ss stoic (.) more open because I will be just as de:vastated." (lines 19-22)—characteristics of dad that son is apparently aware of (lines 21 & 23). Aunt states that dad's being overly ana-lytic (lines 25 & 28) will not work for her as she struggles to cope with these overwhelm-ing and deeply disturbing circumstances, which son also agrees with (lines 26 & 29). By reporting this information to son, aunt thus draws attention to *her* need for emotional sup-port from dad. These are needs that dad also now recognizes: Aunt further reports being "pretty we:ll squar:ed away.", having joked with dad, and finally "We're do:ing- we're do:ing okay." (lines 30-35).

During these moments aunt shifts from reporting what she had said to dad in the past, about being "de:vastated" when mom dies in the future (line 22), to a here-and-now for-mulation of "= It's de:vastating. I mean no matter how [you cut it.] = It's de:vastating. =." (lines 37 & 39). The distressing nature of mom's and the family's cancer journey is thus not limited to only when mom dies, but apparently to the entire process of managing tenuous phases of diagnosis, treatment, and prognosis. These ongoing problems are encapsulated by aunt's "It's", an unspecified and deictic term that aunt employs as an abbreviated resource for referencing a host of unstated, yet assumedly known and oriented-to problems. And these problems are interwoven across time and circumstance. For example, aunt's prior dis-cussion with dad about a dreaded future was inclusive of the present conversation with son in Excerpt 8 (above). And aunt's shift to the present tense, by twice repeating "It's de:vas-tating.", lays claim to both how encompassing the problems are and her entitlement to reporting current my-world (i.e., experienced and lived-out) tribulations. As discussed in a prior chapter (again, see Excerpt 11, Chapter 10), aunt's declarations are next treated by son as not solely hers but personally understood by him as well.

A Fine Line Between Past, Present, and Future

Several phone calls later, prior to Excerpt 9 (below), aunt and son discussed the possibility that mom might die before son had a chance to see her again. Son states a strong preference to get home to be with mom, support dad, and to be with the family. In response aunt assures son that "Yu- you're not (.) not gonna be pushed aside (.) trust me. =", and follow-ing son's "$No hh$ I kn[ow.]", aunt continues:

9) **Malignancy 17: 7-9**

```
 1     Aunt:   [But] we're gonna- we're gonna need ↑every- (0.2) I- I (.) sat
 2             an' talked to your dad for quite a while yesterday about this.
 3             An' I said to him look. (0.8) .hhh I am going to be on my
 4             knees. (0.4) <I know that.> (0.6) And your ↑father's going to be
 5             on his knees. (0.6) And I said Ri:ch (.) pt .hh if we don't cli:ng
 6             (0.8) like glu::e, (0.2) I said >neither one of us is gonna get up.<
 7     Son:    ↑Um hmm.
 8     Aunt:   An' I said (.) ↑I can- I can he:lp:, (.) a lo:t.
 9             (0.4)
10     Aunt:   .hh But you're gonna have to he::lp (.) a lo::t ↑also.
11     Son:    =Yeah. =
12  →  Aunt:   =I said ↑ this is very devastating.
13             (0.4)
14     Aunt:   pt (.) A::nd >↑he an I had a nice long chat about< tha:t, and uh
15             ((sound of banging and moving in background))
16             (0.8) °Ya know° we're gonna a:ll have to pull together.
17             (0.4)
18     Aunt:   An' we really will.
19             (0.2)
20     Son:    Ye:ah. =
21     Aunt:   = This is jus' gonna: knock us for a lo::op uh. =
22     Son:    =$Hhh [hh hh $hh$ ]
23     Aunt:         [ Even thou]gh we've been (0.2) waiting for these days
24             it's ↑still gonna knock us for a lo:op.
25     Son:    Ye:ah.
26             (0.6)
27     Son:    pt hh[ hhh  hhhh   hhhh hhhh hh]
28     Aunt:        [But I- ↑we will be  there,] and you will be part of it,
29             and you will not be (.) pushed aside for a- for even a moment.
30     Son:    pt. .hhhh Well what I told Dad is I will- I will ↑keep things (.)
31             i::n as much ah state uh readiness as possible. =
32     Aunt:   = Ye[ap.]
```

In lines 1-6 Aunt reports to son additional discussions with dad about how future events—likely, the trying experiences of mom's dying and actual death—will bring each to their "knees", requiring each to "cli:ng (0.8) like glu::e" in order to survive the ordeal. Son emphatically agrees (line 7). Aunt then continues by first stating that she had offered her help to dad, but also that dad needed to help "a lo::t" as well. With her next "=I said ↑this is very devastating." (line 12), aunt summarizes the intensity of her feelings by shifting from talk about the future to current here-and-now (though reported from the past) experiences. As with Excerpt 8 (above), aunt's retelling of *past* events initially forecasts future dreaded events as a preview for describing *present* circumstances as "devastating." Again, a fine line is shown to exist between family members' temporal orientations to challenges associated with mom's demise. Concerns and emotions retold from the past, about the future, are shown to have current negative impacts through references such as "It's/this is…devastating."

One grounded and relevant way to describe a "cancer journey", then, is to begin noticing how those involved report that they were, are, and will be preoccupied with what is essentially an expedition through illness: an inherently demanding voyage that, once underway and unfolding, may provide only nominal reprieves and few "time-outs." The more serious the prognosis, the more incessant the work required to monitor, manage, and report on not just what is happening, but how best to cope with and survive many undulating passages. Both individually and as a family, such interactional efforts mirror a patient's well-being, are unremitting, and not infrequently burdensome. Yet the solutions, to have "a nice long chat" as aunt puts it (line 14, above), and "pull together...An' we really will." (line 16), are primary resources for grasping the best possible quality of living in the face of trials and tribulations associated with cancer. As discussed further in the following Chapters 12 and 13, this is but one of many moments when hopeful orientations to troubling circumstances routinely arise. As summarized by an old English Proverb listed in the following Chapter 12—"Hope for the best but prepare for the worst"—speakers' actions can at times reflect what secular reasoning describes in only general terms.

Immediately next, however, aunt's brief glimpse of hope through family support gives way to an abiding recognition: "This is jus' gonna: knock us for a lo::op uh." (line 21; also see line 24). Described previously (see Endnote 1, Chapter 7) as one of many figurative expressions employed by family members when managing troubles, as with son's later "state uh readiness" (line 31), speakers have various interactional resources available for handling the troubles mom's illness continues to regenerate.

HUMORING HAIR: EPISODES OF PLAY

Playing together through talk provides family members the opportunity to replenish depleted resources (emotional and physical), valuable assets when caring for self and others across extended periods of time. As evident in the excerpts below, conversational play can actually build up and edify participants in the game. Humor and play are critical elements of managing troubling circumstances, offsetting the erosion of hope in life, while bolstering the will to endure together as a family.

Whisker Burns and Shaving Mom's Head

Four days and some 20 calls later (see Timeline in Chapter 2), dad had just informed son that mom's condition was "relatively status quo...Situation's about the same.". She is less bothered by pain, though still hurting at times. Dad states that although he's sure mom's condition is "deteriorating" a bit, he really doesn't "know what it's doing.". As mom's hair was lost as a consequence of radiation and chemotherapy treatments, in line 1 son then asks dad the following question about mom's hair:

10) **Malignancy 37: 3**

```
 1   Son:   .hh Is her hair growing back yet?
 2   Dad:   $Heh heh$ No:[:.
 3   Son:             [$Heh heh heh heh.$ =
 4   Dad:   =She does have a little stubble up there, 'cuz I kissed her
 5          goodbye last night and I got whisker burns.
 6   Son:   $Heh heh heh$ .hh Well tell her she should sha:ve. You
 7          >gotta get her one of those electric-< like a- .hh a Norelco or
 8          somethin. =
 9   Dad:      [[ [Yea::h.    ]
10   Son:   = [[ [She could] b'fffph over her hea[d.]
11   Dad:                                    [ Remington.
12   Son:   Yeah yeah, there you go. .hh Or an Epilady for your head
```

13   huh? $Hh [heh heh heh heh.$]
14   Dad: [$Heh heh heh.$] Right. =
15   Son: = Heh. O(h)<u>ka:</u>y.
16   Dad: But other than that I don't have time to do anything else, so

Son's query, and their shared laughter (lines 2-3), knowingly draws attention to mom's baldness as an unfortunate outcome of treatment.[3] Their laughter is hearably endearing, not belittling. Over the next several moments, however, dad and son incrementally transform mom's head and hair into resources for humor and play. In lines 4-5, dad initiates playful action by offering a nonliteral depiction of an event: When kissing mom goodbye on her head, he reports getting "whisker burns" from mom's "stubble." That "whisker burns" are typically caused by men's unshaven facial hair, extended here to mom's head, is an invitation of play that does not go unnoticed by son. In his response (lines 6-8), son's laughter prefaces a next round of exaggeration. He not only encourages dad to "tell her she should shave", but suggests that dad get her an electric (e.g., Norelco) shaver. Produced simultaneously with dad's next "Yea::h." (line 9), son continues by animating the actual "b'fffph" sound that would be produced by mom's shaver. Near the completion of son's turn, dad's overlapped "Remington." (line 11) adds to the trajectory son had been developing, namely, generating name-brand electric razors that mom might employ to shave her "whiskers."

In lines 12-13, son fully acknowledges dad's collaboration, then further extends this playful sequence by not only offering a third name-brand candidate—"<u>E</u>pilady"—but invoking an electric hair remover made exclusively for women. Through repeated efforts, son and dad have essentially worked together to playfully construct a list of name-brand shavers (see Hopper, 1995; Hopper & Glenn, 1994; Jefferson, 1990). What makes this list-construction increasingly outlandish, of course, is that women typically employ "Epilady" for shaving their legs and under-arms, *not* their heads—a not-so-subtle distinction that both son and dad recognize as laughable (lines 13-14).[4]

With "Heh. O(h)<u>ka:</u>y." (line 15), son responds to dad's prior "Right.=" (line 14) as having been not just an agreement, but a sequence closing action designed to terminate the end of their silliness. Son's "Heh. O(h)<u>ka:</u>y." is slightly incongruous (see Beach, 2002c) in that it displays his recognition that dad's movement toward closure treated the prior humor—and perhaps son's final extension to "<u>E</u>pilady"—as being out of place, or inappropriate. And with "But other than that", dad returns to reporting on the lack of change in mom's condition (line 16).

Launched by son's query in line 1, it can now be seen that the humorous "shaving" pursuit was a side sequence (see Jefferson, 1972) that momentarily distracted, but did not derail son and dad from the primary focus on mom's failing health. Such actions in a flurry, evident in Excerpt 10 (above) as well as Excerpt 11 (below), allow family members to construct alternative perspectives: nonliteral activities that become progressively less real, yet increasingly funny (but only up to a point). Though fleeting, these humorous involvements are treated by dad and son as unfolding play in the midst of ongoing troubles. But a break from being serious does not equate to a time-out from meaningful action. Through play, the challenges and responsibilities of directly confronting difficult situations are momentarily put on hold. Though son and dad enliven and animate their talk, laughing and telling an imaginary story together, they remain family members engrossed in a long-term cancer journey requiring perseverance and resilience. Being playful and humorous can be an important resource for bolstering their abilities to remain vigilant, concerned, yet able and willing to be lighthearted when talking and co-authoring stories about mom's condition.

Importantly, however, dad and son specifically design their play to *avoid* being derogatory toward mom (i.e., her appearance, demeanor, or behaviors). The playful solution co-created by son and dad—to shave mom's head with electric razors to eliminate whisker burns—is neither a permanent orientation nor denial of very real and serious cancer circumstances. Rather, their actions embody a respite from what can understandably become a tedious, even monotonous preoccupation with mom's progressive dying. Playful interactions function as life-giving resources, even in the face of dying and death. Playing together can occur whether the topic is shaving mom's head or, as below, when washing and shampooing mom's hair gives rise to polishing her head as if it were a "bowling ball."

Shampooing, Polishing, and Buffing Mom's Head

Less than two minutes prior to Excerpt 11 (below), dad had stated that because he is now caring for mom at home, he more fully appreciates "hospital orderlies and home health care people…the unsung heroes of the hospital." He emphasizes how poorly they are paid (as with teachers and policemen), especially when compared with people such as "TV gladiators" (i.e., professional athletes), "TV evangelists", and even "Watergate conspirators." Son nominates "Donald Trump" as having achieved some noteworthy goals, but further supports dad's concerns by comparing the relative unimportance of Trump's "refinancing an ailing casino" versus "financing a school district." In short, dad and son collaborate in arguing that although many well-known individuals are overpaid, even more persons are not just poorly paid but underappreciated (e.g., hospital care providers).

Following this discussion, son jokes with dad by asking if dad is going to quit his job and become an "orderly." Or, might dad consider taking more patients into his home and create a home health care facility? Excerpt 11 (below) begins with dad's response that he would need more help, followed by a troubles-telling about giving mom a bath. In line 4, with "I bet." son is receptive to hearing dad's troubled story, encouraging dad to elaborate with more details about his experiences with bathing and caring for mom:

11) **Malignancy 41: 5-6**

```
 1    Dad:          [ ↑Probably.   ] I'd have to get some help.=Le- let me
 2                  tell ya: (0.4) just trying to give her a bath yesterday wore me
 3                  out.
 4    Son:    I'll bet.
 5    Dad:    (°Yeah I jus°-)
 6    Son:    You gotta kinda [ practically-   ]
 7    Dad:                     [Get your shoes] an' socks off and yiknow
 8                  >roll your pants up 'cuz you gotta get her in an' out.<
 9    Son:    Mm hm:.
10    Dad:    A:nd $°heh heh°$ fortunately washing her hair is easy.
11                  $°Heh heh°$.
12    Son:    Js- just stick her head under is that- [hh hh $heh heh$. ]
13    Dad:                                           [$°Heh heh heh$ (  ]  ) =
14    Son:    = That's right. = That's ↑right! = That's right, no ha:ir. =
15    Dad:    = I catch myself >doin' that every once in awhile and its
16                  dumb.< Because I mean it's been like this for so long. .hh
17                  But- ya'know I got her ↑in the tu:b, and she had- soap an' a
18                  wash cloth and she was doing a little washin'. = So I said
19                  okay, >hang on a minute I'll go get the shampoo.< And I
20                  walked out the door and I said
21                  ↓$He::hh$, [what a dumb thing.]
22    Son:                     [.hh hh $Y(h)eah. $ ] Although when you ↑said
23                  that I said the same things = > i- why is it- oh I keep
24                  forgettin' she doesn't have any ha:ir. < .hh Ya know? =
25                  Dad:= °Heh he heh.° ↑Yeah. So I went back and I got the wa:sh
```

26   cloth and soap =
27   Son: $Uh hu [heh heh heh heh heh heh heh$ hhh.]
28   Dad: = [(   ) you know. °I said°   ] ↑O:h God (   ).
29   Son: You need a <u>bowling</u> ball washer, huh?
30               $hhh [hhh heh heh.$] =
31   Dad: [$Heh heh heh.$]
32   Son: = Don't tell her I <u>said</u> that,[okay?] =
33   Dad: [No: I] won't (tell).
34   Son: = $Heh heh heh$ .hh hh .pt Bla:h. ((heavy swallow)) Yeah
35   you could just get a- a little p<u>le</u>dge an a- kind a <u>dust</u> cloth an'
36   chika=chika=chika right?
37   Dad: Polish it [up.]
38   Son: [Buf]f it up. =
39   Dad: = Uncle Tom's <u>car</u> <u>buf</u>fer: [an- =
40   Son: [$Yeah heh [heh ha.$
41   Dad: = [Few of those and the-
42   the- then <u>bo:y</u> it'd be shiny! =
43   Son: = Ts:::h::: I:=<u>li:ke</u> it. .hh U:gh.
44   Dad: A::gh:.
45   Son: .hhh So- so what- what's she <u>doing</u> I me:an-
46   Dad: °A:h:°, less and less:. =
47   Son: = Less [and le]ss. = O<u>ka:y</u>.
48   Dad: [U::hm]
49   (0.3)
50   Dad: She got up for a whi:le yesterday. She fe::ll:-
51   (1.2)
52   Dad: O::h: hell <u>F:ri</u>day morning.

In line 10, dad informs son that "fortunately washing her hair is easy.." His utterance is prefaced and followed with "$°heh heh°$", laughter inviting son to rely on his shared knowledge in recognizing the truth and humor of dad's assertion (see Jefferson, 1979). At first son provides a logical connection (line 12) that dad simply needed to stick mom's head under (implicitly) the faucet. But near the completion of his utterance he abruptly displays recognition, with laughter, that dad was not referring to the faucet but to mom's having no hair. In overlap, dad shares son's laughter at the precise moment son solved the puzzle, evident in son's next and repeatedly emphasized "= That's right. = That's ↑right! = That's right, no <u>ha:ir</u>. =." (line 14).

Dad's initial troubles-telling and son's receptiveness thus gave rise to the activity of what might be characterized as *shared forgetfulness*. As dad continues (linies 15-21), it becomes apparent that son was not alone in forgetting about mom's loss of hair due to treatment. Dad reports that he repeatedly catches himself going to get shampoo that is not needed, despite mom having had no hair for some time, actions qualifying him as "<u>dumb</u>" (line 16) and doing "a <u>dumb</u> thing" (line 21). In overlap and with laughter (lines 22-23), however, son is quick to point out that dad is not alone: He too is saying and thinking the "same things." In lines 23-34, son animates his forgetfulness by reenacting cut-off thoughts and even an "oh-prefaced" realization that mom has no hair. Son completes his utterance with ."hh Ya <u>know</u>? =", a solicitation seeking confirmation of dad's shared experience that dad next provides with "= °Heh he heh.° ↑Yeah." (line 25). Dad then continues by again revisiting his humorous bathing/caregiving experience with "wa:sh cloth and soap" (lines-25-26) that son's extended laughter treats as extremely funny (line 27). It is now dad's turn to animate his own reactions by stating "°I said°] ↑O:h God (   )." (line 28): an intoned and oh-prefaced invocation of "God" that, as aligned with many other similar moments across the "Malignancy" phone calls, depicts a troubling situation appearing not to be under dad's full control but in need of some remedy. Repeated experiences at retrieving shampoo, especially when it is not needed, does not qualify as a catastrophe. But the allure of dad's reporting and dramatization of these bathing/caregiving events is further enhanced by depicting an "↑O:h God (   )." moment—the kind of moment that son can, and has, treated as both common and humorous.

Constructing an Imaginary "Bowling Ball"

Thus far (lines 1-28) it can be seen that the troubles-telling nature of Excerpt 11 (above) also involves a related matter: shared commiseration over forgetting that mom had no hair. These forgetful moments were treated by dad and son as humorous in their own right. Each speaker exhibited the ability to laugh at himself and one another as mutually caught up in not fully grasping the details of mom's ongoing physical condition—details that should, by now, be all too familiar. There is a "we're all bozos on this bus" type of orientation created by dad and son that is inherently laughable and, apparently, "par for the course" during this phase of the family cancer journey. Dad, of course, can speak more directly to his actual bathing/caregiving experiences. But son's recognition of dad's curious dilemma, and sharing of his own forgetfulness, allowed for the possibility of laughing through, and with, dad's reporting of a troubling experience caring for mom at home.

Although playful, dad and son's collaborative actions have to this point remained focused on actual (reportable) events: bathing, washing and shampooing mom, and each forgetting that mom had no hair. Next, however, son again initiates play by once again (as in Excerpt 10, above) introducing an imaginary: getting a "bowling ball washer," (line 29) for mom's head.

Though son and dad laugh together at son's proposal (lines 30-31), son quickly recognizes the potential delicacy of his indiscretion (see Bergman, 1993) by requesting "= Don't tell her I said that,[okay?] =." In overlap (line 33), dad next agrees not to "tell", and son follows with an aspirated, heavy swallow ("Bla:h.") that could well have terminated this discussion and topic. But instead, son further elaborates (lines 34-36) about events that will never occur: Applying "pledge" to mom's head and shining it ("chika=chika=chika") with a "dust cloth." Rather than treating son's continued exaggeration as inappropriate by (in various ways) stating so, or withholding support of son's actions by stating nothing at all, dad's "Polish it up." (line 37) confirms and incrementally adds momentum to son's imagined (and envisioned) proposal. And in response to son's overlapped and confirming "Buff it up.=" (line 38), dad extends the playful visualization even further (lines 39-41) by nominating "= Uncle Tom's car buffer: [an- = = [Few of those and the- the- then bo:y it'd be shiny! =."

Dad's shift, from son's hand-shining proposal to utilizing a rotating buffing machine (with implied rotating pad-at-work), is laughed at by son (line 40) prior to a summarized "= Ts:::h::: I:=li:ke it. .hh U:gh." (line 43). In addition to explicitly informing dad that he liked the shift to an electric car buffer, son also moves to close these playful behaviors. His utterance functions as one form of a sequence closing assessment (Jefferson, 1980a), a bid that dad's next "A::gh:." (line 44) is aligned with as the nonliteral, imaginary, head-shining activities get terminated. Immediately, and next, attention is shifted back to what mom is doing and a reporting by dad that "She fe::ll:- (1.2) O::hh hell F:riday morning." (lines 50-52).[5]

Once again, this shift represents a continuing *default preoccupation* with mom's condition. In both Excerpts 10 & 11 (above), talk about matters related to mom's health gave rise to an eventual cascading of collaborative and playful actions about mom's hair and head, moments where son and dad co-created imagined events in ways that neither speaker could produce alone. Once completed, however, the conversations returned directly to mom's status. At times it is difficult to determine what the *business as usual* and *business at hand* might be for dad and son (and other family members as well). Over time, attending to changes involving mom's cancer has become treated by these speakers as not just normal and routine, but the predominant (thus usual) business of their phone calls. Other moments of play and discussions of topics seemingly unrelated to mom's cancer—most frequently cars, dogs, food, and events occurring in son's life (e.g., work, dating, his apartment)—may well be on ways of monitoring and reporting on daily life as it moves forward. But they do not appear to be the primary reason for most phone calls. Rather, talk gets primarily designed to update and commiserate about how, and what, mom is doing.

For this basic reason, another's illness and health condition can literally come to dominate family members' lives—more or less, on a fluctuating yet predictable basis—and thus what counts as "normal" and "usual" can become transformed across time and phase of an illness. It is for this reason that activities such as shaving and shining mom's head, knowingly shaped as unreal yet humorous activities, are both enduring and endearing involvements. Produced by a son and dad who carefully craft their language and talk in order to play together, worlds are momentarily created that are not plausible, and thus not real in their consequences—especially when they won't "tell" on each other! Such fleeting, humorous, and imaginary worlds offer a respite to the business of addressing the stark realities associated with mom's dying.

The End of Play about Mom's Hair

In the final Excerpt 12 (below), less than one minute following Excerpt 11 (above), the predominance of serious attention given to mom, rather than continued humor about her, is further evident. Below, dad continues by informing son about additional troubling events occurring to mom. He reports how mom banged her head on the door when she fell, and son replies with "Wow." (line 5):

12) **Malignancy 41: 6-7**

```
 1   Dad:   And yiknow she ba:nged the back of her head on the door. =
 2          Apparently she was fa:cin' the bed, 'cause she's now got a
 3          hospital bed where her regular bed was. And she just,
 4          yiknow crumbled and went over backwards. So [ there's] =
 5   Son:                                              [ Wo:w. ]
 6   Dad:   = a (.) goose egg on the back of her head.
 7          (.)
 8   Son:   >No hair to cover it.<
 9   Dad:   No::[:.
10   Son:       [Heh heh heh. =
11   Dad:   = Covered it with just a big red (.) raised bump.
12   Son:   Mm hm.
13   Dad:   U:hm.
14   Son:   Wo:w.
```

Mom's fall resulted in a "goose egg on the back of her head." (line 6), which son surmises is apparent because she has ">No hair to cover it.<" (line 7). Both dad's response, an emphasized and drawn-out "No::[:", and son's following laughter, make available to one another the *potential* humor in mom's baldness. But neither pursues more play as dad continues to describe the "big red (.) raised bump." (line 11) on mom's head, a portrayal acknowledged with surprise by son.

This is the last reference to mom's hair or head in the phone call corpus. Through storytelling, mom's hair and head became objects of attention, providing short-lived yet animated topics for discussion. Though spontaneous and thus unmotivated, mom's body became a resource for playful conduct that, however humorous, was not designed to be derogatory toward a dying mom/wife. Instead, her hair and head provided opportunities for son and dad to momentarily rely on language to visualize unreal possibilities that would otherwise not exist. And as mom's condition worsened, so too did these playful opportunities fade away.

NOTES

1. Technically, this is not the kind of moment described by Pomerantz (1980) in her study of how speakers tell about an experience to "fish" or elicit information from recipient. What dad does do, however, is proceed to immediately offer a revelation about his unsettling daily experiences with mom and the kinds of troubling consequences arising as her illness progresses. It is in this specific sense that I refer to his story as a *my-side telling*, immediately following son's "<u>weird</u>." formulation about a present experience.

2. There are a number of colloquial expressions of relevance to family members' unwillingness to find fault, specifically, with a mom who was dying of cancer:

    - To lay bare her potential wrongdoing would be akin to *adding salt to a wound*.
    - By not pursuing mom's actions, speakers participated in *giving a man/woman a break* (which, ironically, is what dad articulated in Excerpt 1).
    - Finally, to go after mom would also be like *kicking a horse when it's down*, which (as has been shown) was actively avoided.

3. Hair loss and baldness is, of course, one common side-effect of cancer treatments (as are nausea, vomiting, and loss of energy). Though troubling, patients' "bald heads" are also a resource for humor, as depicted in the cartoon below from Christine Clifford's *Not now...I'm having a no hair day* (2003):

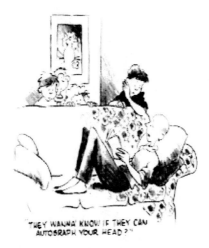

"THEY WANNA KNOW IF THEY CAN AUTOGRAPH YOUR HEAD?"

4. See Beach and Glenn (2009) for a more detailed analysis of how speakers "invite" and respond to "gendered" matters (see also Beach, 2003b).

5. Dad's use of the word "hell" is an emphasis that seems tailored to a troublesome event that dad did not control. And although, it can only be assumed, it is most likely that dad would have preferred that mom did not fall in the first place. In these ways, dad's use of "hell" is not dissimilar to most if not all instances when some "deity" gets invoked in the midst of trouble.

12

SECULAR, SPIRITUAL, AND SOCIAL SCIENTIFIC CONCEPTIONS OF *HOPE* (and OPTIMISM)

In *The Anatomy of Hope*, Groopman (2004) offers a penetrating and moving analysis of the power of hope in cancer care.[1] Relying on nearly 30 years of experience as a Harvard physician and elsewhere, Groopman strikes an intricate balance between two case studies: patients challenged by cancer, and his maturation as a person, care-provider, and friend. Throughout, the practical and scientific importance of *hope* — though long discounted by those in traditional medicine as merely a soft or psychosocial concern, best addressed by professionals such as social workers, counselors, and clergy — cannot be underestimated:

> For all my patients, hope, true hope, has proved as important as any medication I might prescribe or any procedure I might perform . . . a catalyst in the crucible of care [hope] is as vital to our lives as the oxygen we breath . . . the very heart of healing. For those who have hope, it may help some to live longer, and it will help all to live better. (pp. xiv, xvi, 208, 212)

As Groopman argues well, any examination of hope and healing must address complex matters such as why some people rely more fully on hope than others, inevitable fluctuations between hope and despair throughout cancer journeys, and how beliefs and expectations of a better future can actually promote physical improvement (i.e., the "biology of hope"). Hope, it seems, provides persons with greater resources for managing inherently uncertain and fearful events that cannot be fully controlled. And just as hope trumps fear, so too does increasing fear diminish our abilities to overcome what Groopman (2004) describes as "the significant obstacles and deep pitfalls" (p. xiv) universally experienced by those undergoing cancer, as well as those actually providing cancer care.

From the *Anatomy of Hope*, diverse implications arise for enhancing medical education, doctoring effectively, and integrating often dichotomized relationships between primal human emotions, biomedicine, and social scientific investigations of the experience and communication of illness (see also Lamm, 1997; Spiro, 1998; Sternberg, 2000).

FUNDAMENTAL OBSERVATIONS AND QUESTIONS
ABOUT HOPE (AND OPTIMISM)

Examinations of hope (and optimism) require fundamental understandings of the interplay between faith and human conduct in interaction: What do people have (and display) faith in that allows them to be hopeful (or not)—religion, spirituality, trustworthy physicians and medical technologies, family and friends, a "benign order" of everyday life (see below, Maynard, 2003), other worldly affordances? Similarly, if hope is to be considered as more than something people experience individually, that is, as social activities speakers collaborate in producing, *how* are these actions achieved (e.g., see Holt, 1993; Jefferson, 1988; Maynard, 2003)? Is it possible to identify speakers' practices for managing, coping, and simply dealing with cancer (and other demanding life events) on a daily basis? How does hope get socially constructed, both in the clinic (e.g., see Beach et al., 2004; Heritage & Stivers, 1999; Maynard & Frankel, 2006) and throughout interactions among family members and others?

One of the recurring questions I have been asked is "How do people remain hopeful and optimistic in the face of a terminal cancer diagnosis?" And similarly, "Are hope and optimism equivalent terms (and actions)?" As Groopman's (2004) self-reflective journey clearly reveals, these are deceptively difficult questions to address. At least preliminary answers to the first question, involving how family members cope or manage inherently uncertain and difficult situations, are provided in Chapter 13. The second matter, distinguishing hope from optimism, could become a treatise in itself—a conceptual, theoretical, and philosophical inquiry into the importance of expecting and orienting positively toward a bright future—and thus extends well beyond the scope of this present discussion. A more limited focus, though sufficiently critical and complex in its own right, involves attempts to understand the organization of human interactions as anchored in actual circumstances faced by family members. These matters are also addressed in the following Chapter 13, where any identified distinctions or similarities between hope and optimism can be exemplified with actual instances drawn from phone conversations. Put simply, are these equivalent terms when translated into social actions? If so, how? If not, why not?

At least conceptually, I find Groopman's (2004) basic observation—that *true* hope is less delusional than optimism—both intuitive and intriguing. Grounded in a more realistic assessment of any given situation, hope (whatever its foundation) provides resources for overcoming obstacles, making informed decisions, and charting a preferred path. In contrast, optimism is more general and leans toward a rosy (but less realistic) grasp of evolving events and future outcomes. Being optimistic that events will work out fine is markedly different than pessimism, which implies negative and less preferred consequences of expectations, choices, and actions. But, at least intuitively, optimism lacks both the conviction and therefore the resilience offered by hope.

That said, there are of course limitations to my sense of intuition. I initially adopted the term "managing optimism"[2] for an initial paper on these materials (Beach, 2003a). Clear-cut distinctions between hope and optimism were absent then, and to some extent remain vague (even in Chapter 13). What will become evident, however, are moments when speakers explicitly invoke the term "hope/hoping/hopeful." Other, more observable activities occur when speakers do not utter those terms, but do exhibit positive orientations to future time frames and events (e.g., as with shifts from "bad" to "good" topics). So although there may well be worthwhile distinctions between hope and optimism across varying secular, spiritual, and social scientific perspectives, no definitive solution is offered here, nor empirically in the next chapter. And I will (at times) be employing "hope" in a generic fashion, inclusive of diverse optimistic concerns and orientations.

In what follows, I retrace a series of steps taken to address long-standing questions about hope, illness, and (more generally) everyday life. My interests in the possibility of hope in interaction were anchored in initial observations about the first seven moments, identified in calls #1 and #2 and overviewed in Excerpts 1-7 (below). These moments were initially identified on the grounds that family members seemed to be involved in the work of something like being hopeful (or) optimistic. Consider the following seven utterances, each examined in more detail in the present chapter:

1) **SDCL: Malignancy #1:6-7**

   Dad: So .hhh <u>n:o::</u> I would hope by Monday or Tu:esday

2) **SDCL: Malignancy #1:7**

   Dad: .hhh <u>But</u> (0.2) she did have two nice things ha:ppen today.

3) **SDCL: Malignancy #2:2-3**

   Mom: No there's nothin to say. >You just-< .hh I'll? I'll wait to talk
   to Dr. Leedon today.= He's the cancer man, and =

4) **SDCL: Malignancy #2:2-3**

   Mom: My only <u>hope</u>- I mean? (.) my only <u>choice</u>.

5) **SDCL: Malignancy #2:5**

   Son: Well where's our magic wand Mom.

6) **SDCL: Malignancy #2:5**

   Mom: .hh Is find a reason to keep fighting and (.) to keep being

7) **SDCL: Malignancy #2:12-13**

   Son: See, [there] there's a small battle=
   Mom: [( )]
   Son: =that we've won.=

Only Excerpts 1, 4, and 6 reveal "hope/hopeful" as being invoked, and then in similar yet contrasting ways: in dad's reference to medical procedures (1), a personal reflection on mom's ill-fated circumstance (4), and her display of perseverance and tenacity (6). Yet the other instances are also somehow related to hopeful and/or optimistic orientations: As dad lightens prior and serious discussion (2), mom waits and relies upon news from the cancer doctor (3), son invokes and mom responds seriously to "magic," and son's later attempts to edify and simply cheer mom up (7) in response to a story she initiates. From the outset of these phone calls, moments such as these became candidates for managing hope and optimism as a practical matter for family members. Within the Malignancy corpus, this talk emerges in the course of working through varying kinds of troubling illness circumstances.

Before turning directly to these and other instances from the recorded and transcribed phone calls in Chapter 13, this chapter describes how ongoing examinations of these (and related moments) also prompted simultaneous efforts to discover the following: (a) Basic conceptions of hope in society (both secular and spiritual, though limited herein to Judeo-Christian);[3] and (b) social scientific research efforts (both quantitative and qualitative) that have been designed to reveal whether (or not) hope made a practical difference in persons' daily lives. As noted, a third concern involves determining how (or if) these contrasting yet overlapping approaches to hope might be of relevance to understanding what speakers in the Malignancy phone calls *actually do* when communicating together. These data forms the basis for the following Chapter 13.

Returning to questions asked by others regarding hope and optimism, I have tended to respond to others' queries with ample questions of my own: Though intuitive, *do* family members communicate hopefully? *Does* hope get enacted, and if so, in what ways? Is hope even a relevant analytic concept for describing and explaining what speakers do together, in interaction, throughout key moments comprising a cancer journey (and life-in-general)? If hope is something more than what individuals experience, what is the social organization of hope as an interactional accomplishment?

An Ongoing Experiment on Hope

Matters of hope are highly personalized across individuals. As I eventually discovered (as discussed below), very little is known or understood about hope beyond reportings of individuals' experiences (see also Chapter 1). Understanding hope as a set of communicative resources for managing difficult and chronic illness circumstances together is a relatively novel concern for medical practitioners and social scientists alike. So I proceeded to set up an exercise of sorts, an ongoing experiment on hope. Although I had no a priori conceptions that family members' actions on the telephone were driven or constrained by secular or spiritual orientations to hope, whatever they might be, I was curious about what such contrasts might yield. What is it about the human condition that such alternative perspectives reveal? Are there points of intersection, overlaps, that might aid in explaining an otherwise ephemeral notion like hope? How does *this family* manage hope and optimism? As noted, what differences (if any) exist between hope and optimism? Are these closely related conceptions—*family resemblances*, as with Wittgenstein's discussions of category names (1958, 1969)?

Below, an overview of alternative orientations to secular, spiritual, and social scientific conceptions of hope is provided—a backdrop and lens for better understanding how family members organize their interactions with one another.

SECULAR AND SPIRITUAL PERSPECTIVES ON HOPE

Early on in what I now (tongue-in-cheek) refer to as "my search for hope", I ran across an advertisement sponsored by The American Cancer Society (ACS) . The ACS is an organization committed to curing and preventing cancer, but also caring for cancer patients, survivors, and loved ones experiencing this illness. Their concerted advertising and marketing efforts feature *Hope* as a primary resource for maintaining the fight against this dreaded disease (Figure 12.1).

American Cancer Society:
Hope. Progress. Answers.

LIFE

...is a mother who has to tell her little boy that he has cancer.

...is a daughter desperate to get her father to stop smoking.

...is a patient who calms her fears by talking with others.

...is a wife with cancer whose husband has given up hope.

No matter who she is, we can help.

Figure 12.1. American Cancer Society Advertisement.

When I first read these messages, I distinctly recall raising additional questions like the following: How *does* a mother deliver bad news to her young son? What techniques *does* a daughter deploy to persuade her father to quit smoking (e.g., see Beach, 1996)? In what precise ways *does* fear get "calmed" (or does it?) as patients talk with others? Indeed, what does "fear" *look like* in the midst of interaction (see Beach et al., 2004)? Finally, how *does* a husband who has "given up hope" demonstrate such resignation, and how might his wife the cancer patient (and all others in the advertisement above) respond?

Although ACS's advertising messages were compelling, they made reference to but did not provide a communication framework for understanding that these kinds of moments, and the problems they represent, were in the first instance complex, real time, inherently collaborative and interactional involvements. These reactions were triggered by the fact that during that same period of time I was in the very early stages of trying to figure out just how family members in the Malignancy phone calls coped with cancer: Did speakers respond to uncertain and potentially despairing cancer circumstances hopefully and optimistically?

It was the interplay of these kinds of questions, and being engaged in numerous data/listening sessions in which potential hopeful/optimistic moments began to be identified, that prompted further inspections of both secular and spiritual conceptions of hope.

Below I do not offer (by any measure) an exegesis or exhaustive elaboration of hope. Such an exercise is certainly merited and would no doubt yield a vast array of topics extending our current (somewhat myopic) understandings of such a vast concept as hope. Rather, my intention is to provide a basic overview of issues for readers—a comparative framework for yielding enhanced understandings of how family members organize their interactions offered in Chapter 13.

Written and Spoken (Secular) Conceptions of Hope

Consider, first, a series of instances when *hope* emerged as a primary focus for diverse secular writers/speakers (Figure 12.2):

You can't hinder the wind from blowing. Time is a great teacher.
Who can live without *hope*?
(Carl Sandburg)

Have *hope*. Though clouds environ now, And gladness hides her face in scorn,
Put thou the shadow form thy brow–No night but hath its morn.
(Johan Christoph Friedrich von Schiller)

The very least you can do in your life is to figure out what you *hope* for.
And the most you can do is live inside that *hope*. Not admire it from a distance
but live right in it, under its roof.
(Barbara Kingsolver)

Never deprive someone of *hope*–it may be all they have.
(Unknown)

Beware how you take away *hope* from another human being.
(Oliver Wendell Holmes)

Hope is a waking dream.
(Aristotle: 384-322 B.C.)

Figure 12.2. A Sampling of Secular Quotes Involving Hope.

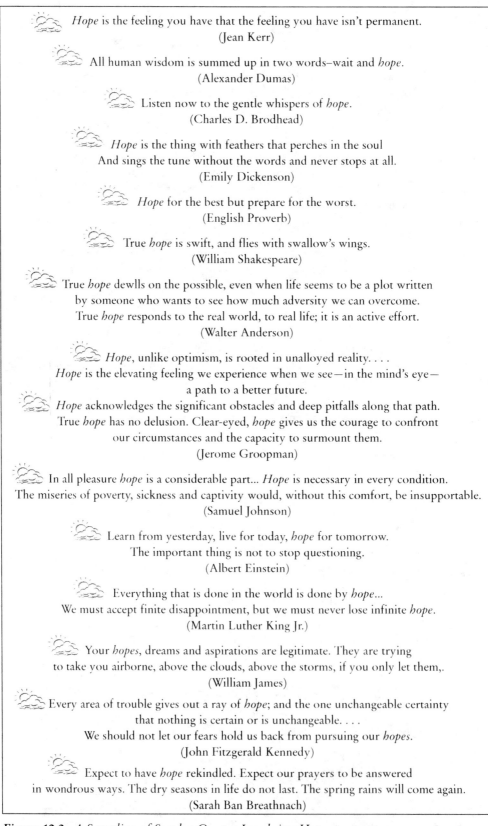

Hope is the feeling you have that the feeling you have isn't permanent.
(Jean Kerr)

All human wisdom is summed up in two words—wait and *hope*.
(Alexander Dumas)

Listen now to the gentle whispers of *hope*.
(Charles D. Brodhead)

Hope is the thing with feathers that perches in the soul
And sings the tune without the words and never stops at all.
(Emily Dickenson)

Hope for the best but prepare for the worst.
(English Proverb)

True *hope* is swift, and flies with swallow's wings.
(William Shakespeare)

True *hope* dewlls on the possible, even when life seems to be a plot written
by someone who wants to see how much adversity we can overcome.
True *hope* responds to the real world, to real life; it is an active effort.
(Walter Anderson)

Hope, unlike optimism, is rooted in unalloyed reality. . . .
Hope is the elevating feeling we experience when we see—in the mind's eye—
a path to a better future.
Hope acknowledges the significant obstacles and deep pitfalls along that path.
True *hope* has no delusion. Clear-eyed, *hope* gives us the courage to confront
our circumstances and the capacity to surmount them.
(Jerome Groopman)

In all pleasure *hope* is a considerable part... *Hope* is necessary in every condition.
The miseries of poverty, sickness and captivity would, without this comfort, be insupportable.
(Samuel Johnson)

Learn from yesterday, live for today, *hope* for tomorrow.
The important thing is not to stop questioning.
(Albert Einstein)

Everything that is done in the world is done by *hope*...
We must accept finite disappointment, but we must never lose infinite *hope*.
(Martin Luther King Jr.)

Your *hopes*, dreams and aspirations are legitimate. They are trying
to take you airborne, above the clouds, above the storms, if you only let them,.
(William James)

Every area of trouble gives out a ray of *hope*; and the one unchangeable certainty
that nothing is certain or is unchangeable. . . .
We should not let our fears hold us back from pursuing our *hopes*.
(John Fitzgerald Kennedy)

Expect to have *hope* rekindled. Expect our prayers to be answered
in wondrous ways. The dry seasons in life do not last. The spring rains will come again.
(Sarah Ban Breathnach)

Figure 12.2. *A Sampling of Secular Quotes Involving Hope.* (continued)

Five general observations about these secular examples might be stated as follows:

1. Only general circumstances, with vague applicability to actual and situated occasions of everyday life, are alluded to across these secular quotes.
2. Difficult challenges are inevitable but not permanent in everyday life. Persons must wait, be patient, and remain hopeful.
3. Hope is a necessary, all-encompassing, primary resource for envisioning positive changes in the future—and must be "rekindled."
4. Hope is something that persons can "live inside . . . under its roof," offering protection and thus providing confidence and peace.
5. Hope has poetic characteristics: It is swift and fleeting, delicate like "feathers that perches in the soul," wondrous like being "elevated" or "airborne," speaks with "gentle whispers," and "sings the tune" ceaselessly, without words.

In addition to these general principles, two predominant themes exist (explicitly or implicitly): metaphorical balances of nature, and tensions between emotional turmoil and triumph. Although these themes are depicted below as a series of bipolarized descriptors, in real life persons simultaneously experience and enact complex combinations of these dimensions (Figure 12.3):

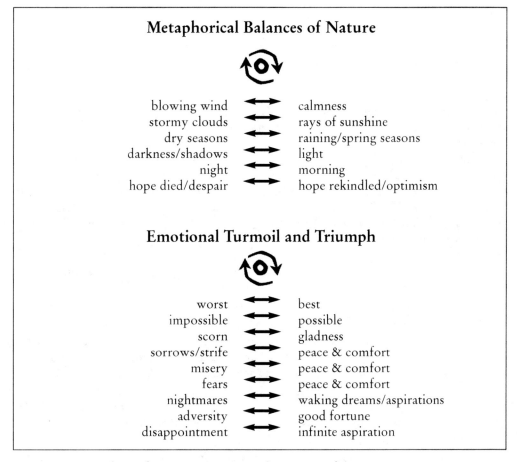

Figure 12.3. Secular References to Nature and an Array of Human Emotions

To summarize, references to nature liken hope and its characteristics, such as calmness and light/morning, as a preferred alternative to storms and darkness/night. Secular quotes also privilege human emotions by giving priority to challenges faced by individuals—*not* within relationships and throughout interactions. Two minor exceptions are included among these secular quotes (the last two listed in Figure 12.2). First, in Breathnach's quote she makes reference to "prayers" being answered, "in wondrous ways" but without acknowledgment to a God or supernatural being. In Huber's verse, it is faith in God that provides ways of ordering and being compassionate about human life. Each presumes spiritual aliveness, being anchored in faith evident in the acts of praying, having positive expectations, and living a life ordered by one's relationship with a God.

Biblical (Religious and Spiritual) References to Hope

Among many and diverse religious orientations that could be discussed, only Judeo-Christian beliefs are overviewed below. Biblically, throughout the Old and New Testaments, relationships among hope and faith are foundational and frequent. The examples below, listed chronologically in Figure 12.4, are only a sampling of possible references.

As with the secular examples in Figure 12.3, hope is made relevant for general circumstances and not for specific, circumstantial events faced by persons on a daily basis. Several recurring themes in the Old Testament are:

- Hope in God promotes security that builds up faith and quiets the soul.
- The absence of hope leads to sickness, in contrast to "a tree of life" from which desires are fulfilled through faith.
- Those who wait on the Lord, and become anchored in his word, will receive steadfast help, love, and mercies.

In the New Testament these themes recur, but there is additional evidence of a new relationship and covenant with God's son, Jesus Christ, sent to this world as the Messiah whose life and ministry fulfills Old Testament scriptures. The life of Jesus Christ reveals God's word to the peoples, teaches others about "faith, hope, and love," and invites discipleship to spread the good news: Through his death on the cross and resurrection, those who believe in him will have their sins forgiven and receive eternal life. Living with this hope is fundamental to Christianity. The sufferings experienced by Jesus, and the hardships of living a good life in an inherently sinful world, are also particularly evident in these New Testament verses. The following themes are prominent:

- Suffering produces opportunities for rejoicing, shaping persons' abilities to have endurance, which yields hope for eternal glory.
- Through the Holy Spirit, lovingly given by God to those who believe in Christ, believers rely on their faith to patiently hope for what they can not see.
- Love is greater than faith and hope. The life and teachings of Jesus exemplify how it is possible to have a personal and loving relationship with a merciful, forgiving, and reassuring God, and to share this love with others on earth.
- Hope put on wealth and possessions leads to uncertainty, whereas hope invested in God yields rich blessings "for our enjoyment." God is the source of all goodness and never abandons us during our trials and sufferings.
- Having hope and confidence in God's grace arises from a conviction that Jesus Christ was raised from the dead and glorified by God.

Old Testament

And thou shalt be secure because there is *hope*.
(Job 11:18)

Why are you cast down, O my soul, and why are you disquieted within me?
Hope in God; for I shall again praise him, my help and my God.

(Psalms 42:5-6)

I wait for the Lord, my soul waits, and in his word I *hope*.
(Psalms 130:5)

Hope deferred makes the heart sick, but a desire fulfilled is a tree of life.
(Proverbs 13:12)

But this I call to mind, and therefore I have *hope*: The steadfast love
of the Lord never ceases, his mercies never come to an end.
(Lamentations 3:21-22)

New Testament

Through him we have obtained access to this grace in which we stand,
d we rejoice in our sufferings, knowing that suffering produces endurance,
and endurance produces *hope*, and *hope* does not disappoint us, because God's love
has been poured into our hearts through the Holy Spirit which has been given to us.
(Romans 5:2-5)

I consider that the sufferings of this present time are not worth comparing
with the glory that is to be revealed to us... For in this *hope* we were saved.
Now *hope* that is seen is not *hope*. For who *hopes* for what he sees?
But if we *hope* for what we do not see, we wait for it in patience.
(Romans 8:18 24-25)

o faith, *hope*, love abide, these three; but the greatest of these is love.
(1 Corinthians 13:13)

continually remember before our God and Father your work produced by faith,
your labor prompted by love, and your endurance inspired by *hope* in our Lord Jesus Christ.
(1 Thessalonians 1:3)

Command those who are rich in this present world not to be arrogant
nor to put their *hope* in wealth, which is so uncertain, but to put their *hope* in God,
who richly provides us with everything for our enjoyment.
(1 Timothy 6:17)

Now faith is the assurance of things *hoped* for, the conviction of things not seen.
(1 Hebrews 11:1)

In this you rejoice, though now for a little while you may have to suffer
various trials. . . . Therefore gird up your minds, be sober, set your *hope* fully
upon the grace that is coming to you at the revelation of Jesus Christ . . .
through him you have confidence in God, who raised him from the dead
and gave him glory, so that your faith and *hope* are in God.
(1 Peter 1:6-7, 13, 21)

Figure 12.4. *Examples of Old & New Testament References to Hope*

A Brief Comparison of Secular and Judeo-Christian Orientations to Hope

There are marked contrasts between secular and Judeo-Christian perspectives on hope. Secular orientations rely on (a) balances of nature as a metaphorical resource for depicting troubles and their hopeful resolutions (e.g., stormy clouds, darkness, and shadows turning into rays of sunshine and light), and (b) how humans manage their emotional lives by remaining hopeful that difficult challenges will eventually give way to positive outcomes (e.g., scorn, sorrows, strife, and misery will give way to gladness, peace, comfort, and healing). The locus of control appears to be with the indomitable human spirit, wisdom to know that all things will change, and a basic belief that (with patience) good will emerge out of bad circumstances.

In Judeo-Christian theology, sole reliance on nature, human wisdom, and perseverance ultimately leads to uncertainty and death of the soul. In the midst of trials and tribulations so common to everyday life, it is faith in a loving God, the creator of all things (including nature) and the giver of life, that provides hope, security, and assurance. Knowing that God is ever-present, believers are encouraged to rejoice in sufferings, which shape character. Perseverance and endurance yields hope for blessings and eternal life. Jews and Christians alike rely on God, not just for their own salvation, but for daily (even momentary) guidance while navigating through a world filled with sinful temptations. Whether faith rests with the God of the Old Testament, and/or Jesus Christ as God's son (and the trinity of Father, Son, and Holy Spirit), hope emerges from a sincere commitment that is anchored in reading, understanding, and following the words of the Bible.

OVERVIEW OF SOCIAL SCIENTIFIC RESEARCH ON HOPE AND OPTIMISM

Nearly 40 years ago,[4] in reference to "different stages that people go through when they are faced with tragic news—defense mechanisms in psychiatric terms, coping mechanisms to deal with extremely difficult situations . . . ," Kübler-Ross (1969b) observed that "The one thing that usually persists through all these stages is hope" (p. 138). In her classic book *On Death and Dying*, Kübler-Ross (1969b) describes how in 1965 she became involved in a research project with four theology students at the Chicago Theological Seminary. The value of hope became evident through a series of interviews and testimonials offered by dying patients. Even for patients not expected to live long, they need to "maintain the *hope* which each and every patient has to keep, including the ones who say they are ready to die" (p. 31). The alternative to being hopeful—hopelessness, despair, loss of feeling valued and the will to live—was to be actively avoided in all cases:[5]

> If malignancy is presented as a hopeless disease which results in a sense of "what's the use, there is nothing we can do anyway," it will be the beginning of a difficult time for the patient and for those around him. The patient will feel the increasing isolation, the loss of interest on the part of his doctor, the isolation and increasing hopelessness. He may rapidly deteriorate or fall into a deep depression from which he may not emerge unless someone is able to give him a sense of hope . . . It was the reassurance that everything possible will be done, that they will not be "dropped," that there were treatments available, that there was a glimpse of hope—even in the most advanced cases. (pp. 35-36, 37)

This seminar eventually grew into an accredited course, for diverse audiences, within both the medical school and theological seminary. It was also a precursor to what is now commonly known as "the hospice movement." Hospice care is based on the fundamental principles that much is to be learned from dying patients and that palliative care (comfort) can be offered when cures are not possible. Patients, family members, and significant others alike can benefit greatly from a peaceful and supportive environment facilitating the acceptance of, and coping with, death and dying (see *www.elisabethkublerross.com* for additional information on hospice and palliative care). Unique and skilled medical expertise is available for these often delicate and tenuous experiences.

In the late 1980s, when I first read Kübler-Ross's *On Death and Dying* (1969b), I began to wonder how phenomena such as "defense/coping mechanisms," "stages," and hope/hopelessness might be evident within specific social actions comprising the Malignancy calls. Her descriptions captured attitudinal orientations by patients and others, but did not offer specific instances of how matters of hope found their way into actual conversations. Then, in 1992, I read a more recent ethnographic study focusing on the "social meanings of death" in three hospital wards in Finland (leukemia, medical, and emergency) dealing with seriously ill patients. In his field work, Peräkylä (1991) identified "hope work" as a predominant set of practices whereby patients are "getting and feeling better" (curative and palliative care) or "past recovery" (where hope per se is dismantled). His interests rested with identifying distinctive interactional processes involved in constructing hope and hopefulness, impacts on medical identities of patients and staff, and ways that "hope work" by medical staff functions to maintain legitimacy of "medical" orientations to treatment, dying, and death.

The particular finding that "What is particular to hope work is that it is accomplished solely through conversation" (p. 430) was supported with a series of examples from field notes and (limited) recordings: "*expectations of a positive development in the patient's condition*" were apparent, and "*the patient's medical identity was constructed in a positive way from an optimistic angle*" (p. 412). For example, utterances such as "The situation is now under control" and "We're feeling better today" favored positive medical developments. Below are some additional examples from Peräkylä's reconstructed field notes from the leukemia ward (Figure 12.5):

---

8) **Peräkylä (1991, p. 413)**

The patient [a 30-year-old woman who had recently contracted leukemia] is talking about her job and at one point says, "if I get better." The doctor intervenes and says, "No, listen, it's always going to be when you get better."

9) **Peräkylä (1991, p. 413)**

(The consultant explains that the cell count of Mr. K, in his 60's, may allow him to leave the hospital—*if* results from his bone marrow sample are good.)

Patient: "So things are looking good?"

Consultant: "As far as the cell count is concerned. Let's hope that the results of the bone marrow examination are just as good."

10) **Peräkylä (1991, p. 413)**

(A physician superintendent and a junior doctor are talking to a young male following a recent bone marrow transplant. His condition seems to be getting better, despite patient's feeling poorly.)

Doctor: "I know it's been no merrymaking for you, but we're doing what's best for you."

Junior Doctor: "You can think of it as an eve of merrymaking."

Figure 12.5. Reconstructed Field Notes from a Leukemia Ward

In each instance doctors construct the possibility of an optimistic future, at times in response to patients assessing or seeking assurance of improvement. Although different social contexts require varying types of "hope work," it is clear that medical staff are routinely involved in being more or less hopeful—competencies underlying the quality of care provided, the nature of relationships between patients and professionals, and ultimately the offering and withholding of assurance so critical for optimism about healing.

In contrast, the Malignancy phone calls reveal not how medical staff work with their patients in institutional settings, nor attempts to legitimate medicine by professionals, but with family members speaking together on the telephone within their home environments (though, as in call #2, mom is in the hospital when son phones from his home). As with Peräkylä's (1991) findings, it is not necessary for hope to be explicitly named for optimistic orientations to be displayed during interactions. Although hope is at times invoked in situated and thus revealing ways in the phone calls, not a single instance of the word "optimism" has yet been identified—even though speakers' actions will be shown to display a sense of expectancy, even assurance, about a hopeful future.

Quantitative and (Additional) Qualitative Studies of Hope

Before returning to the phone call data, one final area of research on hope will be briefly overviewed: a series of interdisciplinary studies focusing on hope and health in the social and medical sciences. In a recent literature review, Crase (2003) suggests that work on hope is simultaneously multidimensional and elusive (e.g., see Bunston et al., 1995; Herth, 2000; Nekolaichuk, Jevne, & Maguire, 1999; Ong, 2001), and that more attention has been given to hope and cancer than other illnesses (see Benzein, Norber, & Saveman, 2001; Chapman, 1994; Herth, 2000). Relying on self-report questionnaires and numerous scaling measures (e.g, see Farran, Herth, & Popovich, 1995; Foote et al., 1990; Herth, 1991, 1992; Miller & Powers, 1988; Nowotny, 1989; Nunn et al., 1996; Obayuwana et al., 1982; Raleigh, 1992; Westburg, 1999), the vast majority of studies focusing on hope (and hopefulness) assume that hope is quantifiable and (more or less) correlated with constructs such as social and family support, coping mechanisms, self-esteem, locus of control, and humor. As noted, the primary unit of analysis is the individual (see also Chapter 1), perhaps best exemplified by the Herth Hope Scale (HHS, Farran, Herth, & Popovich, 1995), in which responses (Never→Seldom→Sometimes→Often Applies to me) are made to 30 "I-prefaced" statements regarding hope. Selected statements from the HHS appear below (Figure 12.6).

Each statement elicits individuals' reactions about their personal and perceptual orientations to matters such as the future, faith, support, assurance about hope, and ability to alter circumstances. Herth (2000) has also constructed a shorter index for clinical settings, complimenting self-report questionnaires with discussion sessions so that "a theory-driven hope intervention program" (p. 1431) might be implemented.

> 1. I am looking forward to the future.
> 8. I have faith that gives me comfort.
> 12. I have support from those close to me.
> 15. I just know there is hope.
> 26. I can't bring about positive change.
> 28. I have hope even when plans go astray.

Figure 12.6. Examples of Statements from the Herth Hope Scale (HHS)

Different qualitative and multimethodological techniques have also been employed, often as interventions to assist nurses working directly with patients and their family members. For example, Hinds and Gattuso (1991) relied on actual quotations of adolescents to help generate open-ended measures for a hopelessness scale. Penrod and Morse (1997) integrated theoretical and autobiographic descriptions of surviving breast cancer patients to identify six phases of hope (recognizing the threat, making a plan, taking stock, reaching out, looking for signs, and holding on). Other studies relied on interviews (e.g., Benzein, Norber, & Saveman, 2001; Farran, Wilken, & Popovich, 1992) to solicit how hope shapes others' experiences with illness. Gaskins (1995), for example, requested that older adults collect photographs of anything that provided hope in their lives, and meaningful descriptions of hope were revealed:

> Hope is a thing longed for . . . something not known, but you anticipate it. It is something good, and it keeps you going when things get really difficult, or sad, or bad. If you have hope, you keep on keeping on. (p. 22)

Across the ten themes that emerged from Gaskins' (1995) study, *spirituality* and *relationships with others* were identified as the most important features of coping with an illness. Indeed, the majority of qualitative research on hope reveals *family* and *interconnected relationships* as primary dimensions of hope (e.g., see Borneman et al., 2002; Herth, 1990, 1993). Related modeling studies, such as Nekolaichuk, Jevne, and Maguire's (1999) creation of a three-dimensional model of hope-related concepts (personal, situational, and interpersonal) have yielded similar findings.

It is clear, then, that even when researchers have utilized various qualitative methods for examining hope (e.g., open-ended interviews, photographs, diaries, and anecdotal stories), the tendency has been to analyze participants' reports about hope rather than actual enactments in interaction (with the partial exception of Peräkylä's 1991 investigation of medical wards, summarized above). As with Benzein, Norber, and Saveman's (2001) findings based on narrative interviews—that patients seek a hope for being cured, a hope of living as normally as possible, a presence of confirmative relationships, and reconciliation with life and death—much is discovered about what is meaningful for individuals. But it remains to be seen *how* speakers interactionally organize their hopeful experiences about the future.

Working to Create a "Benign Order" for Everyday Living

One primary set of findings from Maynard's (2003) work on *Bad News, Good News* is that the delivery and receipt of both good and bad news give rise to shifts in topics and/or attempts to close the conversation. The data Maynard analyzes regarding good news recurrently reveal a move toward closing, as do those of Jones (1997) who examined how various health professionals treat clients' news as "good" en route to topical shifts. These shifts are similar to Jefferson's (1981, 1993) identification of words such as "Yeah", as well as Beach's (1993b, 1995a) analysis of "Okay", wherein recipients design their talk to initiate both speaker and topic shifts.

In contrast, however, Maynard (2003) makes clear that moments involving bad news get organized differently: Transitions, or "good news exists" (p. 177), tend not to occur without recipients first adding some component of good news to the otherwise bad news environment. Three types of prominent social actions are: (a) *Remedy announcements* (i.e., offering of a solution of resolution to a trouble); (b) *Bright side sequences*, initially identified by Holt (1993) as positive evaluations arising out of bad news announcements; and (c) *Optimistic projections*, one set of practices identified by Jefferson (1988) as speakers move to close troubling topics. These are akin to idiomatic expressions analyzed in Chapter 7 (e.g., "↑<u>keep</u> my lesson plans nice and °current°"), though at times a more particular move toward being hopeful is evident (e.g., "it'll iron itself out") (p. 181). As summarized by Maynard:

> Taken together, these interactional patterns make clear that and how participants in interaction structure the social world as a relatively benign one.... After its delivery and receipt, good news can stand on its own as transition is made to other topics and activities, but bad news invariably obtains some kind of mediating good-news exit . . . participants work to sustain an asymmetry in which good news is celebrated and not diminished, while bad news and the accompanying feelings are cushioned and countered. It is in this sense that participants render the socially sanctioned world of everyday life as a benign one rather than a malign one. (Maynard, 2003, pp. 182-184)

The ways these "benign" orientations are employed as resources by family members, managing cancer in part by constructing possibilities for a hopeful future, are addressed in the following chapter.

NOTES

1. Before reading this chapter, some readers may prefer to first inspect the data in Chapter 13 and my analysis of a collection of potential candidates qualifying as hopeful/optimistic moments. By encountering family members' interactions first, as I did as an analyst across numerous data/listening sessions, readers will gain a different (and certainly more grounded and pragmatic) appreciation of how family members orient (in the first instance, by and for themselves) to practical circumstances involving daily choices and actions. In this way, conceptual frameworks for understanding matters such as "hope" will not be overly relied upon as a "template or overlay" pyramided onto the raw interactions, and thus force-fitting what family members actually do into predefined (nonempirical) categories or frames for making sense of the social world (see, e.g., Drew & Wooton, 1988). The conclusion of Chapter 13 also attempts to integrate empirical (interactional) findings with secular, spiritual, and social scientific perspectives overviewed in this chapter. This integration provides another lens for framing the questions and conceptions raised herein.
2. It was my colleague and friend Robert Hopper (deceased; Charles Sapp Centennial Professor of Communication at the University of Texas, Austin) who coined the phrase "managing optimism." This descriptive phrase was employed by him when attempting to depict a wide range of moments for dealing with bad and uncertain news regarding his health condition. It was first uttered (at least to me) within weeks following a diagnosis of colon cancer, during one of a series of phone calls wherein his illness trajectory routinely (though not exclusively) became an explicit topic for discussion. Following his summary of what doctors had told him about ongoing test results, attention was given to the inherent (and often frustrating) uncertainties of medical knowledge, including doctors being unwilling and apparently unable to lay out, in specific terms, just what his prognosis for overcoming cancer's debilitating effects might be. In the face of more basic yet unanswered questions—How long do I have to live? What probability for healing exists? What impacts will further treatments have?—our talking about cancer diagnoses and impacts routinely shifted to being optimistic, reassuring, at times even upbeat about the ambiguities such bad news entails. And it was in response to our being hopeful together that Robert stated something like "Managing optimism. That's what I'm calling what we're doing, as a practical achievement." Later, I adapted this phrase as the title of a chapter I wrote for a festschrift in Robert's name, co-edited by Phil Glenn, Curtis LeBaron, and Jenny Mandelbaum (2003).
3. Matters of hope appear central to the primal human condition, regardless of whether speakers' beliefs are agnostic, atheist, or involve religious beliefs other than Judeo-Christian (e.g., Hindu,

Islamic, Muslim). If the interactions of many families representing diverse belief systems were examined, the central questions would of course focus not just on "Hope in what?" but "*How does hope get done among diverse speakers (and cultural members) in interaction?*" And further: Is hope what they do together when managing serious illness (and other ordinary) circumstances?

4. During this same period of time, Sudnow's (1967) *Passing On: The Social Organization of Dying* offered the first "ethnography of death," a systematic field examination of key social activities through which death and dying were addressed in two hospital settings. Through watching, listening, and intensive nonparticipant observation Sudnow's field notes yielded an alluring portrayal of how staff members handled dying and treatment decisions, including "how members of deceased patients' families are informed of the deaths of their relatives" (p. 3). Attempts to record actual conversations were generally unsuccessful, however, and as a result "only bits and pieces of conversational sequences were transcribed . . . [and marked by] double quotation marks" (p. 6). Regarding hope, Sudnow observed:

> For cancers, it is proposed that there is always the hope of X-ray therapy, and further surgery, for "sudden turns for the worse," and always the chance that he will "pull through." Every announcement in the hospital, save that of a death, can properly have appended to it qualifacatory remarks devised to reduce its apparent seriousness or at least offer some form of "hope." (p. 125)

5. As Byock (1997) observed in his book *Dying Well: The Prospect for Growth at the End of Life*, "Too often and for too long doctors and nurses have referred to dying patients as "hopeless" or "helpless," and that is how people who are dying may feel. . . . By voting with our presence and by doing whatever it takes to provide comfort we demonstrate our conviction that there is no such thing as hopeless or helpless" (p. 44). Addressing how there is "always a chance," Kübler-Ross (1969b) emphasizes the partnership between lay persons and care providers: "it is a battle they are going to fight together—patient, family, and doctor—no matter the end results" (p. 29).

13

"WELL WHERE'S OUR MAGIC WAND MOM...°
BEATS THE HELL OUT OF ME.°"

The Interactional Organization
of Hope and Optimism

Having overviewed secular, spiritual, and social scientific conceptions of hope and optimism in the previous chapter, analysis turns to moments when speakers explicitly reference "hope/hopeful" and in other ways manage various concerns optimistically. The initial seven instances identified within calls #1 and #2, previewed in Chapter 12, are more closely examined. A subsequent search through the Malignancy corpus also yielded a considerably larger collection of approximately 50 distinct moments. A total of 25 of these moments are included herein (see Figure 13.2, below), allowing for a preliminary case to be made that family members routinely exhibit hopeful and optimistic orientations to emerging circumstances and events. Such orientations are critical resources for interactionally managing ongoing problems with mom's (malignant) cancer in a "benign" manner; that is, an overwhelming tendency for family members to buffer difficulties associated with mom's health by talking about positive events and possibilities in their lives.

Fundamentally, this chapter extends and elaborates the observed tendency for "good" topics to arise out of otherwise "bad" and troubling matters (see, e.g., Beach & Dixson, 2001; Beach & LeBaron, 2002; Holt, 1993; Jefferson, 1980a, 1984a, 1984b; Maynard, 1997, 2003; Peräkylä, 1991; Robinson, 2006; Sacks, 1992). The specific criteria for identifying these activities will become evident, on a case-by-case basis and cumulatively, as analysis unfolds. In most general terms, speakers' hopeful and optimistic orientations are best understood as very practical, contingent, and directly tied to managing ongoing problems related to mom's changing condition: seeking information about inherently uncertain medical care, conveying positive and encouraging orientations, shifting from bad to good news, working together to remain upbeat and counter-balance alternative (e.g., despairing) orientations for coping with troubles. These and related activities exemplify family members' concerted efforts to remain hopeful in the midst of challenging circumstances.

The collection of hopeful and optimistic moments is organized into five primary (and overlapping) types of social activities: (a) Managing uncertainty regarding medical care with hope; (b) Shifting from bad and troubling to good, hopeful, and optimistic topics; (c) Balancing hope and choice in circumstances that cannot be fully controlled; (d) Devising resources for fighting the battles together; and (e) Constructing positive futures. This chapter closes by contrasting prior descriptions of hope and optimism (i.e., secular, spiritual, and social scientific), overviewed in Chapter 12, with how family members interactionally organize the social activities noted above. Comparisons clearly reveal how matters of hope are unique communicative expressions, embodying and enlivening more abstract, conceptual, and theoretical depictions of *acting hopeful, ordinarily* (Sacks, 1984b).

HOPE AND UNCERTAINTY REGARDING MEDICAL CARE

Analysis begins with the first identified instance in the Malignancy corpus, approximately four minutes into the call, when dad explicitly mentions the word "hope". In Excerpt 1 (below), dad continues his reporting by offering to son a doctor's description of procedures for treating mom's cancer. In lines 3-4, these procedures include contacting a cancer specialist and conducting "this bo:ne scan thing tomorrow.":

1) SDCL: Malignancy #1:6-7

```
 1     Dad     = .hhh He said he would have somebody else look in on her:.
 2             = He also co:ntacted this cancer specialist so he will be in
 3             Monday. (.) .hhh And they will do this bo:ne scan thing
 4  →          tomorrow. So .hhh n:o:: I would hope by Monday or
 5  →          Tu:esday (0.7) pt they have<pin:ned do::wn>(0.7) the
 6             particulars of what they're after. >Now they may not have<
 7             the course of action all figured out, but [   .hhhh   ]
 8     Son:                                              [°Umhm.° ] =
 9     Dad:    = They'll at least kno:w. (.) .hh  And maybe this is just
10             simplistically in my mind >but they'll know< .hhh what
11             ki:nd? they're dealing with. That way they should know
12             .hhh how quickly does it spread (.) what is- (0.7) what can be
13             done to: to stop it >you know< .hh radiation
14             [ or   chemotherapy   or
```

With "I would hope" in lines 4-6, dad specifies what he considers to be a realistic time frame within which "they" (medical experts) might be able to determine "the particulars of what they're after". Employing "<pin:ned do::wn>", dad depicts the diagnostic need to locate and identify an implied moving target that is difficult to detect: cancer. The inherent complexity and uncertainty of such a diagnosis is evident as dad next and immediately disclaims, ">Now they may not have< the course of action all figured out," (lines 6-7). Following son's quiet and brief acknowledgment (line 8) dad then proceeds by elaborating his lay understandings, "simplistically in my mind", of what he was hopeful about: bottom-line concerns with identifying the cancer and attempting "to stop it" with radiation or chemotherapy. Dad recognizes that the more quickly cancer spreads, the more aggressive the treatment needs to be.

Several features of Excerpt 1 are interesting but not unusual throughout the Malignancy phone calls. First, this excerpt represents the initial display of hopeful conduct in interaction. These actions follow dad's initial and extended delivery and son's receipt and assimilation of bad news regarding mom's cancer (see Chapter 3). Second, a delicate and countervailing balance exists between "hope" and "uncertainty". Dad's expression of hope (line 4) is mitigated with a next-positioned caveat: a "course of action" (line 7) replete with incomplete knowledge. Third, dad must inevitably rely upon and report about what doctors have told him about their specialized knowledge (see Chapters 8 and 9). It is clear that dad's source of hope is anchored in the involvement of assumedly competent medical providers, professionals who are expected to do everything possible while devising a plan for halting the insidious progress of mom's cancer.

Put simply, the sooner mom's cancer is located, identified, and appropriately treated the better the likelihood of a good prognosis. And therein lies the primary basis for dad's invoking of "hope by Monday or Tuesday" in line 4. He provides a realistic yet intrinsically uncertain expectation, replete with numerous and necessary medical procedures that (in dad's view) must be performed.

His attempts to describe doctors' suggested treatment options to son (e.g., "this bo:ne scan thing" in line 3, and later to "simplistically in my mind" in line 10) reveal dad's lay attempts to understand complex medical procedures, including the technical expertise comprising bone scan procedures. Throughout the chapters, it has become evident that family members have little choice but to offer lay constructions of medical experts' work and knowledge (see Beach, 2001a). Attempting to describe, figure out, and exhibit some confidence that upcoming events will be managed effectively (i.e., to mom's advantage) is routine in all cancer journeys. Indeed, the hope for healing outcomes is a critical feature of most all illness journeys.

Although the activities comprising future medical episodes cannot be controlled, they can be framed in advance as possible (even likely) positive experiences. Such orientations are drawn from, and provide essential sustenance for, one interactional engine for hope and optimism: mechanisms designed to remain upbeat about not-yet-delivered news. At times, as in Excerpt 2 (below), looking forward to receiving new information can be noted even when the valence of such news (i.e., positive and/or negative) remains unknown:

2) **SDCL: Malignancy #37:2**

((Dad had just reported that when he went to visit mom in the hospital, he eventually located her in the "nuclear medicine ward".))

1	Dad:	Uh I had no idea of what they fo̱und, or what they were
2		lo̱oking for 'cause there wasn't any of the doctors there
3		yesterday, except ya know for emergency on ca̱ll. So
4		obviously I didn't see one of 'em.
5		(1.2)
6 →	Dad:	**But I hope to fi- ((clears throat)) hope to find out this**
7		**morning so,**
8	Son:	**Umkay.**
9	Dad:	**Maybe I will learn some more.**
10	Son:	But other than that looks as though things are re̱latively
11		sta̱tus quo, huh. =
12	Dad:	= Yeah they're just about the same. U:m, (1.2) still y'know
13		gettin' up and down she'll get up sit in a chair, get up go to
14		the bathroom with a little assistance.
15	Son:	Well that's good. =
16	Dad:	= U:hm (.) pa̱in doesn't se̱:em to be bo̱thering her quite so
17		much. I mean- y'know when she gets up it hurts, but (0.7)
18		she doesn't seem to be compla̱ining of the pa:in just la̱ying
19		like she was there last week so, =
20	Son:	= Mm hm.

Though the results from mom's recent visit to the "nuclear medicine ward" are uncertain, dad's hope is anchored in receiving forthcoming news. He does not specify that he seeks to hear *good* news. Rather, dad prioritizes a need to "learn some more" as the basis for constructing subsequent assessments. That this occurs during call #37 also suggests that the essential bad news about mom, even her likely terminal prognosis, is known and oriented to by dad. Expectations about remission of mom's cancer are not articulated in the later calls of this phone call corpus. And as mom has no doubt visited the "nuclear medicine ward" multiple times in the past several months, yet another visit may be treated by dad as increasingly routine. This is not to say that dad in any way trivializes another test and/or round of treatment for mom. He does state that he hopes to find out more later this morning. But one might speculate that his range of expectations may well be more constrained during this phase of mom's treatment, and he behaves accordingly.

Fortunately, however, the data themselves provide constant reminders that dad was speaking directly to his son. In next turn, it is son who does not treat dad's reporting and "hope to learn more" as a cause for alarm. Instead, in lines 10-11, he quickly moves past dad's update and queries as to whether "things are relatively status quo," which dad next confirms. Subsequently, son treats mom's status quo as positive news with "Well that's good." (line 15). In the final moments of this excerpt, dad reports that mom's pain is not bothering her as much, adding to the good rather than bad nature of the news dad provides (see also Excerpts 10-12, below).[1]

Waiting to hear news (good or bad) is exceedingly normal. By *staying in the loop*, as it were, a family member (friend, and/or coworker) retains his/her status as informed and therefore consequential for managing ongoing events and circumstances. In line 9 (below), referring to a phone call from dad that she did not receive, aunt states she "was hoping that was him," so that she might hear about doctor's report on mom's condition:

3) SDCL: Malignancy #17:1

```
1     Aunt:  [ $Hu]h$ No ↑I'm not <puz:zl:ed.> I- ↑I have not talked to
2            Dr. Wylie. ↑I  haven't talked to your dad.
3     Son:   O::hkay. =
4     Aunt:  = I sent 'em in (.) °ya know.° =
5     Son:   = ↑Yeah he jus' called me <like- like> (.) thirty seconds
6            a[g o.]
7     Aunt:  [<We]: :ll> (.) [  I- the lin ]e was busy.
8     Son:                 [ Ah minute.]
9  →  Aunt:  An' I was hoping that was him, so: =
10    Son:   = Yeah. =
```

Her reference follows son's reporting that he had just spoken with him/dad (lines 5-6). Because dad's line was busy when aunt called (line 7), she had not been able to receive updated news son now possesses (i.e., from dad). And it was her search for such information, in the midst of uncertainty, that prompted her "hoping" in the first instance.

Waiting to Hear What the Doctor Has to Say

As discussed in Chapter 12, the word "hope" is not always explicitly invoked when speakers refer to possible future trajectories. This is especially the case when a minimal basis for being hopeful is apparent. Excerpt 4 (below) was examined previously (in Excerpt 7, Chapter 4). During call #2, mom has just informed son that her cancer has been diagnosed as a very fast growing "adenoma type." This is an update from call #1 (see Chapter 3), in which dad was not aware of the general cancer classification, nor whether mom's cancer was slow or fast growing. She has also just reported that because very few people respond well to treatment, and those who do live five years or less, "It's r(h)eal bad". Below, a revealing glimpse of mom's construction of her own cancer dilemma is evident as she relies on medical procedures and providers as sources of information and thus attributed (but not named) hope:

4) SDCL: Malignancy #2:2-3

```
1     Mom:   And uh: >I don't know what else to ↑tell you.<
2            (1.0)
3     Mom:   ((coughs))
4     Son:   .hh hhh Yeah. (0.2) um- ((coughs)). Yeah, I don't know what
5            to say either.
6  →  Mom:   No there's nothing to say. >You just-< .hh I'll I'll wait to
```

7		talk to Dr. Leedon today.= He's the cancer man, and =
8	Son:	= Um hmm.
9	Mom:	See what he has to say, and (0.4) just keep goin' forward. I
10		mean I might be real <u>lu</u>cky in five years. It might just be
11		six months.

It appears, at least initially, that mom and son collaborate in dropping the topic of cancer. Both speakers utter "I don't know" (see Beach & Metzger, 1997), first in line 1 as mom claims she has nothing further to tell, and next in lines 4 & 5 as son affirms that, as recipient, he does not know what to say. In this sense there is indeed "nowhere else to go" (Jefferson 1984b, p. 191), and lines 1-5 bring closure to further talk about the seriousness of mom's prognosis.

Yet lines 1-5 also demonstrate a transition to talking with her cancer doctor, which mom initiates in line 6. As the conversation unfolds, it becomes clear that the insufficient knowledge they claim and display an inability and/or unwillingness to talk further about, is tied only to mom's prior diagnosis (most notably the anguish mom's immediately prior news makes available) and not her ongoing treatment.

In line 6, mom's "No there's nothing to say." is one form of an extreme case description (see Edwards, 2000; Pomerantz, 1986), employed here to emphasize her position and to terminate her diagnostic update for son's hearing. Next, mom's "I'll I'll wait to talk to Dr. Leedon today.= He's the cancer man," (lines 6-7) implicates her having cancer without explicitly stating it. This is but one instance representing a larger collection where the word "cancer" is either noticeably absent or, as with this instance, treated with some sensitivity (see Jones, 2005a) as mom attributes doctor's professional identity but does *not* identify herself as a cancer patient. In this moment, when mom clearly has been diagnosed with cancer but fails to directly state it, she is nevertheless left with the task of formulating herself as a sick person. One practice for doing so, which mom employs here, is to make reference to a provider-patient relationship in which she is involved. Thus, the professional expertise of "cancer man," provides one solution to directly stating "I have cancer." And by stating "See what he has to say" (line 9), mom situates herself as recipient for obtaining any new information the doctor might impart. Only the doctor has the expertise to announce any new, potentially good, and more or less definitive news regarding her acute medical condition. Mom is not revealing her expectations about what the doctor might say, but does offer a hint of patience and hopefulness through her willingness to "See what he has to say."

A central feature of her next "just keep goin' forward." (line 9), therefore, involves waiting for the doctor and whatever news he might disclose. As updates about mom's terminal illness evolve, this is but a single instance of how faith in one's doctor is grounded in moments in which "waiting" is explicitly stated, whereas the possibility of hopeful news is only implied. There is, of course, no guarantee that any update of her condition will amount to whatever good news might imply. This is revealed straightforwardly through mom's "I mean I might be real <u>lu</u>cky in five years. It might just be six months." (lines 9-11). When five years is considered fortuitous, just what might constitute good news is an altogether relative notion. (As noted previously, and apparent in the Timeline in Chapter 2, mom's death occurred 13 months following diagnosis.) Mom demonstrates her resolve in the face of subsequent humbling and uncertain news: a five year to six month window for living. Akin to a doctor's prognosis, she also describes a best to worst case scenario for son's hearing. It is not known how mom may have received this information (most likely from a doctor), but it does contain a dose of realism. Mom's hope rests, it would appear, in being "real <u>lu</u>cky", and then only if she were to live a full five years. Not exactly a vote of confidence in her chances for a long life, mom nevertheless leaves open the possibility that some good news might arise from talking with her doctor (see also Excerpt 13, below, an extension of this discussion between mom and son).

SHIFTING FROM BAD TO GOOD NEWS

For approximately one minute following Excerpt 1 (above), dad continues by describing to son how mom's original neck problem (some 35 years ago, at 25 years of age) was a slow growing lymphatic cancer. He then raises the possibility that mom's current cancer may also be slow growing, which bone scan results will aid in determining. In Excerpt 5 (below), dad summarizes what is essentially a bad news description of how mom was doing. His portrayal (lines 2-11) escalates in its telling, from mom's "co:nfirmation and res-ignation" to "I just hurt too b:ad to be anything else" to "something drastic." to "problems with pa:in" whose medications were "hardly slowin' it down":

5) SDCL: Malignancy #1:7

```
 1    Dad:   A:: yeah .hhh (.) But she seemed to be doing (.) >as I said<
 2           pt .hh at this point it was mostly (0.5) co:nfirmation and
 3           resignation.
 4    Son:   [ Mm hmm:. ]
 5    Dad:   [ Cause   she] said, .hhh I just hurt too b:ad to be anything
 6           else (0.2) >ya know.< It ha::d to be som- (0.7) something
 7           drastic.
 8    Son:   Mmhm.
 9    Dad:   And she was really having some problems with pa:in today.
10           She had .hh one and a half (0.2) >percodans< in her and it
11           wasn't hardly slowin' it down.
12 →  Son:   °Mmm wow.°
13 →  Dad:   .hhh But (0.2) she did have two nice things ha:ppen today.
14           She was on her way do:wn and .hhh and was ↑kinda,
15           depressed or  concer:ned I guess with having >to go down<
16           for these needle biopsies and Will? showed up.
```

In Line 12, following dad's progressively distressing update, son's "°Mmm wow.°" displays a shift from acknowledging dad's description in progress (i.e., with "Mm hmm:" and "Mm hm") to quietly assessing it as troubling news. This response is treated by dad as son's unwillingness to comment further and consequently, *not* inviting dad's further elucidation of mom's painful condition. This is one form of a sequence-closing assessment that initi-ates transition out of a troubles-telling by dad (see Jefferson, 1980a, 1984a, 1993). Immediately following son's "°Mmm wow.°", dad initiates transition to a new but related topic with his pre-announcement "But (0.2) she did have two nice things ha:ppen today." This "conversation restart" (see Jefferson, 1984b, p. 193; 1996; Sacks, 1992) is responsive to son's prior "°Mmm wow.°", treating son as having initiated a closure implicative action. It also reveals how dad's insertion of good news is on topic, yet designed by him to ease the burden of previously articulated grievous circumstances about which enough had been said (at least for now). In this way, dad essentially cloaks the bad news in favor of exposing good news (see Maynard, 2003, Ch. 6). By transitioning to positive events that occurred (i.e., a visit by mom's acquaintance, Will), dad mitigates her problems with pain in favor of a more benign topic.

Dad's "↑kinda, depressed or concer:ned" (lines 14-15) was inserted following his pre-announcement, before announcing the good news that "Will? showed up." Here, as with how dad and son collaborate on reporting bad news as a prelude to announcing good news, the close proximity of mom's reported mood, immediately prior to an old friend showing up for a visit, reveals how everyday life is comprised of tightly interwoven relationships among bad and good circumstances. The valence of social occasions are subject to change and alteration, literally on the cusp of interactional time (see Maynard, 1997, 2003).

The shift from bad to good news evident in Excerpt 5 (above) is similar to Holt's (1993) previously discussed findings involving death announcements by tellers, particularly to recipients not especially close to the deceased. In each of the ten instances she examined, the tendency to treat the death of an intimate or acquaintance as bad news nevertheless eventuated in movement to a "bright side sequence" revealing some positive stance toward the news (e.g., deceased persons worked until the time of death, died peacefully, and in so doing solved problems associated with prolonged illnesses and caregiving tasks and/or had the opportunity to say goodbye to people, thus providing for a funeral that is less dismal). Holt observed that "there seems to be a strong link between bright side sequences and topic termination" (p. 208), not uncommonly termination of a phone call. In Excerpt 5 (above), two exceptions can be noted. First, dad transitions not just to a closely related topic, but to a decidedly positive orientation to updating news. His actions reveal how the shift from bad to good news is an apparent resource for facilitating closure to a discussion that son initially, and next dad, treated as a delicate matter. Second, not only is good news about friends' unexpected visits elaborated, but the phone call continues for more than 15 minutes. This is not surprising, however, because this is the first phone call between dad and son regarding mom's malignant diagnosis.

Approximately three minutes later in call #1, son has reported to dad that it's nice to hear good stories about those diagnosed with cancer, not just bad outcomes. One example he provides, to support his view that people tend to focus on bad experiences, involves how women commiserate about how awful their pregnancies were:

6) SDCL: Malignancy #1:12

1	Son:	[<u>Oh</u>] you're <u>pregnant</u>? Let me tell you how <u>awful</u> my
2		baby was. Oh my Go:d I thought I was gonna die .hh You
3		know how how =
4	Dad:	= Su:re:. =
5	Son:	= people are always so helpful in that way. .hhh
6		(1.5)
7 →	Dad:	We::ll unfortunately (.) y- you're right. But >ya know<
8		medication .hhh and- and <u>methods</u> have, impro::ved (0.7)
9		<u>gre:at</u>ly for cancer and that kinda stuff in the last few
10		years (continues)

Following an extended pause in line 6, however, dad's "We::ll"-prefaced response initially aligns with son's position. But he then shifts toward how both medication and methods for cancer treatment have improved "in the last few years." In this way, dad counters son's prior negative characterization, emphasizing good rather than bad health outcomes. For the next 17 lines of transcript, son further pursues and dad eventually collaborates on several "horror stories" involving medical care. But as apparent below, dad again refocuses discussion by realistically assessing that mom's prognosis is not good, but "a hell of a lot better than >ya know< some of the alternatives." (lines 2-3):

7) SDCL: Malignancy #1:13

1	Dad:	Yeah:. hh So: (0.6) .hh It <u>see::ms</u> like the prognosis while it is
2 →		not (0.4) <u>good</u> is (.) **a hell of a lot better than >ya know<**
3		**some of the alternatives.**
4	Son:	Mmm hmm.
5	Dad:	.hhhhh But tha::t's as <u>much</u> as I know about her condition at
6		↑<u>thi:</u>s point. >°So I thought°< we::ll i:t's-

```
 7 →  Son:     pt Well I'm (.) glad to kno:w somethin' (.) anyways. [°It's° ]=
 8    Dad:                                                          [Yea::h.]
 9             (0.2)
10    Son:     =better than =
11    Dad:     = The unknowing is is as you said is is °so° da:mnably
12             frustrating. An- and maybe ya don't wanna kno:w but (.) I
13             don't wanna no:t know either. (.) [Because  bo:y  I] could=
14    Son:                                       [  °Um   hum.°  ]
15    Dad:     = co:njure up some re:al wi:ld nightmares. So-
16    Son:     Yeah tssh:::.
17    Dad:     .hh S:o I probably will no:t have a lot more information until
18             Monday night.
19             (0.4)
20    Son:     °Okay.° Well I'll probably (0.6) go up (0.2) °Sunday.° (0.6) .hh
21             I gotta work all day tomorrow.
22    Dad:     [(Ye:ah.)]
23 →  Son:     [ I'm go]nna take Pa:tty out tomorrow ni:ght.
24             (1.0)
25    Dad:     Oh you're takin' her ou:t?
```

Son responds by acknowledging that it's better to know something than remain uninformed (line 7 & 10). This is followed by dad's affirmation that *not* knowing can lead him to "co:njure up some re:al wi:ld nightmares." (line 15). In stepwise fashion, dad and son then talk about schedules before son announces "[I'm go]nna take Pa:tty out tomorrow ni:ght." in line 23. This is another, off-topic shift toward a good-news event.

In both Excerpts 6 and 7 (above), then, a dialectical tension exists between attempts to focus on negative/bad vs. positive/good aspects of people, medical care, and mom's condition. Like an interactional pendulum constantly in motion, son and dad each counterbalance the other's orientations to bad and good topics. At least from the moments examined thus far (Excerpts 5-7), it would appear that there is somewhat of a *tolerance threshold*, particularly for negative/bad topics, and especially at the outset of bearing and hearing bad (but not hopeless) news about mom's cancer diagnosis (see also Chapter 10). A fine line seems to exist between exhibiting realism, venting frustration, yet not expressing too much pessimism or jadedness. Understandably, such actions would contribute negatively to a cancer journey that has only just begun.

These orientations persist as the cancer journey unfolds. In Excerpt 8, for example, dad brings closure to a humbling news update by first stating that mom is struggling, overly thin, and not eating well:

8) SDCL: Malignancy #25:4

```
 1    Dad:     But uh (1.0) she's still strugglin' she still looks (1.2) thi:n.=
 2             A:nd you know she's not eat:ing (.) a whole lot.
 3    Son:     Mm hm. =
 4 →  Dad:     = Uh well, she does eat you know (       ).
 5             (1.0)
 6    Dad:     Spi::rits beenbetter the last two days or so.
 7 →  Son:     Okay.        .hhh Well I guess that's about all we can hope for =
 8    Dad:     = Yeah.=
 9 →  Son:     =at- at this point.
10    Dad:     > It's as good as it gets. < And I told her the other day after I
11             talked to you she can't (.) get into serious trouble next week
```

12		cause you said that's not a good week for comin' so. =
13	Son:	= ↑Yeah not next week. And ↑certainly not finals week. (.)
14		Any time in between is okay or after.

Yet in line 4 dad quickly clarifies that mom has not stopped eating altogether. Then, following a (1.0) pause and son's withholding of response, dad shifts to "Spi::rits been better the last two days or so." (line 6). This reorientation by dad exemplifies one incremental practice for pursuing a response (see Beach, 1996; Pomerantz, 1984b). The upgraded information he provides also demonstrates that when a specific topic (such as food/eating) has run its positive course, other possible and more encouraging topics can be raised and thus nominated for consideration.

That son heard dad as working to be encouraging, that is, as avoiding excessive negativity and making the most of an otherwise dire situation, is evident in his response: "Okay. .hhh Well I guess that's about all we can hope for=at- at this point." (line 7). His invocation of "hope" was tied directly to a realistic, yet heartening attempt by dad to emphasize what is available and worthy of appreciation. This is but another instance of how family members commiserate together, optimizing a distressing set of circumstances. Or as dad states simply, "It's as good as it gets." (line 10). This utterance adds finality to a sequence in which inherently bad news was not ignored, but somewhat mitigated with the recognition that some good things (i.e., mom's spirits) remain alive and (reasonably) well.

There is one final increment that dad provides, namely, a humorous shift to a prior event between dad and son: son's (tongue-in-cheek) informing dad, at an earlier date (see Chapter 6), that mom can't die "next week" because he'll be too busy at work. Mutually recognized as an absurd but joking position to take, son stoically adheres to it by reasserting his untenable demeanor in lines 13-14. So doing lightens the moment, and ability to cope with mom's imminent death, by extending the boundaries of known, acceptable behavior. An episode is initiated so that dad and son might play at not being responsible in the midst of an otherwise serious and entangled situation (e.g., see Glenn & Knapp, 1987; Hopper, 1995; Hopper & Glenn, 1994).

Managing Mom's Pain

In Excerpts 2 and 5 (lines 16-19 and 9-11, above) pain management is a prominent concern that gets increasingly addressed as mom's cancer progresses. Indeed, as dad reports, mom experienced problems with pain as early as call #1:

9) SDCL: Malignancy #1:7

9	Dad:	And she was really having some problems with pa:in today.
10		She had .hh one and a half (0.2) >percodans< in her and it
11		wasn't hardly slowin' it down.

Not surprisingly, then, family members closely monitor how mom's pain level is being minimized (or preferably, alleviated altogether) as time passes. The following three excerpts—from calls # 30, 37, and 39—are examined in the order they occurred and in the ways talk about pain management gives rise to hopeful and optimistic concerns.

The first instance from call #30 addresses whether mom's "pain medicine" will be sufficient to "keep it calmed do:wn" (lines 2 & 4)—"it" being her pain—and if so, raises the possibility that she will be able to come home from the hospital. The emphasis on "we" (lines 4-5) implies that dad, and assumably a team of caregivers (family, friends, and hospice staff), will be able to care for mom if her pain can be managed:

10) SDCL: Malignancy #30:9-10

((Dad had just reported that mom was receiving "intervenous antibiotics" for an infection she was fighting.))

```
 1      Dad:    =If- if she is balanced out as well as (.) can be expected
 2              o:n the pain medicine to where she does not need any kind of
 3              sh:ots. = She's now taking it in a (.) yucky tasting liquid form.
 4              (1.5) But if (.) ya know if we can keep it calmed do:wn with
 5              that then maybe you know we can deal with it here? = So she
 6              may be comin' home (.) Mo:nday afternoon or Tuesday.
 7      Son:    Okay.
 8      Dad:    Okay.
 9  →   Son:    Well (.) that's good to know.
10  →   Dad:    Yeah, (.) you know it might be nice for her to be home for a
11              while [and you]=
12      Son:          [ Y e ah- ]=
13      Dad:    =know.
14  →   Son:    =yeah even if she ends up goin back and forth at least there's
15              something to be said about sleepin in your own bed and
16              (0.5) [havin a (.) you  know-]
17  →   Dad:          [Oh sure and   hav:ing] your own surroundings and it's
18              quieter and maybe a little ↑too quiet sometimes.=
19      Son:    =Um hm.=
```

Son treats dad's informing as good news (line 9). Dad next agrees by highlighting that it would be nice to have her home for a while (lines 10-11), allowing mom to sleep in her own bed and live in her own quiet surroundings (lines 15-18). Though some uncertainty exists—as with "might be nice" (line 10), the possibility that mom may go "back and forth" (line 14) between the hospital and home, and that it "maybe a little ↑too quiet sometimes." (line 18)—the general orientation is toward good rather than bad news. Rather than belabor the problems with mom's current infection or the delicate balancing of "yucky tasting" (line 3) pain medication and disease, dad and son work together to construct a set of positive future benefits.

In the second excerpt from call #39, mom reports "it hurts" four times in lines 3-5 before stating "Nothin' I can do." Son's response draws a logical conclusion, confirmed by mom, that "everything hurts" (lines 6-7):

11) SDCL: Malignancy #39:26-27

```
 1      Son:    Mm hm. (.) pt So what are ya doin' with yourself during the
 2              day mostly sleeping.
 3  →   Mom:    Yeah. .hh eh Oh jeez it hurts uugh. It just hurts when I do
 4              things like lay down- lay down. An' it hurts when I do this,
 5              it hurts when I do that. Nothin' I can do.
 6  →   Son:    Huh .hh Just everything hurts, huh.
 7      Mom:    Yeah.
 8  →   Son:    Have they gotcha on something that- that
 9              ke[eps that down I hope].
10      Mom:      [Oh yeah. Oh  yeah.]
11      Son:    Oh that's good.
12      Mom:    Yeah for sure.
13      Son:    Otherwise it would probably drive you nuts, huh.
14      Mom:    It would certainly.
```

It is to pain medications that son next turns, referencing "they" as anonymous medical staff (see Chapters 8 & 9) administering some form of drug that "keeps that down I hope." (line 9). In overlap, mom assures son that she is indeed being adequately cared for, which son is relieved to hear. Mom's "Yeah for sure." (line 12) ensures that her twice stating "Oh yeah.", in prior turn (line 10) but in overlap, was nevertheless heard and understood by son now that her speaking is in-the-clear (see Jefferson & Schegloff, 1975; Schegloff, 2000). In this way, and despite having stated there's "Nothin' I can do." (line 5), mom seeks to minimize son's worrying that without pain medication, "it would probably drive you nuts" (line 13). It can now be seen and understood that son's prior statement of "keep that down I hope" was specifically designed in consideration of mom not being driven crazy by pain. This is an inherent uncertainty and dreaded possibility that causes steadfast reliance on care provided by medical experts. Even more than reliance, however, the management of one's own or another's pain facilitates the building of alliances with experts as persons who are able and willing to responsibly ease distress triggered by chronic aches and pains.

A third instance involving pain medication, occurring ten calls later, begins with Gramma reporting that mom's vomiting occurred because "they weren't getting' enough of the (.) morphine down." (lines 4-5):

12) SDCL: Malignancy #49:5

```
 1      Gramma:  An' uh I called him last- I called him last night
 2               because .hh one day your um Carol said well that
 3   →           she was having trouble she was vomiting all the time
 4               So they weren't keeping enough of the (.) morphine
 5               down.
 6      Son:     Mm hm.
 7      Gramma:  And uh so they gave her liquid morphine anyway.
 8   →           So the next day she was- she came out of it and she
 9               was eh- talkin to Carol and (.) an' an' was- seemed
10               a whole lot better except that they knew that (.) if she
11               didn't have the morphine that pain would come back
12               again. [So=
13      Son:           [Mm hm.
14   → Gramma:  =yesterday the pain started again. But .hh um (.) the
15               nurse called and said to give her some of the liquid
16               morphine, so that .hh when the nurse comes over to
17               give her a bath it won't be so painful.
18      Son:     Mm hm.
```

There is no explicit reference to "hope" throughout these moments. But as Gramma continues her reporting with "mom seemed a whole lot better" (lines 9-10), it is clear that her improvement was made possible by "what they gave her," noted in her prior utterance (line 7). And as the pain would come back without additional morphine—and it did—a call from the nurse instructed further liquid morphine as an effective intervention for mom's discomfort. Through these procedures, and knowing that mom's pain could be managed effectively with liquid morphine and helpful nurses, it can be seen that Gramma's reporting is not filled with alarm or despair. Although hope for cure is unrealistic during this phase of hospice involvement, confidence is exhibited that mom's pain will not be out of control and not closely attended to by medical professionals. With such assurance a different kind of optimism is displayed: an enacted faith, rooted in palliative care, that can at least safeguard mom from (most) physical suffering in the latter stages of her life. And despite mom's vomiting and other maladies, the possibility of pain management is good news.

A DELICATE BALANCE BETWEEN HOPE AND CHOICE

Family members facing cancer are routinely embroiled in circumstances that cannot fully be controlled. When radiation and chemotherapy are determined to be the only viable treatment options, for example, a choice can be made to undergo such therapy or not. If the choice is made to move forward with these regimens, the hope for remission or cure is invested into these medical options.

As evident in Excerpt 13 (below), when limited choices are available an inherent tension exists between treatment constraints and hopefulness. Returning to call #2 between son and mom, in line 24 mom's reference to "hope" quickly gets repaired in favor of "my only choice":

13) SDCL: Malignancy#2:2-3

```
 6    Mom:   No there's nothing to say. >You just-< .hh I'll I'll wait to
 7           talk to Dr. Leedon today.= He's the cancer man, and =
 8    Son:   = Um hmm.
 9    Mom:   See what he has to say, and (0.4) just keep goin' forward. I
10           mean I might be real lucky in five years. It might just be
11           six months.
12           (0.4)
13    Son:   Yeah.
14    Mom:   °Who knows.°
15    Son:   Phew::.
16    Mom:   Yeah.
17    Son:   .hh hhh (0.4) Whadda you do: with this kind of thing. I
18           mean- (.)
19    Mom:   >Radiation chemotherapy.<
20           (1.2)
21    Son:   Oh bo:y.
22    Mom:   Yeah.
23           (0.5)
24 →  Mom:   My only hope- I mean (.) my only choice.
25    Son:   Yeah.
26    Mom:   It's either that or just lay here and it'll kill me.
27           (1.0)
28    Mom:   And that's not the human condition.
29    Son:   No. (1.0) I guess [not.]
30    Mom:                     [ No.] (.) So that's all I can tell you.
```

In lines 12-15 (and 20-23, discussed below) uncertainties surrounding such an illness trajectory make it problematic for son and mom to do more than employ few words while assimilating and commiserating about the quandary they are caught up within (see Chapters 3 & 10). In response to son's query in lines 17-18, "Whadda you do: with this kind of thing. I mean-", mom immediately and quickly replies ">Radiation chemotherapy.<". By proposing medical procedures as forms of treatment regimen, mom also avoids addressing what son may very well have been pursuing with his "I mean-" : more personal issues involving her coping (e.g., fears, anxieties, anger) with what appears to be a terminal diagnosis. It remains unclear whether son was in fact soliciting and thus inviting mom to talk further about her feelings. What is apparent is that by responding in this manner, mom exhibits steadfast reliance on medical protocol that, for now, is put forth as critical to "just keep goin' forward." (line 9).

It is both her resoluteness and the recognition of the looming inevitability of these treatments that son's delayed "Oh bo:y." seems to address (lines 20-21). As discussed at the outset of Chapter 10, his "my-world" display of surprise also treats mom's predicament as remarkable and troubling. And in response, mom's "Yeah." simply and elegantly claims knowledge of her dilemma in ways son cannot experience. It is at this moment, following a personal revelation of owned experience, that mom makes fleeting reference to "hope": "My only hope- I mean (.) my only choice." This is a curious self-repair, in which "hope" and "choice" are at once treated by mom as interwoven yet distinct, an explanation for which might be gleaned from prior discussion: In light of her five year prognosis as a best case scenario for life expectancy, any hope emerging from radiation and chemotherapy is limited. Such treatment options offer little certitude nor assurance of healing her cancer. Thus, in this utterance, "hope" appears to give way to "my only choice.", which is itself clearly restrictive and further legitimizes her decision making. It is not really a preference, but rather an ill-fated necessity, that mom is orienting to. Addressed in no uncertain terms in lines 26-28, mom displays an essential unwillingness to be passive while allowing the cancer to "kill me. (1.0) And that's not the human condition." Through reference to basic human instincts for survival, mom therefore expresses her willingness to be treated through radiation and chemotherapy—a series of moments intertwined with hope *and* choice, each informing yet constraining the other.

In the final utterance of Excerpt 13 (above), mom's "So that's all I can tell you." (line 30) exhibits departure from a storytelling her cancer experiences entitle her both to reveal and to terminate (see Sacks 1984b, 1992).[2] It is clearly mom's story to tell. As cancer patient and as decision maker, mom does not solicit son's advice. Rather, she makes known to son how she will chart the course of her own treatment and what, if anything, she will remain hopeful about in the face of restricted choices such as radiation and chemotherapy.

Within the next minute of conversation, the consequences of her informing are evident. Though not examined here, son initiates his own story and informs mom that he is aware of how the medication she is on can make her depressed. Mom then informs him that her diagnosis is "very serious" because the cancer has metastasized. As examined in Chapter 4 (Excerpt 7), mom next apologizes and son's response is marked by confusion, surprise, and a reciprocal apology for the bad news mom (and the family) needs to address. And in Chapter 10 (Excerpt 4) the aftershocks of these delicate moments are further evident, as son and mom exhibit difficulties employing few words when sharing commiserative space yet claiming epistemic knowledge. Following this revealing one minute, additional key moments are analyzed in Excerpt 15 (below).

First, however, it is important to briefly recognize that other family members are also faced with circumstances they did not choose but are nevertheless impacted by. The excerpt below begins as mom's sister (son's aunt) invokes "with: any lu:ck at all", an optimistic reference to a chance occurrence that she will reach son before he gets to the airport and boards the plane (see also Excerpt 17, below):

14) **SDCL: Malignancy #10:14**

((Following son's calls to the airlines, examined in Chapter 5, his next call is with his aunt to discuss details of his traveling plans.))

```
1  → Aunt:  = I will- I will (.) with: any lu:ck at all I will get to you
2             befo:re then.
3    Son:   pt Oka:y.
4    Aunt:  Oka:y.
5    Son:   .hhh We:::ll ti:ll then .hh
6    Aunt:  'Til then my dear.
7    Son:   Ha:ng in there.
```

```
 8  →  Aunt:  I:'m hanging.
 9     Son:   Oka:y.
10  →  Aunt:  I have no cho:ice.
11     Son:   Thanks for the call.
12     Aunt:  Oka:y hon:ey. >I'll talk to you tomo:rrow.<
13     Son:   Alright. >Bye bye.<
14     Aunt:  Bye.
```

As the phone closing unfolds, her response to his encouraging "Ha:ng in there." (line 7) reveals yet another hope-choice dilemma. The phrase "hang in there" is not uncommonly uttered when it is known that another is dealing with some difficulties or troubles (see also Endnote 9, Chapter 7). It is in this sense quite fitting that son would offer such a statement. And it is equally fitting that aunt's "I:'m hanging." (line 8) clearly affirms that she is, indeed, fully caught up in somehow managing mom's cancer diagnosis and its aftershocks (e.g., coordinating son's travel plans to arrive home before she is expected to die).[3] This is further evident with her added "I have no cho:ice." (line 10), a defining moment revealing how little control she has over uninvited and unwanted external circumstances.

Yet to "hang in" is not to give up or give into undesired events, but to cope as best possible when moving toward a possible bright and improved future. In this way, mom's being steadfast and resolute about treatments (Excerpt 13, above) is not that dissimilar to her son and sister's efforts to encourage and support one another as the trying journey unfolds (Excerpt 14, above). Each set of orientations speaks directly to some presence of hope (i.e., in radiation and chemotherapy, and in waiting and managing together), efforts designed to ward off the domination of despair even when choices are not the most favorable.

INVOKING AND RESPONDING TO "MAGIC": FINDING REASONS TO KEEP FIGHTING

As noted previously, approximately one minute following Excerpt 13 (above), other key actions occur offering yet another perspective on how family members work to manage hope and optimism. Below, son shifts orientation by querying "Well where's our magic wand mom." (line 14):

15) SDCL: Malignancy #2:2-3

```
 1     Mom:   Yeah. See it's already metastasized. It's already gone
 2            ↑°someplace else even.°
 3     Son:   Mm hm.
 4     Mom:   That's what makes it >that's partially what makes it< so: (.)
 5            ve:ry serious.
 6     Son:   Mm hm.
 7            (1.4)
 8     Son:   .hhh hh
 9            (1.2)
10     Son:   pt Sh:i:t. hh
11     Mom:   Yeah $I know.$
12     Son:   $Heh.$
13     Mom:   I kno:w.
14  →  Son:   Well where's our magic wand mom.
15  →  Mom:   $It he$ (.) °Beats the hell out of me.°
16            (1.2)
```

17	Mom:	I guess the o:nly thing: (.) <u>I:</u> can do: is (.) after I'm done
18		<u>ree:</u>ling from this,=
19	Son:	Mmhm.
20 →	**Mom:**	**=.hh is find a reason to keep fighting and (.) to keep being**
21		**hopeful. (0.5) You know that- that's about all you can do.**
22		**>That's all a person can do.<**
23	Son:	**How can you <u>do:</u> that. (0.2) That's [gotta]=**
24	Mom:	[We::ll]
25	Son:	=be tough. >I mean< I don't <u>mean</u> to sa:y that sounding like a-
26	Mom:	Here comes your Pa<u>pa::</u>.
27	Son:	A:hhh.

In line 14 son's reference to "our" assumes ownership of mom's illness predicament, not only as a dilemma both mom and son are affected by, but as problems that can be faced together (see also Beach, 1996). This move toward inclusiveness is but one relational and commiserative display of being "with" (see Goffman, 1963, 1971; Mandelbaum, 1987, 1989), yet another exemplar that cancer journeys involve family members and not just cancer patients (see Kristjanson & Ashcroft, 1994; Chapter 1). Next, with "magic wand" son invokes a fairy tale image akin to Tinkerbell in Disneyland pictures, or the source of Merlin's and Harry Potter's wizardly powers. As Webster's dictionary describes it, "magic wand" is a slender rod used by fairies, or other beings, to achieve supernatural feats (e.g., turning a prince into a frog, a troll into a rabbit, or a beast into a harmless bird).

It is not coincidental that son raises "magic wand" at this particular moment. His reference is precisely tailored to commiserating, with few words and extended silences, about immediately prior bad news. This state of affairs seriously diminishes hopeful possibilities for healing. Through the supernatural power of "magic", however, even a metastasizing cancer can be held in abeyance. In the best-case scenario, cancer can be eliminated altogether through the slightest touch of a "wand." These possibilities are expressed within son's out-loud, wishful thinking. It is also clear that he does not offer his expression as literal truth, but by subtly injecting a sense of humor and brightness into a serious health scenario. With $It- he$, his actions are next treated by mom as a laughing yet troubling matter. Based on prior actions in call #2, mom was caught up in revealing a set of dire circumstances and thereby constrained from being capable of uplifting herself (even momentarily).

In responding with "$It he$ (.) °Beats the hell out of me.°" (line 2), mom accomplishes two key actions. Her initial attempt at laughter ($), though quickly aborted, thus treats son as having made an effort to invite such laughter through his magical reframing of such critical topics. Curiously and next, however, mom acts as recipient of her own telling situation by producing a despairing and "recognizably serious response" (Jefferson, 1984a, p. 346). Appearing unable and/or unwilling to take the trouble lightly, she enacts a troubles-resistant response (Jefferson 1984b, 1988) to son's prior invocation of magic and attempted humor. Understandably, she demonstrates being engrossed in (and ensnared by) her diagnostic dilemma.

But there is more here, a poetic and delicate preoccupation evident in her unwitting and quietly tailored "°Beats the hell out of me.°" (see Beach, 1993a, 1996, Ch. 5; Hopper, 1992; Jefferson, 1996; Sacks, 1992).[4] The word "°Beats" adds pragmatic force to mom's description, a lexical choice reflecting the kind of power required to drive cancer out of her body. This description stands in marked contrast to how magic wands are typically employed (again, through a simple waving or light touching, which are sufficient to achieve magical consequences). Her extended utterance also precisely characterizes an unintentional sensitivity to the very troubles at hand: If a "magic wand" could heal an illness approaching hopelessness, it would literally exorcise a dark and foreboding force from "hell" that stifles rather than improves living.[5]

Following his humorous attempt to uplift mom's condition, son next withholds further commentary (line 16) to her quiet, yet foreboding response. But the despair evident in her reply is only momentary (see also discussion of Excerpt 16, below). As revealed in mom's next "I guess the o:nly thing: (.) I: can do: is" (line 17), she continues by specifying that there are uncertain and limited options for coping with cancer. Her utterance is consequential in three key ways. First, it prefaces her insertion "after I'm done ree:ling from this.", a bewildering formulation referencing her here-and-now reaction to a malignant diagnosis (what dad had earlier portrayed as "co:nfirmation and resignation." in Excerpt 5, lines 2-3). Second, it also sets up mom's ".hh Is find a reason to keep fighting and (.) to keep being hopeful." (lines 20-21). Framed as an ongoing and practical matter, mom sketches out a procedure for living with and through her cancer, exemplifying basic survival instincts underlying the "human condition" (see Excerpt 13, line 28, above). As she constructs it, remaining hopeful requires motivated fighting, two interwoven yet distinct actions facilitating the search for reasons to live. Finally, a key portion of mom's "I guess the o:nly thing: (.) I: can do: is" (line 17) is repeated two more times in lines 21-22: "You know that- that's about all you can do. >That's all a person can do.<". As "can do" gets repeated, mom's attempt to inform her son evidences a movement from "I" to "you" to "person". In unison with her use of "me...I...I'm" in lines 15-17, mom's description becomes progressively less my-world centered as she endeavors to manage bad diagnostic news.

This stepwise shift, beginning with a revelation of her experiences yet ending with a generic "person" (see Sacks, 1992), accomplishes additional critical and interrelated actions. Although falling short of magic, mom reveals herself as doing "all" she can (line 22) within her challenging circumstances. Having first disclosed her dilemma, she moves to normalize her lived reality as an ordinary feature of illness management—an orientation common for others dealing with cancer predicaments and a category of persons she is now qualified to be a member of. Once again, as Sacks (1992) observed, by invoking such a third person characterization, " 'you' means that 'you' can in fact be a way of talking about 'everybody'—and indeed, incidentally, of 'me.' For 'you' stands as a pronoun for the set of terms: 'everyone,' 'someone,' 'people,' etc." (p. 349). Through third person references such as "you", mom distances her illness problems in a manner allowing her to more easily manage her diagnosis when coming to grips with future uncertainties, particularly dying, is inherently threatening. Yet at the same time, she treats herself as one of many cancer patients undergoing similar trials and tribulations.

Mom is also designing her talk in consideration of son's hearing, and even protection from having to directly confront a hopeless terminal illness. She is not altogether avoiding his prior and attempted lightening of the dire situation (line 14). Rather, as best possible, mom is being responsive to his uplifting efforts. Although her current disposition can be explained as "reeling," it is only temporary: Mom's orientation reveals that her confusion will give way to a more determined and hopeful condition, a "fighting" (line 20) perseverance that son can himself be hopeful about.

Excerpt 15 draws to a close as son continues by further pursuing just how mom can remain hopeful (lines 23 & 25), a solicitation that is preempted with mom's announcement that "Papa::" has just entered the room.

A Story and Its Consequences: Fighting the Battle Together

As mom stops talking (not shown in Excerpt 15, above), dad and son continue talking for nearly five minutes about fixing cars together and an upcoming chili dinner son has prepared for when mom returns home from the hospital.[6] Son then requests to speak with mom once again and announces his dinner plans to her. It is at this juncture that mom initiates the following story, about a "sign" the son had placed in her hospital room:

16) SDCL: Malignancy #2:12-13

1	Mom:	>By the way< your sign 'Do not take me' really worked.
2	Son:	$Did it?$
3	Mom:	Totally confu:sed one girl. She looked, and she looked, and
4		she looked. Now this is a little oriental gal. =
5	Son:	= Mm hm.
6		(0.4)
7	Mom:	<And ah> (1.0) [she went out]
8	Son:	[Do not] ah (.) take oh (.) me (.) [ha]
9	Mom:	[She]
10		went out and she brought in >ya know< those things have
11		liners?
12	Son:	Mmm hm.
13	Mom:	She brought a li:ner of like a of clear water in to set it there.
14	Son:	Mm hm mm hm [°hm°]
15	Mom:	[She] didn't she couldn't quite figure that
16		who:le thing out. >But she wasn't gonna touch it.<
17	Son:	Mmm. (.) Good.
18	Mom:	°So that was kinda funny.°
19 →	Son:	See, [there] there's a small battle=
20	Mom:	[( )]
21 →	Son:	=that we've won. =
22 →	Mom:	$Right, [right,] right.$
23	Son:	[hhh]
24		An(d) that's all ya can do is jus just
25		[rack up the] sma:ll battles.
26	Mom:	[Ri:ght ri:ght. Um hm.]
27		°Well,° .hhh well okay. I'm gonna let you go:.
28	Son:	O[kay.]
		((Mom & Son move to phone closing.))

That mom even initiated such a humorous story displays her attempt to lighten what had become, prior to son and dad's conversation, a very serious discussion of both her diagnostic condition and orientation to coping. She also acknowledges son's thoughtful effort to meet her needs by placing a "Do not take me" sign on her bed. This stands in contrast to her prior and momentarily despairing response to his "Well where's our magic wand mom." (Excerpt 15, line 14). Taken together, the actions built into this shift in topic mark a contrast in mom's demeanor. They are remedial in just the ways mom's initiation of this particular story appears designed to invigorate her earlier displayed unwillingness and/or inability to take her troubles lightly. She also displays appreciation for son's ongoing concerns with her illness.

This marked shift in mom's disposition does not go unnoticed by son. In response to her reference to "little oriental gal." (line 4), son collaborates by personifying the girl's scenic reaction with a stereotypic "[Do not] ah (.) take oh (.) me (.) [ha]", a voiced switch enacting an Asian identity (see Beach, 2000b; Holt, 1999; Holt & Clift, 2006), and an action he treats as humorous with his final "[ha]". Next, when mom brings the story to a close with "°So that was kinda funny.°" (line 18), son relies on mom's initiated, humorous story to revisit yet extend their earlier discussion in Excerpt 15. He retopicalizes and reframes mom's immediately delivered story by connecting mom's earlier "keep fighting" with "small battle", and "our magic wand" with "we've won". In these ways, son shows sensitivity to mom's "keep fighting and (.) to keep being hopeful." while simultaneously treating this as a moment for reemphasizing that they are indeed facing the problems together.

Following mom's aligned recognition and their shared laughter (lines 22-23), son's "An(d) that's all ya can do is jus just[rack up the] sma:ll battles." (lines 24-25) offers a moral to the story by reinvoking mom's prior "That's all a person can do (Excerpt 15, line 22). He reenacts mom's own demeanor toward her cancer problems, essentially mirroring the actions she had previously generated (i.e., by extending a story of appreciation and humor, initiated by mom). Though certainly well intended, son's actions are treated by mom as having overextended an otherwise well-taken point. In line 26, she interjectively moves to close down son's contribution and transition to bringing the phone conversation to a close (lines 27-28).

A brief comparison of Excerpts 15 and 16 reveals that when mom initiates talk about how she will fight her cancer battle and a story about son's sign "Do not take me", she is more tolerant of discussing her dilemma than when son revisits and reenacts her orientation. As cancer patient, mom is well positioned to employ her *epistemic authority* in this manner (see Chapter 10), displaying in these last moments an unwillingness to talk further about any "small battle that we've won." In this important sense, it can be seen that there are limits to just how benign one's set of circumstances might be constructed to be, and just what shifts from bad to good news might be allowed to occur (or not) by the primary figure facing the bad news. (See also a similar move by son to terminate discussion and bring a phone call to closing, in Excerpt 18, below.) Though son attempts to align with and further encourage mom's determination and resolve, mom demonstrates that at times more is not necessarily better. Indeed, as the cliché goes, "good enough is often best left alone."

CONSTRUCTING POSITIVE FUTURES

As evident in the analysis above, hopeful and optimistic moments arise predominantly when the focal concern rests with mom. For example, in a previously examined call between aunt and son (see Excerpt 14, above), aunt's "with: any lu:ck at all" (line 1) offers an optimistic possibility (but with no assurance) that she will contact son before he departs the airport. A similar moment appears below, as son's "I- I've got a day at least I hope." (line 5) refers to whether he will have sufficient time to kennel his dog before departing for home. His "hope" specifically addresses a desire to arrive before mom dies:

17) **SDCL: Malignancy #3:7**

((When working out travel scheduling with dad, son had just remembered that he had forgotten about taking his dog to the kennel.))

1	Son:	Yeah I don't think that's expen<u>sive</u> anyway. (.) I just the only
2		thing is I- I probably coul<u>dn't</u> leave till tomorrow. Because I
3		have to take him there in the morning you know. (.) um-
4	Dad:	I don't- I don't see that as a problem.
5 →	**Son:**	**Okay. I- I've got a day at least I hope.**
6	Dad:	Yep.
7	Son:	Okay.
8	Dad:	(I would think so.)
9	Son:	Allright I'll stay by the phone.
10	Dad:	Okay. =
11	Son:	= Let me know. ((continues toward phone closing))

In line 6, though dad's "Yep." initially confirms son's "I hope.", he quickly adds "I would think so." (line 8). Dad cannot definitively predict, and thus guarantee, that mom will live until son arrives. And it is this doubt that prompts son to state that he will remain by the phone (line 9)—a displayed state of readiness evidencing emergency preparedness (see Chapter 7). Indeed, it is the urgency of such timing that son's prior "I hope." is designed to address.

A related instance occurs over 50 calls later, as son again prepares to travel home to be with mom and family before she actually dies. (As described in Chapter 6, mom lived through earlier crises.) Below, a friend offers his assistance, support, "An:: good luck...whatever that means." (lines 4 & 6):

18) SDCL: Malignancy #55:2

1	Greg:	Okay. Now if there's anything at a:ll I can do for ya Doug,
2		lemme kno:w.
3	Son:	.hhhh Okay.
4 →	Greg:	**Ya know, anything. (.) An:: good luck. We're bo[th-] =**
5	Son:	[Thanks.]
6 →	Greg:	**= whatever that means.**
7 →	Son:	**Ya know whatever it means. A- at this point it just means**
8		**let's hope we all (get) through this reasonably well.**
9	Greg:	Ri:ght. Right.
10	Son:	Okay. Well thanks. =
11	Greg:	Okay. Take care.
12	Son:	Bye bye.
13	Greg:	Alrighty. Bu' bye.

In response, son repeats with "Ya know whatever it means." (line 7). He then moves direct-ly to define "good luck" in practical terms: "It just means let's hope we all (get) through this reasonably well." (lines 7-8). His shift from luck to hope was not based on mom's miraculous recovery, but more realistically on reasonably coping with "this"—the unnamed but clearly recognized reference to mom's inevitable dying, how her death will come about, and consequences for how the family will manage her passing. Even in the face of unavoidable death of a loved one, "hope" can still exist; not about *curing* mom's disease, but maintaining healing relationships providing needed comfort and support (e.g., see Barbour, 1995; Engel, 1977; Groopman, 2004; Kubler-Ross, 1969b, 1974).

It is this recognition that Greg's "Ri:ght. Right." acknowledges (line 9), and the call moves quickly to closing as son (like mom in Excerpt 16, above) displays an unwillingness to talk further about these delicate matters.

Hope About Dating, Friends, Careers, and Finances

Life goes on in the midst of cancer journeys. Many events occur that seemingly have little or nothing to do with cancer. Hope also arises in the midst of these otherwise benign (but by no means trivial) circumstances, when talking about details of everyday life having lit-tle if anything to do with illness or other (possibly urgent) health matters.

Prior to Excerpt 19, for example, son had been informing mom that he had met a woman he was considering asking out for a date. They had been talking for hours, and son states "and we just got on like peas in a pod.":

19) SDCL: Malignancy #39:32

1	Son:	An' it made me feel good. I thought AH HAH ya know.
2		.hh I'm feeling all this terror and panic about uh .hh
3		ya know, how would I ever meet anybody. And ya know
4		'cuz I don't like to go to ba:rs an- [.hh] =
5	Mom:	[Yeah.]
6	Son:	= ya know there's really not that many people in my
7		department that I could ever even think about. And I think
8		[geez how yucky. .hh Um pt =
9	Mom:	[Mm hm.
10	Son:	= But I- I met this- this woman and I thought I- I could ask
11		her out and I think she'd maybe go.
12	Mom:	Mm hm.
13 →	Son:	**So there you can- you can know that- that at some point uh**
14		**pt there's hope for me yet. Heh heh heh heh.**
15	Mom:	You're not really just a straight um ju- straight across u:m
16		(2.0) Oh I know what ya mean by golly, but I can't repeat it.
17	Son:	Heh heh. Well I'm not gonna turn into a monk.
18	Mom:	Well that's what I mean in a way.

In contrast to the "terror and panic" (line 2) son had been experiencing because he may not ever meet anybody, he next reports "And I think geez how yucky." (lines 7-8). Here, as with numerous identified prior instances in previous chapters, "geez" is uttered as a derivative of invoking the deity "Jesus". Not uncommonly, "geez" emerges in troubling environments not fully controlled, as with son facing the possibility of not meeting a woman he could date.

It is this good news that son immediately announces to mom in lines 10-11. This is followed by his summary of the point of his story: informing mom that "there's hope for me yet." (line 14), as if mom might be concerned that following his divorce, he may not meet (and spend time with) other women. As his subsequent laughter indicates (line 14), he has touched on a delicate matter for a mom he treats as interested and caring. And though mom next attempts to be receptive to son's hopeful story about dating, reassuring him that he will be fine with other women, she is unable to coherently do so as she is heavily medicated for her pain. Son's laughter-prefaced uptake, "Heh heh. Well I'm not gonna turn into a monk." (line 17), reveals how son translates mom's prior incoherence into a summarized version of his own fears about not meeting or dating other women. In turn, mom's "Well that's what I mean in a way." (line 18), acknowledges that although son's version is not exactly her own sentiment, it will suffice. As their discussion unfolds, however, coordinating exactly what the other "means" is treated as less important than a more primary and shared recognition: That "hope" is alive (at least regarding son's meeting and dating other women), and that son and mom give priority to assuring one another that a positive future is unfolding (again, at least for son's relationships).

As an enrolled doctoral student, son's career aspirations are also important throughout mom's illness. Below, in lines 1 & 3, dad now offers assurance that his hard work invested in graduate school will "pay off.":

20) SDCL: Malignancy #43:3

((Discussion had focused on a friend completing graduate school and seeking employment by a university—similar to what son will be facing in four years.))

1	Dad:	Ya gotta pay the piper first [and uh-] and then =
2	Son:	[That's right.]

```
 3      Dad:    = Ya get the re:ward. So tha:t's alright. It'll pay off.
 4  →   Son:    Hmm. I hope so. It- it damn well better that's for sure.
 5      Dad:    <What is he: loo:king to do:,> te:ach?
 6      Son:    Yeah. [Ex- exa:ct]ly =
 7      Dad:          [As far as- ]
 8      Son:    = Exa:ctly wha- what [I'm doing.]
 9      Dad:                         [Get into ] academia not back
10              [into industry.]
11      Son:    [   Ri:ght.   ] Right. He- he is me in four yea[ rs.   ] =
12      Dad:                                                   [(Yeah.)]
```

Son's response to dad's encouragement, "Hmm. I hope so. It- it damn well better that's for sure." (line 4), begins with reflection then moves to a statement of "hope" about the rewards he will receive (i.e., a teaching position in academic, lines 5-10). With "it damn well better," son claims the right to emphasize (even demand) an apt reward, or pay-off, pressumably (though not stated) because of his hard work, commitment, and investment in his emerging profession. By comparing himself with a friend and fellow graduate student, son's "hope" is more clearly envisioned: His colleague will soon receive his doctorate and therefore be interviewing for university positions, just as son will be: "He- he is me in four years." (line 11).

Dreams and aspirations about positive, often distant futures are centrally important for hopefulness. So too are more immediate plans. Slightly over one minute later in call #43, son and dad continue to talk about son's colleague:

21) SDCL: Malignancy #43:5

```
 1      Dad:    Sounds like a de:lightful human being.
 2      Son:    He is. He's a re:ally nice fellow. I really enjoyed going I-
 3  →           I'm hoping to .hh get together and do a few more things
 4              with him before he va:nishes, and uhm and we become .hh
 5              ya know contacts through BitNet or one a these $things.$
```

Dad's summary of son's prior and complimentary descriptions of his colleague are confirmed and even upgraded as son continues to elaborate. In lines 2-3, son's "I'm hoping" emerges as a progression from "He's a re:ally nice fellow. I really enjoyed going I- I'm hoping." Spending quality time together with friends and colleagues is an ongoing source of hope for most people. (And readers might also note that on line 5, son's reference to staying in touch via "BitNet"—an early precursor to more recent e-mail technologies—was portrayed by son as one means of retaining contact with valued persons.)

Six minutes later in the same call, discussion had shifted to a related topic of finances, specifically, son's ability to pay bills following his recent divorce. Below, he sketches how his monthly rent is paid, and his plans for renewing his lease "with just me on it" (line 4):

22) SDCL: Malignancy #43:11

```
 1      Son:    [But ] no i- it just shows up here and I just send 'em a check
 2              like always I don't think they even know. And then my
 3              le:ase- when I renew my lease in January .h I'll just renew it
 4              with just me on it. .hh And uh ya know get all of that
 5  →           changed over. pt And uh I'm ho:ping that there isn't gonna
 6              be a problem with that. (.) .hh Because ya know I don't
 7              know that technically I make enough money.
```

In a time of financial transition (i.e., shifting from dual to single income), son's "I'm hoping there isn't gonna be a problem" (lines 5-6) previews his next and explicit concern that he doesn't "make enough money." (line 7). It is clear that taking care of the basic necessities of living—for example, food, shelter, and clothing—cannot be overlooked despite surrounding circumstances requiring emotional and practical investments of time and energy. Hope, then, is equally important for managing routine daily affairs (such as paying bills and rent), envisioning the possibility of gainful employment, and seeking the ability to cope well with a loved one's dying when possibilities for physical healing no longer exist.

COMPARISON OF ALTERNATIVE ORIENTATIONS TO HOPE AND IMPLICATIONS FOR RESEARCH

Faced with a serious and uncertain cancer diagnosis, and thus in the very midst of emergent troubles and possible despair, family members have been shown to construct hopeful responses to a variety of events tied directly to cancer and everyday life. Living with and through cancer and an array of other chronic and life-threatening illnesses (e.g., see Packo, 1991), creates diverse circumstances in which the interactional achievement of hopeful conduct is apparently needed and appropriate. Dealing with and attempting to ease burdens is a primary preoccupation in social life. Whether burdens arise from the often harsh and restrictive impositions of illness and/or routine worldly problems, considerable time and effort is invested by speakers to manage hopeful conduct in interaction.

We are now in a position to compare contrasting orientations to hope: secular, spiritual, and social scientific perspectives overviewed in Chapter 12, and the series of moments analyzed in this chapter as family members interactionally engage in arguably hopeful and optimistic activities. Implications for future research on hope will also be raised as this chapter is brought to a close.

In the order they were analyzed, Figure 13.1 lists 15 specific utterances involving *Explicit*[E] references to "hope/hoping/hopeful" and 12 *Implicit*[1] orientations to hopeful possibilities.

Speakers' *Explicit* references to "hope/hoping/hopeful" exhibit orientations toward positive outcomes for future time frames and events:

- Receiving news about diagnosis and related medical information from doctors.
- Acknowledging the importance of medical personnel by steadfastly relying upon medical protocol and treatment procedures (see also Chapter 9).
- Mom putting faith in treatment options and keeping fighting, even in the midst of restricted choices.
- Mom's being able to eat, being in better spirits, and receiving adequate pain medications are positives that (at least to some extent) ease a progressive and terminal cancer journey.
- Son having adequate time to travel, meet and date other women, being able to pay rent, rewarded by his investment in graduate school, looking forward to seeing a friend, and (with his family) managing mom's passing well.

Across these moments, some hope prevails in the face of adversity and ongoing challenges. Hope persists even though medical news may not be good, treatment options are limited and may not be successful. And despite mom's failing health her eating, good spirits, and medications counter her troubles by providing some good news. For son, burdened by traveling and coping with mom's passing, a brighter future is constructed in which he will be involved with other persons, meet his expenses in the near future, and be gainfully employed in years to come (i.e., following graduate school).

Explicit/Implied Reference to Hope/Hopeful Possibilities (E=Explicit, I=Implicit)	Excerpt#/ Call#	Interactional Work Displayed
Dad: So .hhh n:o:: I would hope by Monday or Tu:esday **E**	1/1	seeking realistic time frame for diagnosis
Dad: But I hope to fi- ((clears throat)) hope to find out this morning so, **E**	2/37	looking forward to receiving new information from doctors
Aunt: An' I was hoping that was him, so: **E**	3/17	waiting to speak with dad about what the doctor said
Mom: I'll- I'll wait to talk to Dr. Leedon today…I mean I might be real lucky in five years **I**	4/2	awaiting possible good news from doctor
Dad: But (0.2) she did have two nice things ha:ppen today. **I**	5/1	shift from bad → good news
Dad: medication .hhh and- and methods have, impro::ved (0.7) gre:atly for cancer **I**	6/1	shift from bad → good news
Dad: the prognosis while it is not (0.4) good is (.) a hell of a lot better than >ya know< some of the alternatives. **I**	7/1	realistically acknowledges prognosis is not good but better than some
Son: I'm gonna take Pa:tty out tomorrow ni:ght. **I**		shift from bad → good news
Dad: = Uh well, she does eat you know ( ) …Spi::rits been better the last two days or so. **I**	8/25	emphasizes what can be appreciated in the face of mom's failing health
Son: Okay. .hhh Well I guess that's about all we can hope for = **E**		responsive acknowledgment
Dad: it might be nice for her to be home for a while **I**	10/30	emphasizes what can be appreciated in the face of mom's failing health
Son: Have they gotcha on somethin that- that keeps that down I hope. **E**	11/39	seeking assurance that adequate pain medication was available for mom
Gramma: she came out of it and she was eh- talkin to Carol and (.) an' an' was- seemed a whole lot better **I**	12/49	emphasizing mom's brief recovery and stabilization
Mom: My only hope- I mean (.) my only choice. **E**	13/2	putting faith in radiation and chemotherapy in the midst of restricted choices

Figure 13.1. *Summary of Interactional Work Achieved Across Twenty-Five Hopeful Moments*

Aunt: with: <u>any</u> lu:ck at <u>all</u> I will get to you befo:re then. [I]	14/10	expressing need to contact son before he travels
Son: Well where's our magic wand mom. [I] ing	15&16/2	subtly and humorously invoking
		supernatural powers for healing
Mom: find a reason to keep fighting and (.) to keep being hopeful [E]		expresses basic survival instinct in the face of limited choices
Son: See, there there's a small battle...that we've won. [I]		extends mom's prior 'fighting/ hopeful' with a moral to the story she has told
Son: Okay. I- I've got a day at least I hope. [E] has	17/3	seeking confirmation that he
		adequate time before traveling to see mom
Greg: An:: good luck...whatever that means. [I] midst	18/55	offering best wishes in the
		of uncertainty regarding mom's dying
Son: it just means let's hope we all (get) through this reasonably well. [E]		realistic assessment that mom will not recover, but that the family will manage her passing well
Son: at some point uh pt there's hope for me yet. [E] will	19/39	stating a likelihood that son
		meet and date other women
Son: I hope so. It- it <u>damn</u> well better that's for sure. [E]	20/43	references gainful employment in the future – a reward for his educational investment
Son: I'm hoping to .hh get together and do a few more things with him before he <u>va:</u>nishes, [E]		looking forward to spending more time with a friend
Son: I'm <u>ho:</u>ping that there isn't gonna be a lease, problem with that. [E]	22/43	stating desire to extend his
		even though he doesn't make enough money

Excerpts Listed In Order of Analysis
[E] = Explicit References to "Hope/Hoping/Hopeful"
[I] = Implicit Orientations to Hopeful Possibilities

Figure 13.1. *Summary of Interactional Work Achieved Across Twenty-Five Hopeful Moments* (continued)

Speakers' *Implicit* references utilize various resources for creating and maintaining positive orientations without using "hope/hoping/hopeful". Through topical shifts from bad to good news, but also in other ways, these actions are designed to manage bad news by emphasizing that some positive occurrences are notable and reported as such:

- Nice things happened on an otherwise difficult day.
- Methods for treatment have improved, even though people can be negative about cancer-related events.
- Son can meet and date someone as mom's cancer progresses.
- Mom can await possible good news from the doctor.
- Matters of "luck" can facilitate critically important events such as living a longer life and managing mom's passing, as well as aunt's comparably less important (but not trivial) need to get in contact with son before he travels.
- Acknowledging positive aspects of prognosis and coping (e.g., eating, being in good spirits, home for a while, and temporarily feeling better).
- Invoking supernatural wishes ("magic wand") and winning small battles.

Activities such as these comprise ongoing efforts by family members to simply survive, day by day, by making the most out of otherwise oppressive illness circumstances. Together with *Explicit* references, they represent balancing mechanisms mitigating the dominance of bad states of affairs. Dark, foreboding, and despairing modes of existence can be mitigated when survival and a more comforting future are actively pursued. Activities such as "fighting" are basic survival instincts even when resistance to troubles may be diminishing. Though now apparent, it is important to reemphasize that it is not necessary to employ words such as "hope/hoping/hopeful" to maintain some sense of stability and equilibrium in daily life.

The Explicit and Implicit references analyzed in this chapter are recruited by family members to address emerging troubles (actual, possible, and anticipated). Through interaction, hopeful aspirations get continually bolstered, and in extremely practical ways. When navigating through inherent cancer uncertainties — "the significant obstacles and deep pitfalls" noted by Groopman (2004, p. xiv) and discussed previously in Chapter 12 — each instance is contingently tied to managing specific, moment by moment, and consequential matters treated as important and even critical. Close examinations of these enactments allows for key contrasts to be made between actual family phone calls and secular, spiritual, and social scientific orientations to hope described in Chapter 12.

Revisiting Secular Perspectives on Hope

In society, written and spoken conceptions of hope were revealed as generic depictions having only vague applicability to actual and specific moments in everyday life. Fundamental features, such as accepting the inevitability of conflict/struggle, the need for patience and endurance, and the importance of not abandoning but relying on the uplifting power of hope, are central to alternative secular philosophy and modes of thinking. The American Cancer Society, for example, routinely employs visual images to instill the power of hope (Figure 13.2). These and other images are powerful reminders that hope can prevail despite challenging cancer circumstances.

In secular reasoning about hope, it was also shown that the human condition is likened to (a) balances of nature (e.g., clouds and sunshine, night and morning) as the seasons of life pass by, and (b) the dialectical tension between emotional turmoil and triumph (e.g., fears and peace/comfort, nightmares and dreams/aspirations). In these ways, a framework for conceptualizing hope is advanced, while specific communicative rules for operationalizing hope remain unspecified.

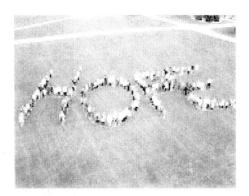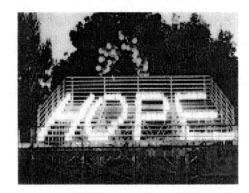

Figure 13.2. *Visual Reminders of the Power of Hope*

Basic similarities emerge when comparing these generic depictions to family members' interactions. In real time, when family members face terminal cancer together, hopeful orientations recurred and were shown to be critical resources for balancing obstacles and pitfalls. For these family members, the pendulum of interaction predictably moved from bad to good/positive news. In various ways, survival (e.g., through "fighting" and winning "a small battle") was emphasized throughout different stages of mom's progressive cancer. A patient, at times methodical demeanor was also exhibited when engaging in activities such as awaiting medical news, seeking positive aspects of daily events, and not giving in to extended stretches of despairing talk. Even when chronic uncertainty was apparent, and the likelihood of negative health outcomes for mom were imminent, a hopeful rationality reigned over despondency. Indeed, viewed as a whole, the Malignancy phone call corpus is far more hopeful than desperate. Considerably more attention is given to how to live (as best possible) through the dying process, than to the inevitability of death itself. As noted in the Introduction to this volume, mom does not actually pass away until following the last call in the phone corpus.

Analysis makes clear that speakers' practices constitute a markedly different language than the language of secular (hopeful) reasoning. Regarding words alone, and with few exceptions (e.g., "good/worse", "nightmares"), the language of secular philosophy does not resemble the lexicon of conversational participants involved in navigating through practical circumstances in everyday life. In these phone calls, the idealism and grandeur of many secular depictions of hope are replaced with sensible, matter-of-fact, no-nonsense displays of hopeful conduct—about medical information, positive daily events, assurances of care, a future to look forward to—all of which, and more, occur by family members doing their best to cope with ongoing difficulties associated with mom's cancer.

Even more importantly, in writing and during inspiring and motivational speeches by orators, matters such as the need for hope, the cycles of living, the turmoils and triumphs of lived experience do not get built for, nor require immediate next response from copresent interactants. Musing, ruminating, and reflecting about hope need not occur in a vacuum, of course: In both writing and public speaking, specific kinds of messages may get designed for particular purposes, persons, and audiences (e.g., see Atkinson, 1984; Clayman & Heritage, 2002a). Yet the envisioning evident in writing and public speaking are constrained by individuals' expectations and preferred outcomes (if any) for more general circumstances. In contrast, within talk in interaction any positive or hopeful attempt to shape events must be tailored with particular recipients in mind, made available to unique next speakers who themselves have the option of commenting on, elaborating, or even disconfirming prior speakers' well-intended movements toward hope. These collaborative possibilities—such as encouraging another to remain patient and hopeful and leaving it for the recipient to respond in ways that the initial speaker must somehow address next (e.g., see Excerpts 14-16, above)—are commonplace in ordinary interactions. From the 25 excerpts examined above, these moments are most frequently plain and pragmatic, yet meaningfully understood as resources for not allowing here-and-now problems to silence the many voices of hope.

Putting hopeful conceptions and secular philosophy into action is the problematic crux of affairs for social life. It is not an easy task to articulate the essence of hope in discerning and authentic ways, no matter the mode of expression.

For these family members, however, despite being lay persons possessing minimal technical and medical expertise, a capacity was revealed for producing interactional solutions for managing potential despair by constructing hopeful possibilities.

Revisiting Biblical and Spiritual Perspectives on Hope

A brief review of biblical scripture, from both the Old and New Testaments, makes clear that hope is anchored in faith about a living and loving God. For Jews and Christians alike, God is merciful, filled with wisdom, and capable of helping persons regardless of their circumstances, even unto death. For Christians, the death and resurrection of Jesus Christ—God's son sent to earth to live, experience, and ultimately die for humans' sinful nature—forms the basis for faith, forgiveness, and eternal life. Believers find hope by knowing (in heart felt ways) that joy can emerge from suffering, good will overcome evil, and the Holy Spirit (Christ's presence on earth) will guide and comfort believers who are never abandoned by God.

Though Judeo-Christian theology is predominant in Western American culture, and a primary worldview for religious beliefs (e.g., see Pearcey, 2004), this particular family did not explicitly or implicitly rely on God, Jesus Christ, or any other supernatural deities to manage their uncertainties and minimize their sufferings.[7] Not a single moment was identified where family members exhibited purposeful faith in biblical texts or assured one another that God or Christ was ever-present and will shape something good out of present trials. Encouragements and offers to pray for, and thus edify one another, did not occur. For Jews and Christians, this may be both surprising and puzzling. For those sharing other belief systems, including agnostics and atheists, this family handled cancer through normal and commonplace patterns of communication—practices and techniques that are known, familiar, and used across their and others' family structures.

Over the years numerous students and colleagues who have heard and/or read transcriptions of various portions of the Malignancy corpus, have commented on how they (and/or their family) might have managed such a cancer journey on the telephone. In numerous cases, these persons have directly experienced cancer (or other chronic/terminal illnesses) in themselves, family members, and/or significant others. They have also participated in local and long-distance phone calls in the course of their own or others' illnesses. Their perspectives and positions might be summarized as follows:

- Some are puzzled about the lack of faith and spiritual hope in these particular calls. They report that their own experiences are anchored in prayer and explicit discussions of God's plan, actions that would have occurred from the very first call and throughout the course of mom's illness (and beyond). An over-reliance on self-control, fighting one's own battles, doctors, medications, luck, magic wands, and more—worldy affordances and random occurrence—do not give God a chance to work and even perform miracles. Such a lack of faith will ultimately restrict healing outcomes (of the body, mind, and spirit).

- Others report that despite being involved in families and friendships espousing Judeo-Christian beliefs, their faith remains private and is not (or only rarely) raised during actual conversations as a resource for hope and acceptance. The majority of these persons have reported, however, that they have or would consider praying for themselves and/or others. Prayer makes a practical difference for coping, healing, and living a higher quality of life.

- Still others identify strongly with this family, noting familiarities in strangers' voices who have encountered serious challenges. For them, the absence of God or Christ is neither noticeable nor bothersome. They generally do not believe in supernatural beings, nor in eternal life, and thus treat matters of this world as appropriate and adequate resources when facing life's challenges.

These contrasting and at times irreconcilable perspectives trigger a series of key questions: In *what* to persons invest their faith? *How* is faith communicated across diverse families with different religious and spiritual beliefs during times of struggle (including illness)? What (if any) practical differences do answers to these questions make when encountering life's traumas and triumphs? These and related questions are certainly easier to raise than answer.

At the very least, however, this family's nonbiblical orientations exemplify that hope needn't be tied to spiritual and religious beliefs. For the vast majority of persons, hopeful activities are critically important for counter-balancing seemingly unsurmountable troubles occasioned by the affairs of everyday life.

Revisiting Previous Social Scientific Investigations of Hope

As previously discussed, regarding coping with (and through) difficult situations, it was Kübler-Ross (1969b) who first observed that "The one thing that usually persists through all these stages is hope" (p. 138). The data analyzed herein confirm what her interviews and field work made apparent. From the first call and throughout (see Figure 1, above), family members produced hopeful actions by re-orienting to positive futures across diverse occasions. At least for these family members, being hopeful—in all its manifestations and across time—was fundamental to coping with life in the midst of cancer.

Though Peräkylä (1991) focused on "hope work" in Finnish hospital wards, there is also an affinity with his basic findings (see Excerpts 8-10, above) and those emerging from these family phone calls. The emphasis given to positive developments in patients' medical conditions—for example, that better control was achieved, patients were feeling and would get better, and through expressions of hopeful expectations—were also apparent across calls and family members. Speakers gave priority to such activities as shifting from unpleasant to pleasant topics, acknowledging hopeful possibilities for (as yet) undisclosed medical news, and recognizing that some positives occurred (or will occur) despite an inability to halt the spreading of mom's cancer. Of course, rather than medical staff offering encouragement and hopeful assurance to patients in clinical settings, family members were shown to not only support one another by being hopeful, but to portray their own aspirations for a future filled with life-affirming possibilities. These brief comparisons make clear that relationships among clinical and family interactions require further exploration and integration, rather than treating them as distinct institutional and casual/ordinary domains of everyday interactions (see also Beach, 1996).

In general terms, key findings from quantitative and additional qualitative studies of hope were also confirmed through analysis of the 25 excerpts in this chapter. Indeed, as mechanisms for coping, the interactional work involved in being hopeful regularly appears to be aligned with what might roughly be characterized as offering and receiving social and family support. Movements toward positive events could also be understood as resources for managing trying circumstances and controlling adverse events. But in all cases, what counts as social/family support and control are inherently empirical matters. Indeed, a chasm can exist between extant theories, and the details of interactional involvements comprising interconnected relationships. It has been observed that "research on the connections between hope and social psychological functioning" is minimal in cancer research and that "maintain[ing] a sense of control" is an essential determinant of how cancer patients cope with their illness hopefully (Bunston et al., 1995, p. 79). So too can it be noted that this chapter only begins to address hope (and possible relationships with control) as interactionally organized moments of practical action.

Similarly, although it could be assumed that family members are socially constructing their identities in and through being hopeful, it remains unclear just what impacts these behaviors might have on speakers' self-esteem and self-concept (see Jones, 2005b). Insights about the use of humor as a coping strategy also remain vague. Instances such as son's invoking a "magic wand" (Excerpt 15, above) and mom's story about son's sign for the nurse in the hospital (Excerpt 16, above) provide preliminary evidence that certain forms of humor may well play important roles in coping with cancer as a family (see "hair" excerpts in Chapter 11), especially as efforts are made to draw attention away from negative and toward positive events (see also Endnote 1). This makes intuitive sense, but cannot be substantiated from the data in this chapter alone. The study of humor and play is also altogether normal, yet deceptively complex. Just as the many instances of laughter examined throughout the chapters of book reveal delicate and often troublesome interactional work, so does any examination of relationships among humor and hope require careful studies of moments where such actions seem to be occurring.

Hope: Is That What Makes a Family, a Family?

Many would assume that families are primal habitats for hope. The query "What makes a family, a family?" (e.g., see Gubrium & Holstein, 1990) is particularly deserving of substantive, interactionally grounded answers regarding hope. Such matters as how hope, support, coping, and commiseration get interactionally managed become evident (in part) as family members' work as a team. These efforts are noticeable during moments when family members refuse to give up hope, take turns at being hopeful, inject humorous concerns into troubling circumstances, identify with others' concerns, and work to protect one another from fears and anxieties so often associated with difficulties.

Among other findings, this chapter has also revealed that "bright side sequences" are only one type of response available for family members dealing with bad news (see Holt, 1993), that the proximity and interwoven nature of good and bad news is indeed omnipresent (see Maynard, 2003), and that hopeful actions directed toward others are resources for taking on another's problems. Working to be hopeful together can also produce its own interactional dilemmas, however, most notably in the midst of talking about other "dreaded issues" (Peräkylä, 1995). Further investigation is needed into how the management of hope in relationships is itself an ongoing and often problematic achievement, including moments of (a) Doing the work of moving away from troubling topics (e.g., dad's shift to good from bad news precipitated by son's display that enough had been said); (b) Moving talk forward even though family members express that they do not know what to say (e.g., mom and son rely on few words when assimilating the news together, as addressed more fully in Chapter 10); (c) Initiating, pursuing, and responding to intimate and personal topics (e.g., son twice querying mom about how she copes with her condition); (d) Uplifting and compensating for responses to such edification efforts (e.g., son's invoking "magic", and mom's delayed telling of a funny story to counter her prior lacklus-ter response to his displayed concerns); and (e) Attempting to encourage another (e.g., by making the point that small battles can be won together), which gets dismissed as mom interjectively initiates closure by moving to end the call.

Finally, with regard to talk about troubles (e.g., see Jefferson 1980a, 1980b, 1984a, 1980b, 1988), these family members appear remarkably sensitive to limitations on serious topics, yet at times proceed to enact topic shifts without necessarily terminating talk about cancer per se. Understanding how (or if) being hopeful gets constructed during these shifts merits ongoing examination (but see Figure 1 in Chapter 10). Similarly, environments need to be more fully inspected when, following moments when mom's ability to resist troubles essentially fails, she nevertheless "rebounds", that is, attempts to muster the energy required to rally her appreciation for son's concerns and to remain hopeful. As a practical achievement, even though actions involving endurance, patience, and resilience are critical-ly important for coping and healing, little is known about their interactional character.

NOTES

1. Within the next two minutes, following dad's reference to mom's condition "deteriorating", a humorous shift to mom's hair, and later dogs, is initiated—both lighthearted exchanges that are eventually extended by more good news. Below, son announces news that he had "one nice thing happen." Following dad's response, he elaborates that he'd received an invitation to a dinner he had last night:

   SDCL: Malignancy #37:4

   1 → Son: [heh heh heh .h hah] .hh Well had one nice thing happen.
   2   Dad: What's that?
   3 → Son: I got another <u>dinner</u> invitation and I- I went to <u>dinner</u> last
   4   night.
   5   Dad: O:hh.
   6   Son: Some- some <u>fellow</u> that- uh is in the office across the hall from me. (continues)

2. Schegloff's (1998) analysis of "word repeats at turn endings" reveal a similar resource: Tellers dis-play their entitlement to initiate closure to stories only they are capable of narrating.
3. Like other moments noted throughout the Malignancy corpus, "hang/hanging" seem poetic in this sense: That in the midst of mom's uncertain yet anticipated dying and the inherent problems of arranging son's travel to be with mom and family, son and aunt are suspended and dangling in doubt. Pushed further, aunt's "I:'m hanging." could be taken even more literally—i.e., as with "at the end of a noose." Of course, neither son nor aunt display awareness of these deeper (possible) preoccupations where their language is precisely tailored, in parallel but meaningful fashion, to the very circumstances they face together.
4. Extending the discussion of figurative expressions described in Chapter 7, the phrase "°Beats the hell out of me.°" may be added to the collection of idioms as Drew and Holt (1988, 1998) have analyzed them (e.g., "it's gone tuh pot", "down the tubes"). Mom's utterance clearly occurs in a sequential environment involving "complainable matters" (i.e., a serious cancer diagnosis). However, this interactional moment is unique in this sense: whereas Drew and Holt (1988) have shown that such complainable matters are routinely directed to others' treatments of them, here mom's utterance is not treating her son as the source of the trouble, but rather the illness she is enduring, including potentially dreaded consequences that can neither be fully controlled nor pre-dicted.
5. Viewing "hell" as a domain of dark forces, the opposite of heaven, it is seen how invoking the deity can occur in negative, troubling moments as well as positive, hopeful orientations to present circumstances.

6. Although it may appear that "fixing cars together" is of little relevance to understanding the interactional management of cancer predicaments, quite the contrary is the case. It is revealing to examine just what everyday topics find their way into the midst of "cancer topics" and how and when they appear and are terminated. For example, in this instance of "fixing cars together", is it coincidental that dad and son talk together about something they are both knowledgeable about—that they can thus (with some confidence) diagnose together—in stark contrast to technical matters of cancer diagnosis and treatment (see also the family interview in Chapter 15)? Ongoing analysis of a larger collection of "car stories", not included in this volume, suggests otherwise.

7. The exceptions, noted repeatedly throughout prior chapters, are moments when speakers invoke "deities" unintendedly, spontaneously, and thus without awareness that uttering "Jesus", "Holy Christ", "geez", and the like routinely occur in environments of trouble over which speakers have minimal control.

VI

PAST, PRESENT, AND FUTURE PERSPECTIVES

14

EPILOGUE

Journeying Through Cancer Interactionally

A broad horizon of possibilities now exists for ongoing empirical investigations of families talking through cancer, as well as innovative educational applications designed to address how family members navigate their way through circumstances defining cancer journeys. So too can the "Malignancy" materials be further integrated with collections drawn from diverse ordinary conversations and institutional interactions, as research continues to dis-cover discover distinctive and fundamental patterns of human social existence.

Though previous chapters have examined only a sampling of one family's phone calls, it should by now be clear just how rich and revealing such interactions can be about the omnipresence and critical importance of communication in everyday family life. This is particularly the case when illnesses such as cancer are encountered, varying crises emerge, and routine orientations get established through key social activities. Previous chapters have examined the organization of a wide range of defining moments, including: updating and assessing news, being stoic, claiming epistemic knowledge, reporting and responding to ongoing troubles, making the case for airline compassion fares, monitoring and resolving ambiguities about mom's stability, displaying frustration, maintaining a "state of readiness," referring to and evaluating doctors and medical care, producing "lay" diagnoses of biomedical information, sharing commiserative space, telling and retelling stories, being humorous and playful together, and constructing hope as an alternative to despair. Though routine, until now these involvements have remained largely taken for granted as the kinds of interactional involvements arising throughout family cancer journeys. With recordings and transcriptions of such naturally occurring events, it becomes possible to identify the organizing features of whatever moments family members collaborate in producing.

EXTENDING RESEARCH ON FAMILIES, COMMUNICATION, AND CANCER

Now that a preliminary empirical foundation exists for understanding how a single family communicates about and through cancer, there are several obvious next moves that can be initiated. Most importantly, analysis can be extended to more diverse families, experiencing varying kinds of cancer and phases of illness. A broader sampling of ethnic, demographic, socioeconomic, and spiritual backgrounds can yield distinct similarities and differences as family members communicate with one another and care providers. The communicative challenges inherent in managing varying cancer diagnoses, coping with treatment modalities, enacting strategies for survival, and maintaining quality of life can be identified and compared as practical, interactional achievements.

Cancer is not restricted to particular settings. Because the routine cycle of daily family life requires mobility in and out of different relationships and settings, efforts should be made to track these encounters and determine their interdependence and communication significance. Systematic attempts can be made to generate understandings of how family members communicate about cancer in home, clinical, work, and related environments. Research has a tendency to artificially separate the contexts shaped in and through human interaction—what Drew (2002, 2003) refers to as "membranes" across diverse personal and institutional interactions—and by so doing, only partial glimpses of the interwoven fabric of everyday social life get generated. For example, previous chapters have begun to examine how family members report on what doctors have informed them and how family members hold concerns only doctors can address. But what might be learned if it could be shown that in meaningful ways, family members' talk at home (including phone calls) shapes how they structure their problem presentations during subsequent medical encounters? How do different family members actually participate in these medical interviews and attempt to raise concerns addressed out of the clinic? And when attempting to describe their lives at home—their lifeworld and psychosocial experiences anchored in family life and their lay diagnoses of biomedical aspects of cancer—how do care providers respond to different family members' concerns (e.g., see Beach, 2009)? These are only a sampling of the kinds of questions that could be addressed if communication activities could be collected and examined across the social settings families navigate in and out of, cross-situational and relational networks within which cancer is discussed over extended periods of time.

These kinds of possibilities require, of course, that ongoing emphasis be given to the collection and analysis not only of longitudinal data, but the formation of interdisciplinary research teams that can devise ways to creatively utilize alternative methods (including ethnographic field work, interviews, audio recordings of phone calls, video recordings of face-to-face interactions, transcriptions, document analysis, and self-reports such as surveys, questionnaires, diaries, and related techniques for gathering information). Fundamental questions about family members' experiences could be developed and tested to better determine how such activities are socially constructed through interaction, and how these encounters impact the management of cancer and family relationships in social life.

To my knowledge, the best exemplar of such an interdisciplinary approach is UCLA's Center on the Everyday Lives of Families (CELF).[1] Their concerted focus rests with documenting and discovering how working parents and their children encounter and attempt to resolve diverse challenges inherent to the simultaneous existence of work, school, and family life. The innovation of this long-term project rests with the ability to bring together diverse researchers addressing, each in their own way, the fundamental details of ordinary family life. Routine activities, such as making dinner and doing homework, reveal key insights about the kinds of problems inherent in the fast-paced, multitasking, short-on-time lives experienced and enacted by family members.

What CELF has created is an innovative and viable model for drawing close attention to otherwise taken-for-granted activities comprising daily family life. How might such a "centered" approach be adapted to the systematic investigation of cancer and other major illnesses (e.g., heart disease, diabetes, or Alzheimer's Disease)? Perhaps even more elemental, how is "stress" manifest in and through daily interactions comprising family relationships? What impacts do "stressful" communicative environments have on sickness and healing? These are monumental yet basic questions awaiting systematic investigation.

It is already clear, however, that the possibility and need for creating interdisciplinary centers, designed for the explicit purpose of studying and working toward resolving major social and wellness problems, also creates a paradoxical reminder: The complexity of social life—a thick, dense tapestry of collaboratively achieved activities—can only be dissected when taking "the ordinary" seriously. And through context-stripping methods, the historical tendency has been to initiate investigations that either ignore "the ordinary" on its own merits, or inadequately sample from the rich and cyclic texture of everyday existence.[2]

IMPLICATIONS FOR SELECTED FINDINGS

In the Introduction to this volume, the phone calls examined herein were described as both ordinary yet extraordinary, unique and universal in scope and application. As summarized in Chapter 2, both context sensitive and context-free operations shape conversational organization. Family members were shown to organize their talk in interaction as sensitive displays to specific and unfolding (i.e., local) moments. Attention can now be given to whether and how these particular kinds of social actions generalize across more diverse speakers, topics, activities, and cultures. Just as close examination of one set of family interactions gives rise to noticing how numerous conversational practices are recurrently employed by those family members, work remains to determine how other speakers, in diverse circumstances, organize their interactions. Though each chapter identified many viable candidates for continued empirical investigation, only five are discussed below: epistemic rights, figurative expressions, invoking deities, references to "they," and intoned "okays."

Claiming and Defending 'Epistemic Rights'

It has been show that (and how) family members are constantly involved in claiming and defending their epistemic rights to know and act upon what they assert to be the most updated news, best decisions, and reasonable ways to progress through mom's cancer (both in her treatment and staying together as a family). These territorial matters occur not only despite the presence of cancer, but as a worked-out remedy for actually navigating through the need to be accurate, informed, and responsible for mom's ongoing care. Family members caring for loved ones understandably desire and act upon what is "right" (at least for them) and construct their opinions and positions accordingly. Although such epistemic actions may indeed cause their own troubles—the family is, after all, the primary social and political institution—they also provide opportunities for families to establish intersubjective agreement on emerging and contingent matters (e.g., dad's ability to report what the doctors had told him, mom's disclosing a six-month to five year time-frame for her prognosis, mom's choice for no life support, son's decision to visit mom "now" rather than attend her memorial service, son and aunt's asserting of their rights as primary and consequential family members impacted by mom's cancer). Familial roles and hierarchies are constantly being reachieved by negotiating who knows what, and best, about matters impacting family life. By claiming and responding to authoritative knowledge (i.e., deferring and/or re-asserting one's own rights), the course and trajectory of a family cancer journey gets shaped moment by moment. To do otherwise would be tantamount to behaving passively, as though no influence or control can be imposed on the runaway train of cancer.

Employing Figurative Expressions

When examining how family members worked together to maintain emergency preparedness, and a chronic sense of urgency tied to mom's imminent yet unpredictable death, figurative expressions (or figures of speech) were one primary resource for organizing these interactions. These included repeated references to activities such as "keeping one's bags packed," "lesson plans current," "lists up to date," and "staying by the phone." Twenty-six of these expressions were analyzed to reveal the interactional work involved in achieving readiness, resolve, and references to cancer impacts. This collection of moments unequivocally supports extensive prior research on sequential environments involving topical transition and closure, but also extends understandings of speakers' diverse methods for organizing moments involving disagreement, disaffiliation, and lack of alignment. That such troubles occur in the midst of managing delicate moments involving cancer reveals how the trials and tribulations of a family cancer journey are comprised of interactional remedies for uncertainty, flux, urgency, and hope.

Invoking Deities

In environments of troubles over which there is apparently little control, family members repeatedly invoked deities and their derivatives (e.g., God, gosh, gol, Jesus Christ, gee, geez). Speakers were no doubt unaware of these usages as deity-invoking. The utterances examined are not designed to be literally prayerful as with, for example, "Oh my God" or "Jesus Christ." Throughout the "Malignancy" phone calls, there are no obvious indications that this family held strong religious or spiritual convictions that triggered such words, derivatives, and actions. But is it just a coincidence that deities get invoked in trying circumstances? And how might these kinds of moments contrast with other types of acknowledgments (e.g., surprise), response cries, and expressions? An earlier manuscript (see Beach, 2000a) can now be revised by relying on the diversity of these "Malignancy" instances, as well as a broader collection of ordinary conversations, to distinguish particular sequential environments in which speakers do or do not invoke various deities.

Who Are "They"?

Family members frequently referred to medical experts as "they/they're/they've," anonymous yet known others playing important roles in mom's care. By noticing these kinds of moments throughout the phone calls, a related inquiry was initiated that extended (but did not yet rely on) these family cancer materials (see Beach, 2006). Understood as a prerequisite for social organization, numerous speakers' "they" references are examined from a collection of several hundred casual/ordinary conversations and institutional interactions (e.g., during counseling, therapy, 911, and legal encounters). It has been discovered, for example, that there are interactional consequences for speakers relying on "they" yet producing vague or absent references to others: Recipients/next speakers will not allow interaction to proceed until who is being referenced, and his/her relevance to particular occasions of ongoing talk, are sufficiently clarified. Basic sequential positions are identified within which speakers rely on "they": within same turn/utterance following antecedent referent, following minimal response (or transitional relevant pause), and as next speaker responds to referent in prior utterance. Instances involving simple and more implied (or marked) references are examined across these three primary positions. Attention is then drawn to how speakers deploy "they" to differentiate between singular and plural references, manage ambiguities, and shift foci (and meanings) within and across speakers' utterances. One upshot of this investigation suggests that despite the tendency for "indexical" or "deictic" expressions to remain resistant to inquiry, speakers routinely and systematically rely on 'they' as an efficient resource for unambiguously linking prior referents, and thus for promoting coherence and understanding in social interaction.

Incongruous "Okay" Usages

In prior chapters, various interactional environments were identified where speakers prosodically rely on "okays"—for example, "O::ka:::y?" or "↑Ok:a::y."—to display that something is "not okay," that is, that some prior actions are heard and understood to be somehow incongruous with "okay producers'" position toward those actions. These moments have become integrated into a large collection of instances that I have characterized with a rather crude and catch-all categorical description: "prosodically marked" and other "odd" instances (see Beach, 2002b). Upon closer inspection, however, it is apparent that by deploying vocal prolongation and stretching, emphasis, volume, and intonational contour—and by simply repeating "okays," prosodically or not—stances are enacted that treat prior actions discrepantly and incongruously, as perplexing, inappropriate, or even as grounds for mistrust and incredulity. A combination of one or more of four displayed orientations, in diverse interactional environments, seem to be apparent: (a) Treating some prior action as curious, odd, or strange; (b) in the midst of, and thus accomplice to, taking an alternative and perhaps adversarial position; (c) Being imposed upon to comply with anothers' requests or commands, and/or reluctantly "giving in" to another's wishes; and (d) At times, quite proactively, in shift-implicative ways, en route to moving to closing troubling topics, and thus to next-positioned matters and "agendas," which may briefly acknowledge yet nevertheless ignore others' expressed concerns.

TOWARD MEANINGFUL EDUCATIONAL INTERVENTIONS

Family members facing cancer must manage ongoing interactional predicaments. These problems require communication to make choices and initiate actions, designed to coordinate the needs and concerns of not only cancer patients, but also all involved in the journey. For brief and extended periods of time, there is little or no "time-out" for those journeying through cancer. The simultaneous coordination of changing health conditions, diverse relationships, and other demanding obligations (e.g., work, finances, and remaining healthy) only begin to exemplify the concerted efforts involved in working through cancer diagnosis, treatment, and prognosis (e.g., see O'Hair, Kreps, & Sparks, 2007). Whether caught up in a whirlwind of tumultuous events or humorously playing together, such pragmatic actions are often characterized as "getting by," "hanging in there," "coping," and "doing the best you can" to deal with whatever situations must be addressed (e.g., shifting bad news, urgent but ambiguous travel, figuring out how to best care for mom at home, or waiting to speak next with the doctor).

For these reasons and more, family members have limited time, energy, or resources for reflexively making sense of what they are doing or how they are doing it together as a family. Cancer patients and families are coping on a daily basis with cancer, and thus are typically not in a position to understand the communicative journey they are undertaking. It is therefore not surprising that family members, as well as care providers and other medical experts—all embroiled in the events themselves—remain largely unaware of the very actions and patterns they collaborate in producing. The time, effort, materials, and guidance required to generate alternative orientations to communicating about cancer (including the providing of cancer care) have not been readily available.

But with the "Malignancy" phone calls as resources for ongoing education and care, it is possible to more closely examine actual events made available only through recordings and transcriptions of real-time interactions. Although family support groups and counseling may provide important opportunities to share and commiserate about cancer experiences, knowledge about actual communication patterns and practices could become an additional and valuable resource for better understanding and managing often troubling illness predicaments. Similarly, doctors and medical staff could benefit by grounded understandings of how patients and family members comprehend what they informed them within the clinic, including what positive and/or negative impacts such informings might have on the daily lives of lay persons. Typically, from the time patients leave the clinic and return for a scheduled appointment, doctors do not have access to patients' lives. Knowing what and how talk about cancer gets done, practically and over time by family members, may well promote renewed appreciation for communication in home environments. This information could enhance providers' sensitivities about the lived experiences of patients and family members, thus giving rise to communication techniques tailored toward patient and family-centered discussions during clinical interviews.

Triggered Enactments of Everyday Cancer Experiences

As this volume is completed, and in response to the encouragement from many individuals impacted directly by cancer (including patients, family members, cancer professionals, medical educators and administrators), we are beginning to consider how basic empirical findings might be disseminated through innovative instructional modalities.[3]

One such modality is assessing how the "Malignancy" materials might be employed to actively engage learners in hearing and responding to actual phone calls and transcriptions. It has become evident across classroom environments, research conferences, and community events in which the "Malignancy" calls have been played and inspected that these materials trigger spontaneous and chained stories, produced by participants, about their own (and others') cancer experiences. These reactions are anchored in their own daily lived experiences and are deeply imbued with personalized and meaningful memories of notable family and illness events (e.g., a son disclosing a story of how he spoke with his mom about her cancer diagnosis; a mom, who is a cancer survivor, explaining how difficult it was to talk with her children about a potentially serious cancer diagnosis; stories about participants' caregiving experiences and relationships with their cancer doctors). These narratives often promote discussions about contrasting perspectives and raise key questions about alternative orientations to communicating and coping with cancer across families, settings, and cultures (e.g., see Kreps & Kunimoto, 1994). Throughout these interactions, routinely taken-for-granted features of daily family life, and the role of communication when managing cancer, become explicit topics available for further discussion and reflection.

The details in patients' and family members' triggered stories are rich in texture and extremely pragmatic. Much can be learned about communication and cancer by analyzing reactions to hearing the "Malignancy" phone calls, as well as reading the transcriptions and research reports. Varied topics arising from these discussions can be incorporated as essential elements in the learning process. By integrating these rich and diverse narratives about real-life cancer events, unique opportunities could arise for facilitators to link these narratives and discussions with key learning priorities (and expected outcomes) related to specific domains (e.g., not taking for granted the importance of ordinary communication activities, generating alternative ways of talking about what doctors have told them, working to support family members' needs, talking through grieving, resolving conflicts, and recognizing the availability of different "hopeful" resources for managing difficult events).

Throughout any emerging curricula, workshops, and learning activities prescriptions about communication comprising cancer journeys (i.e., how activities should be organized) will be minimized. Rather, emphasis would be given to making available rich descriptions of family communication activities, soliciting hearers'/readers' reactions, and channeling their responses toward enhanced appreciation and viable alternatives for organizing and addressing the trials and tribulations of their unique family cancer journeys.

Learning modules could be developed from and anchored within selections of digitized audio recordings of family phone calls. As noted, accompanying transcriptions of these phone calls would compliment these recordings, providing a visual representation of ordinary conversations between family members, and curricula materials could be generated from chapters in this volume. In addition to playing audio recordings to initiate the learning sequence, it has also been recommended that dramatizations, re-enactments, and oral performances (that is, having participants read and role-play selected excerpts from the Malignancy corpus) could also be employed as launching points for instruction. Video recordings of these discussions and performances, available for repeated viewing, can supplement learning—yet additional triggers for elaborated discussions about real-life events.

Theatrical Production as an Educational Resource

In 2002, I directed a master's thesis by Lanie Lockwood (2002), who began to explore the possibility of adapting the "Malignancy" transcriptions into a theatrical performance. Over the years, the considerable dramatic potential of these phone calls had been discussed with many colleagues,[4] and the thesis provided an opportunity to begin the long process of adapting these materials into a workable script. From 2005-2006, collaborations with theatre professionals extended these efforts,[5] resulting in staged workshop readings and, eventually, a more developed theatrical production at an exploratory theatre on campus.[6] Across all performances, it was an explicit understanding that no dialogue would be added that was not initially uttered during family members' actual phone conversations. To date, more than 1,000 individuals have seen these readings and performances. Based on the written and verbal comments from diverse audience members and responses across the community, this new theatrical genre has already touched many peoples' lives.

Either live or recorded performances of some future production, focusing on "conversations about cancer," could also be integrated into the curricula (only sketched above). Following live performances, we conducted "talk back" sessions allowing audience members to respond and ask questions about the production. This format allowed for additional insights to be generated about ways these family phone calls are similar to, and different from, their own and others' experiences with cancer. Taken as a whole, these sessions added significantly by providing unique opportunities for diverse individuals to engage others in discussion (and at times, constructive debate) about communication and cancer.

ENVISIONING THE FUTURE

The "Malignancy" materials hold considerable potential for positively influencing attention given to communication, families, and cancer. Is it possible to affect change by promoting more effective, compassionate, and supportive interactions throughout cancer journeys? What criteria will be employed to make these assessments? Can conversation analytic findings (and materials) be effectively transformed into meaningful educational interventions for cancer patients, family members, and medical experts? At this early stage, it is premature (and perhaps even presumptuous) to assume that any such interventions might make substantive and positive differences in the daily lives of diverse populations of individuals and groups somehow involved with cancer. At the very least, such an undertaking is sufficiently tenuous to proceed with caution and careful planning.

Given the very nature of family interactions examined in this volume, however, it may well be shortsighted to not envision and pursue innovative educational programs. The possibilities for meaningful translation of basic research findings into grounded strategies for better understanding communication and cancer in everyday life are too heuristic to ignore. Any efforts to foster mutual influence between lay and professional communities intent on healing the adverse effects of cancer should be enthusiastically pursued. It would be wise to not forget that all major paradigm shifts occur on the periphery of disciplines. Meaningful dialogue among community members, communication researchers, and cancer and health professionals represent only one historical example of where alliances should be formed. It takes many gifts to accomplish goals that, by definition, could not be achieved in isolation. Ultimately, the successes and failures of any attempted interventions will become evident through careful program evaluations. Any necessary adjustments can be made as time passes.

Though the future is inherently uncertain, as with families facing cancer, plentiful resources exist for remaining hopeful that the matters addressed in this volume will not die on the vine.

NOTES

1. Directed by Elinor Ochs in UCLA's Department of Anthropology, CELF is funded by the Alfred P. Sloan Foundation (http://www.celf.ucla.edu/). Several years ago, when CELF was in its early formation, I was invited to present a colloquium on the emerging work on these family phone calls. One discussion that arose involved how phone calls (not collected in the CELF project) provide insights about family life not captured through fieldwork or video recordings of family interactions. Similarly, this volume focuses only on phone calls and not copresent interactions in family homes. Though an extensive undertaking, the integration of phone calls with ethnographic fieldwork and digital video recordings would provide an even more encompassing framework for understanding families and their daily challenges, including the trials and tribulations of health and illness.
2. I recall, for example, the ways a documentary filmmaker described how the film he was using captured 24 frames per second. Subsequent discussion led to how easy it was to examine only single or limited frames—snapshots of everyday life—that, however revealing, provided only frozen and myopic images of fluid, dynamic, and well-orchestrated social activities.
3. Initial efforts have involved working with David Dunning at the University of Nebraska Medical Center and a variety of health and education professionals who foresee a considerable need to integrate communication research into ongoing medical curricula.
4. Prominent among them was Robert Hopper (deceased, University of Texas, Austin), who had been involved in developing what came to be entitled Everyday Language Performances (ELP). In collaboration with colleagues and graduate students (e.g., Paul Gray, Nathan Stuckey, and Phil Glenn), Robert had students read and "perform" transcriptions of naturally occurring interactions to sensitize them to the details of ordinary conversations. Actual public performances also occurred, both in Texas and at Southern Illinois University.
5. Most notable among these theatre professionals were Patricia Loughery, Carla Nell, and Marybeth Bielawski-DeLeo. Various individuals associated with SDSU's School of Theatre, Television, and Film also contributed in significant ways.
6. Generous on-campus support has been provided by SDSU's President's Leadership Fund, the Fund for Excellence within the College of Professional Studies and Fine Arts, and a Research, Scholarship, and Creativity Award. Generous support has also been provided by funding from the Arthur and Rise Johnson Foundation, and the Sallah Hassein family, allowing for continued development and application of these important materials.

15

RETROSPECTIVE INTERVIEW WITH FAMILY MEMBERS

Eighteen Years Following Diagnosis

The interview below was conducted with son, dad, and aunt—three of the primary family members participating in the original corpus of the "Malignancy" family phone calls. This discussion also occurred on the telephone, but as a conference call that was digitally recorded. A subsequent and simplified transcription was produced. The following excerpts have been edited from the longer interview (2:13:02 in length). Deleted material within, and between, turns at talk is denoted with '…'. To facilitate ease of reading most repeats and repairs, dysfluencies, laughter, and words such as "um", uh", and "you know" have also been removed from this edited version.

The chronology of the interview, that is, its emergence from beginning to end, has not been altered apart from certain excerpts ('…') not presented in the transcript below. Within the transcription, I have provided topic headings of primary themes addressed. It is hoped that these headings will aid readers in understanding what matters were discussed as the interview unfolded.

One final comment. A decision was made to not analyze the interview, for example, by comparing what family members reported with actual recorded moments examined in previous chapters. Though a close reading of the interview provides numerous possibilities for such contrasts and overlaps (e.g., when reporting key events analyzed in previous chapters, or alternative styles for managing mom's cancer, and thus the inherent epistemic nature of family relationships), the primary purpose for conducting the interview was not analytic in nature. Rather, this volume draws to a close with family members' retrospective understandings, in their own words, to gain a fuller appreciation for an alternative set of perspectives on *their* cancer journey.

THE FAMILY INTERVIEW

1 <u>**Making Sense of 1988-1989**</u>
2 WB: In September of 1988, that's now over eighteen years ago, your mom, wife,
3   and sister was diagnosed with cancer. Thirteen months later, in November
4   of 1989, she died. How do you now make sense of that period of time in your lives?
5   …

6   Aunt: I don't know if you can ever make sense of it. I think you just live through
7   it.
8   ...
9   Dad: She went through the original cancer surgery at age twenty-five, went
10   back through it again at age thirty...So it was just kind of an ongoing
11   thing. And in eighty-eight, when we hit that diagnosis, ya think well,
12   okay, here we go again. But the finality of it was not apparent to me at
13   that point...we've beaten this at least two or three times already...it's just
14   another iteration of going through that. And then as it begins to slide
15   downhill, you start to think oh my goodness, now what? And it's just a
16   long slide...it is almost insidious until it overtakes you. And then you just,
17   all of a sudden, get to the end and ya think how the hell did I get here
18   without noticing? And you think oh shit. But eighty-eight was to me just
19   another milestone...not anymore or less than the earlier ones had been. So
20   I guess, you know that I guess-
21 Son: You almost want to be using the same mental template you used the
22   other times.
23 Dad: Sure, if those work.
24 Son: Without necessarily knowing that this was going to be-...Once you've been
25   told somebody's gonna die, and they don't, the next time you're told
26   they're gonna die you don't necessarily think about it the same way I
27   guess...And so it was just a monumental complication in the midst of a
28   number of other truly monumental complications. One of which was the
29   inevitable demise of my first marriage, and then the fact that I was in
30   graduate school...in my last term, as I recall, and getting ready to move to
31   Texas.
32 WB: Aunt, what do you think, in retrospect?
33 Aunt: Well I come from a unique perspective because I was raised with this
34   woman. And having watched her with her illnesses all my- all my life, my entire life,
35   I knew the history of her particular thyroid cancer. I knew
36   what it did, where it came from, why it was there. And knew that she had
37   healed well after whatever occurred...This time, she had dental implants,
38   and they went awry. Now I had worked for an oral surgeon, and I looked
39   into this, and I realized that this had to be something else. When we all
40   managed to get this diagnosis, I had a I- I don't know, an experience—I
41   don't know what other word to use—that said this is different. And I was
42   then in a state of panic the entire time, until she died. Because I always
43   knew that she was going to die, and I couldn't save her.

1   **Different Ways of Handling Mom's Diagnosis**

2   WB: The future is entirely uncertain, and you often don't know what's coming.
3   You're saying that you had a sense of discernment, that you did know
4   what was coming?
5   Aunt: Oh yeah, yes.
6   WB: How did you deal with dad and son, who maybe did not know it was
7   coming?
8   Aunt: Well knowing both of them, and loving both of them...I know their family,
9   I know how they operate, and what they do in tragedy. And I just simply
10   walked around it, and through it. Because you can't- couldn't change it.
11 WB: And what was "it"?
12 Aunt: How they handle things, how- what they do...
13 Son: I think that it is safe to say that my father and I do tend to respond to

14   things like this quite similarly…I think he and I handle adversity very
15   much the same way. But I think it is completely different than the way
16   aunt handles things. And I think they are both legitimate approaches. But
17   sometimes I think some of our challenges…came from clashing
18   paradigms…When you talk about sense making…the way you make
19   sense out of things don't always line up with other people's sense
20   making…it creates difficulty in talking. And I think we went through a
21   few of those over the years.
22 Aunt: …that is how I approached this…this is what we needed to do, and that's
23   what you do.
24 Dad: I suspect aunt did more investigative and intuitive stuff. I tend to be a
25   stoic plotter…I will figure out what I think the target is, and I will just
26   keep grinding until I get there or don't…
27   …
28 Dad: Anyway that is the reality of it…as I said, when I got through the nineteen
29   eighty-eight diagnosis, I thought well, okay, I know the path, been down
30   it several times. I will just keep trotting until things get better again. My
31   mother used to say if everything else fails, emulate the turtle. Just put
32   your head in and go.
33 Aunt: You're talking to two turtles.
34 Dad: Yes. Yes.
35 Aunt: There are two turtles on this conversation.
36 Dad: Yes.
37 WB: And one rabbit?
38 Dad: Probably.
39 WB: Okay.
40   …

1 **Cancer Impacts the Entire Family**
2 WB: It is increasingly known, understood, and accepted that cancer affects not
3   just the patient but, of course, the entire family. Would you agree with
4   this assessment?
5 Aunt: Absolutely.
6 Dad: Oh boy, yes.
7 Aunt: Certainly.
8 Dad: Anybody that cares is involved in some regard. Because I remember her
9   talking about some of the friends that she had, who would now stay at a
10   distance. They wouldn't hug her, they wouldn't touch her. They felt, in
11   some cases, uncomfortable talking to her. And they just kinda went by
12   the wayside, because either they couldn't deal with it, or they wouldn't
13   deal with it for whatever (reason). So the whole unity of people that you
14   have in your life have some effect, and obviously the closer to the patient
15   they are, the more effect it has.
16 Son: So one of the names that very seldom comes up in any of these
17   conversations to this date is- I'll just call her my sister. And it was pretty
18   much right at the point that mom was diagnosed that she disappeared.
19   And for the most part, was almost completely gone. I didn't see her again
20   until the funeral…she said she couldn't handle it and so she just
21   disappeared. Much to my mother's dismay. But-
22 Aunt: And heart break.
23 Son: Yeah. Absolutely.
24   …
25 Dad: My daughter walked out probably two weeks, or there abouts, after the

26   diagnosis. She went out for a hamburger one night and nobody knew

27   where the hell she went until we found her two or three months later.

28   …

29   Dad: …she came back for a "let's see if we can make peace and resolve this"

30   kind of meeting. And they talked for several hours, and she disappeared

31   back into the woodwork again. And the next time anybody saw her was at

32   the memorial service.

33   Aunt: And she came back one more time (dad).

34   Dad: Oh, did she?

35   Aunt: Yeah.

36   Dad: Okay.

37   Aunt: She was there the day that the diagnosis came back, that it was in the

38   brain.

39   Dad: Oh, okay.

40   Aunt: And she did not handle that in any form of okay. And I took her to a bus

41   stop, and that was the last time any of us saw her until the memorial

42   service.

43   …

Physical, Emotional, and Practical Challenges

1

2   WB: What physical, emotional, and practical challenges have you faced?

3   Aunt: Well I- I remember having to deal with hundreds and hundreds of phone

4   calls that went to doctors across the country. I spoke with some of- many

5   cancer patients that had similar or close diagnoses…to try to come up

6   with a direction…And in fact that particular aspect was not only

7   financially very expensive but emotionally expensive, because I often

8   heard you can't do anything. But I did not- my intent was to not quit until

9   there was no way of ever conceding, and I did not. Emotionally, it was an

10   unusual circumstance because it provided me with an insight that I would

11   be the matriarch. I had always been the matriarch, but I was the baby that

12   was the matriarch…My sister was a talented artistic individual. I had

13   absolutely zilch in artistics- I am a business head. And with the diagnosis,

14   and the inevitability of this, I realized that this was the last person on the

15   planet who would remember me. She was there when I was born, and

16   there was no one else left. That was a very difficult concept to wrap my

17   arms around. It frightened me because I didn't know how one handles

18   that, because I've never been that before. And I managed to get my arms

19   around it that- that it was my sibling. This was the closest relative I could

20   ever have…And I was watching her die, and when she was gone, I had no

21   one left that knew me as a child. Kind of an odd place to be.

22   WB: Yes. And at the same time, dad of course was married to her, and son was

23   watching his mom die.

24   Aunt: Absolutely.

25   WB: You all had very intimate, close relationships with her. I think for most

26   families, it's difficult to know who's been impacted the most.

27   Son: Well yes, that is the truth…When you asked the question, my mind went

28   a whole different way. The thing that I struggled with at the time, that I

29   still go back and forth over, is that the timing of this was such that I

30   finished my masters degree and went to Texas to get my PhD. Now Texas

31   is a heck of a long ways away and of course, being a graduate student

32   doesn't pay especially well. And I was putting myself farther away,

33   farther (rather) than closer, at a time when logic would have dictated that

34   I do differently. And I remember actually talking to my mother at length

35   about this. And her persistence in insisting that I go. Her logic was that

36   she spent her whole life trying to have things, to get where I wanted to go,

37   and if right at the end she became the obstacle to my being there she

38   would not be able to forgive herself for it…But they came to Texas, my

39   father and mother, and she came in with a picture frame and she hung it

40   on the wall by the door. And it says in it "A frame of place". She told me

41   that this was going to be for my diploma to go in. And she stuck it on the

42   door- next to the door, so that every day going out I would see it…And

43   incidentally, as I'm speaking, I'm looking at it because I did not put my

44   diploma in it. I searched all over the place to find an identical frame for

45   my diploma, because I kind of like thinking that my mother is always

46   looking over my shoulder. But it- it is still on the wall next to the

47   diplomas. I just remember struggling with whether or not I should try to

48   go forward with my own life or wait.

49 Aunt: Well one of the things that I find most interesting in not only the journey

50   that we took, but the journey that I have watched others take, is that… if

51   you discuss this with each one of the family members, as we are doing

52   today, you will discover, almost with out failure, that each member made

53   their own level of sacrifice for the issue. And one of the things that I know

54   about this family is that we did indeed each make sacrifices for the issue.

55   And I have always said that, and looked at this with great pride. Because

56   I watched my nephew make sacrifices, I watched my brother-in-law make

57   sacrifices. Doesn't matter whether they were large or small. They were

58   sacrifices to them, and they did them willingly. This to me was

59   extraordinary. It was then, and it still is.

60 WB: Dad, what physical, emotional, or practical challenges come to mind, in

61   retrospect, for you?

62   …

63 Dad: Well I- I guess, because I was closer in some ways, some of these

64   memories that jump out at me are- I remember trying to give my wife a

65   bath in the bathtub. And at this point she could barely stand, did not have

66   a lot of strength to help, and she was not tiny. And to pick her up and get

67   her into the bathtub, and wash her, and get her back out and dry her, took

68   probably two hours. I was soaking wet, she was embarrassed. She was

69   pissed beyond anything you can think of. Because the only thing worse

70   for her was when she would go to the restroom and I would have to wipe

71   her bottom. She wanted to kill anybody and everybody. She didn't care

72   who, she was so mortified. The indignity of the whole damn thing just

73   frosted her buns.

74 Aunt: And we-, the father and I, went through that with regularity.

75 Dad: Oh yes.

76 Aunt: And it was very difficult. Toward the end, she needed morphine when

77   (serviced)…rather than taken orally. And I remember one particular time,

78   she came- rose up in the bed, and said "What are you doing?!". And you

79   could see the humiliation. And as I inserted the morphine, I wept

80   copiously. Because there was no option…it had to be done.

81   …

82 WB: To what extent did the hospice facilitate that?

83   …

84 Dad: Go ahead.

85 Aunt: Well, my recollection is that they were kind…they would come in and

86   they wouldn't sit. But the primary responsibilities were between my
87   brother-in-law and me.
88 Dad: Yeah, they did a nice job of informing us of things as they were
89   happening. And as aunt said, they were a help, you know, but you have to
90   realize they're only there a few hours a day.
91 WB: Yes.
92 Dad: So you know that's nice they could come in and- and sponge bathe her. Or
93   they could do things. But one of the...you get hung up in guilt on a lot of
94   things...one of the things I remember is...as her brain tumor progressed,
95   she lost more and more use of the right side. And we were standing...at
96   the kitchen counter, and just talking...You don't stare at someone
97   constantly...so you have to say okay, they gotta have a little space for a
98   little dignity. So I turned, and I don't know what the hell we were talking
99   about, but I looked out the window. And the next thing I hear is crash!
100   And I think oh shit! And she had collapsed on the right side, and had just
101   fallen and hit her head on the...floor. And you think, I can't watch her all
102   the time cuz I'm not fast enough to catch all of this.
103   ...
104 WB: Well I think those experiences are not only humbling, but they are
105   exceedingly common, unfortunately...family members are going through
106   this cancer journey as well, not just the cancer patients. And it does take
107   many people, with many gifts and many resources, to manage the full
108   cancer journey, from diagnosis to death.
109 Aunt: One of the things that the family goes through, that we all went through,
110   was the feeling of helplessness. You knew what the problem was, you
111   could watch it, but you could do nothing. And to stand back and watch
112   her dignity was always a fine line...there was always a fine line.
113   ...

1 Control Over Cancer?: Choices, Suicide, and Being Overwhelmed

2 WB: Well in what ways, then, did you have control?
3 Aunt: I don't believe you ever...it is a controlless, if there is such a word.
4 Son: I think that is one of the things you learn from this, is just how much of a
5   myth having control even is, in the first place.
6 Aunt: Well there are a couple of things that I have learned over my lifetime with
7   these particular events. And one is that I have no control. And one is that
8   there is no closure. I think closure and control are some of the greatest
9   myths in this world. You get past it, but it is never gone. My sister is
10   never gone from me. Never. September comes and I remember her
11   birthday and their anniversary. Christmas comes, and there has never
12   been a Christmas in eighty years, probably, where tears haven't run down
13   my face. Missing those who were so important in my life. So yes, you
14   walk beyond these things, but you don't ever have control of it. It has
15   control of you.
16 WB: And by "it", you mean the cancer or disease?
17 Aunt: The cancer. This kind of tragedy has control of you. It will do what
18   it does. And you are required to stand and watch it. And do the best you
19   can to assist who ever is ill, or dying, or both.
20 WB: Do you believe that there are choices you can make as family members
21   that can help the journey out?
22 Aunt: Such as?
23 WB: Well I guess that's my question to you.
24 Aunt: The choices are, you can do the very best you can to find a cure, to find a

25		solution. That I know I did. I assume my brother-in-law did the same, and
26		if I remember correctly, he did. And then there is suicide...my sister very
27		poignantly asked me to assist her in dying.
28	WB:	Well I know on the recordings, she asked for no life support at one point.
29	Aunt:	Yes, but she was asking me to go further than that. And when she asked
30		me for permission, I couldn't do it. That was probably the most difficult
31		time of my life.
32	WB:	And how far along in her cancer was that?
33	Aunt:	A few days after the diagnosis, and then numerous times throughout the
34		journey.
35	WB:	So- she didn't even want to face the possibility of these kinds of
36		treatments, and the possible hopes that might come from the treatments?
37	Aunt:	Those were fleeting. Those were fleeting.
38	Dad:	That's mostly smoke and mirror stuff.
39	Aunt:	Yes.
40	Dad:	Because my wife and I went through that discussion on several occasions
41		too. And I also did not have the will at all do that. To end her life.
42		...
43	Dad:	You know making peace with that situation was tough...I am more a
44		detail and a lesson and goal person...it becomes a reaction to everything,
45		no matter how minute. Going to the bathroom was a challenge, getting
46		her washed was a challenge. Trying to keep her mind off the ultimate
47		demise was a challenge. Every day is kind of a laborious challenge that
48		you try to work your way through...You hope you're doing the best you
49		can at the time. And yeah, you can look back and say oh my gosh, what I
50		didn't I think to do, what ever in the hell it is. But it's like being in a sand
51		trap where you're sliding. It would be nice to say well hell, if I wouldn't
52		of walked over the edge I wouldn't be here. Except you're so busy
53		scrambling in the sand, I can't even see the edge.
54	Aunt:	That's correct.
55	Dad:	And I would just get overwhelmed...the struggle to just get through every
56		day would wear you out. And in my case to say well, had I fought my
57		way through all of this, I probably could have made her a little more
58		comfortable, a little more whatever in the heck it was at the time. But I
59		don't think like that. And I didn't think like that. And just keeping up
60		with things, keeping the house running, cuz while you're going through
61		this, the world doesn't stop. The plumbing still goes to hell. I had a job to
62		maintain so we could pay the bills. The roof leaks. Things go on-, I mean
63		you have to say wait a minute, I gotta steal an hour out of time between
64		her bath, and her next set of pills, to go fix whatever the next disaster is.
65		And it's just endless.
66		...
67	Aunt:	It is-, it is indeed overwhelming.
68	Dad:	Oh my yes. You would come to the end of the day and you would just
69		collapse. And you would think oh my god I cannot do this, and then you
70		think that I have no choice, I have to do this.
71	Aunt:	There are no options
72	Son:	I think that is where a lot of that guilt comes in. Because to me, those are
73		the things that are for the people that are going to go on living. And so at
74		the end of the day, if the roof leaks, you say what the heck. Except hey, a
75		year from now, I'm still going to be living under the leaky roof, and its
76		going to be a huge problem. So I should fix the roof. And then you think

77   oh how petty that seems, when you contrast that with dying. And then
78   you feel bad for even giving it a moment's thought...you go around and
79   around, and it's this constant struggle to find the point of balance
80   that doesn't exist. And every day, everything changes. So you have to try and
81   reestablish that point of balance. And you fail on every point...You think
82   well, today I stopped the roof leak, but my wife fell over and hit her
83   head in the kitchen. Tomorrow, maybe your wife doesn't fall over and hit her
84   head in the kitchen, but the roof leaks. No matter what.
85 Dad: No matter what...You say wait a minute, you have to have facilities here.
86   I've gotta have plumbing. I've gotta have-
87 Son: Money.
88 Dad: Whatever the hell- yeah...She died on the 22nd of November. That's the
89   same day President Kennedy was shot, just in a different year... The
90   inevitability of it doesn't necessary dawn on you, but it wears on you.
91   And you just- I keep plotting as best I can, and trying to cover all the
92   bases...

1   **The Question of 'Hope'**
2   WB: What did you all turn to for hope?
3   Aunt: I didn't have any.
4   Dad: Yeah, I guess there wasn't any...You're standing up thinking well jeeze, if
5   I wouldn't've walked off- There's no hope out there...I was so busy with
6   the details of taking care of her, and me, and my world around me...I
7   guess didn't even really cross my mind.
8   Aunt: And with me it was taking care of my sister. And trying to figure out how
9   I could be mother to my two children...and 'Mombeck' to my niece and
10   my nephew. And support my brother-in-law in the process. And one of
11   the things that occurred is after her death, I realized that I had been given
12   no time to me, in that length of time, and to this day cannot remember a
13   single thing... because I had given all I could give, and in my own ways, I
14   suppose I was thinking of being Hercules, which no one can do. It
15   affected me very deeply and it took over a year for me to get back to a
16   point where I actually went back on my seat and could think.
17 WB: And Son, was there hope for you throughout this cancer journey?
18 Son: Yes I guess. Here's a place where I'm going to be very different from both
19   dad and aunt. I think at the time I wasn't ready to do it quite so soon. But I
20   think just about every person, when they hit adulthood, it dawns on them
21   that they are going to watch their parents die. So you have sort of a
22   mental template for that. It's in the cultural ethos that this is something
23   that we all go through. So the idea that my mother was going to die was a
24   difficult idea, but I don't think it was the same kind of shock that I saw on
25   both my father and my aunt...But the other differences, remember dad
26   was talking about this started at twenty-five. I grew up in this. I didn't
27   have it happen, I grew up in it. It was always there. I don't ever
28   remember my mother not having this sort of big "C" stamped on her
29   head. And it would go away, and it would come back. I remember the
30   first job I ever talked about having...I wanted to grow up to be...a
31   biological chemist. And I wanted to find a cure for cancer. I remember
32   saying that when I was in the second grade.
33 Aunt: Yes.
34 Son: So it was always there. So you know when you asked the question, I think
35   it was a little different question for me. But the answer is I guess not hope,
36   but...just the ability to get through. My answer was simply the turtle

37   thing, head down. You know, all I gotta do is move one foot in front of
38   me, and then I'm good. And then I'll reassess. And so that's where I'm
39   like my father I think, in that we- what I did was I handled things by
40   focusing on the details that were in front of me, and allowing myself to
41   get lost in them. I won the award that year for best graduate student in the
42   program. So I- I got a publication out that year...I had a good year, cuz it
43   was the one thing I could do. If I sat down at the computer, I could
44   work...
45   Dad: Idling without dwelling.
46   Son: Yeah, the stuff I could actually do, I would do that. And it would just give
47   me a little rest...
48   WB: So it sounds like your mom wouldn't have had anything else happen to
49   you.
50   Son: No she would not have. No...when I suggested the possibility of staying,
51   I won't say she got hostile, that's too harsh. My mother was forceful, and
52   she would simply not hear of it. It would've been just an awful thing if
53   I'd've stayed, because she would've just never forgiven herself, or me, for
54   it. So I guess part of what I wanted to do was make it worth it.
55   WB: Yes.
56   Aunt: When you talk about hope, my lack of hope was in the diagnosis... I was
57   always, always aware that this was likely not going to have a good
58   ending. The difference between the father, and the son, and the aunt is
59   the aunt moves faster and will continue to move faster and faster and
60   faster in order to try to find a solution. Try to figure it out, or make it
61   better, or make it work.

Turtles, Rabbits, and Coping

2   Aunt: And that is the difference between the three of us.
3   Son: That's right, because I go the other way. I slow down.
4   Aunt: Both the father and the son slowed down, and got occupied in something
5   else. Whatever that may be. Primarily woodshop, tools. And I have
6   never been someone that does that. I don't know why, and it doesn't
7   matter why, but I move faster.
8   WB: Well I do know that, at least between the dad and the son in their phone
9   conversations, there was quite a bit of attention paid to cars, to food, and
10   to dogs.
11   Dad: The details.
12   Aunt: Yeah, the details. This is, and I don't say this out of anything other than
13   reality, it is an avoidance. It is a security method. It is, if I don't think
14   about this, it is not going to hurt so bad.
15   Dad: It is a coping mechanism.
16   Aunt: It is, yeah, a coping method. I was trying to come up with that word-
17   Son: The avoidance. I'm not so sure that's its...avoidance. What possible
18   purpose would be served by dwelling on the fact that my mother has
19   cancer, given that absolutely nothing I do will change a thing? Whereas, a
20   little more pepper would make the roast better...
21   Dad: What you can fix, and one you can't.
22   Son: Yeah, so I-
23   Aunt: Cope.
24   ...
25   Aunt: Yeah, the word cope was the one I was trying to find in my little pea brain
26   here. And that is truly how they cope...I don't do that.
27   WB: Well clearly, part of the challenge that is faced by families in their

28   communication is to somehow accommodate alternative styles and
29   approaches to coping.
30 Aunt: I think if you have a close family, and we have had one. I consider my
31   brother-in-law, although he has remarried, he is my brother-in-law. I
32   have no other words for him. And so that remains a close bond.
33 Dad: Same for me
34 Aunt: And I answer for no one else, but I am saying for me, because of who I am.
35   And I am the investigator. I am the one who thinks outside of that little
36   box. How they coped was not surprising to me, nor out of the ordinary.
37   We didn't need communication of how do we do it. I know how they
38   would.
39 Son: And in the grand scheme of things, I'm not sure it was non-functional
40   either. I mean-
41 Aunt: No, not at all.
42 Son: At the end of everything, there were still things pointing forward. I think
43   here is a point of contrast, I guess...aunt's experience with going at it, with
44   the intensity that she did, I would think is probably partly why she
45   doesn't remember the year that follows.
46 Aunt: Exactly.
47 Son: I think they're more like sprinters than marathoners. And so your turtle
48   and rabbit from earlier...And I think that maybe that the family piece of
49   the puzzle that's good, is that even though we often were at odds with
50   each other, in terms of our approaches, I think
51 Aunt: The goals-
52 Son: the combination of those things made us fairly functional. Because we had
53   resources for the minutia, and resources for the emotions, and resources
54   for all the other points as well. And uh I think that was probably
55   something that we didn't appreciate fully at the time. But in retrospect, I
56   think back on it and I think as a group we covered the bases pretty well.
57 Aunt: One of the reasons I was able to go faster and faster, and devote whatever
58   it was I did devote to, was that my beloved late husband was a rock.
59   There were never any questions when I was not home, because it was not
60   uncommon for me to get up at five-thirty or six in the morning to be at my
61   sister's home. And then my brother-in-law would leave for work, and I
62   would be there. And this went on for a long time. And he would come
63   home and I would go home.
64 Dad: The night shift kind of thing
65 Aunt: Pretty much.
66   ...
67 Aunt: My thought process was that it needed to be done, and therefore I would
68   do it. Not out of any other thought process. This is what needed to be
69   done. My husband was extraordinary throughout this, because I would
70   come home and the laundry would be done. You also need to realize we
71   performed a business together during that period of time, my husband
72   and I. And it was a very thriving business, and so that had to be operated
73   also, and two children...But I could not have done this, had it not been for
74   his magnificence and it was nothing short of that.
75 WB: Again, the extended family comes to bat here.
76 Aunt: Well my late husband considered my brother-in-law his brother...This
77   was a family. I moved to California. My sister, and her husband, and their
78   two children followed after, so we wouldn't be separated.
79 Son: It was cheaper than the phone bills and all the plane tickets.

80	Aunt:	Well that's sure true.
81	Dad:	We threw them together, since it was the last of the Mohicans here. So
82		they wanted to be together, and I did have the option to transfer so I did.
83		But one other little point I was going to make...you were talking about we
84		were talking about cars and cooking and other things. One of the coping
85		skills that I think has to be found...is you have to have a few successes
86		along the way of ultimate failure. It tends to preserve your sanity. So if
87		you put a little extra pepper in the roast, and it makes it taste better, that's
88		a success. If the car isn't running right, and you can find an hour to go
89		work on it and it now runs better, that's a success. You have to score a
90		few points here and there.
91	Son:	The word impotence comes up here...
92	Dad:	Yeah, I know, I know.
93	Son:	You do feel so impotent.
94	Aunt:	Yes, we were all impotent.
95	Son:	During this process...I agree.
96	WB:	In the very first call, dad referred to his feelings about what was
97		happening, even right at diagnosis...he felt so "damnably impotent".
98	Aunt:	And that is awful.
99		...

Reflections About Phone Calls

1		
2	WB:	Yeah it is interesting that, uh, in fact I'd like to kinda shift gears here and
3		start back and kinda trace some things through. And I wanna start with
4		the first phone call that was recorded by the son...Dad, I believe the son
5		knew he needed to call home, and he called you, and you delivered to him
6		the news that the tumor was diagnosed malignant. Do you have any
7		recollections about that first phone call?
8	Dad:	Well I am afraid, to be quite honest, I have none...I think some of this stuff
9		gets blurred, and in the beginning, this is eighteen years ago.
10	WB:	Exactly.
11	Dad:	You know I can remember hearing the diagnosis, and it sinks in but it
12		doesn't. And then it sinks in a little more, just the enormity of it gets kind
13		of overwhelming. And as I said, one of my coping abilities was thinking
14		well okay, this is another challenge, we get to try and figure out how in
15		the hell we'll get around this one.
16	WB:	Were you referring to hearing the diagnosis from the doctor?
17	Dad:	Yes.
18	WB:	And was that in the hospital?
19	Dad:	To the best of my recollection, yes. We were- she had gone in for a biopsy.
20	WB:	Yes.
21	Dad:	Of a lung tumor, and they came back and said it was, I don't know, some
22		kind of wheat whatever the heck they called the thing.
23	Son:	Oat cell.
24	Dad:	I'm sorry?
25	Son:	Isn't it oat cell?
26	Dad:	Oh, it could be.
27	Son:	You're saying wheat but you mean-
28	Dad:	It could be wheat or barley or whatever, but anyway, only thing I knew
29		was they said was okay, well you have several pipes and this is one of
30		them, and it is fairly (viral) and a quick one. And I think at that point
31		they said you have about twelve to eighteen months. And I think that part
32		kinda of slipped by in the register of things at the moment. I guess in

33   disbelief or whatever you want to think of it as, I just heard the first part
34   that says okay you have a malignant tumor. And I thought okay this is
35   now number seven or nine or twenty-five, or what ever in the hell it was,
36   and okay we'll deal with this one. And you know...ambling off with a
37   diagnosis in mind...I dropped down into my mode of self alarm. And I
38   say, we go back into caregiving mode and we'll just keep on going.
39 WB: Yes. And son, do you have any recollections of that first call?
40 Son: I can, did it begin with something like "Hola" or "Que Paso"?
41 WB: Hola, como estas.
42 Son: Okay do you want me to tell you where I was standing and what I was
43   wearing? Cuz I can remember it like a photograph. I lived in a little
44   apartment downtown, just off of the park. I was in the
45   bedroom...Actually, that was literally moments after I had just for the first
46   time installed that equipment. I wasn't even sure it was working yet...
47   And as I recall, I was sitting on the edge of a futon.
48   ...
49 WB: Now did you remember, did you anticipate that the news was going to be
50   bad about your mom's cancer diagnosis?
51 Son: Yup. I guess I didn't anticipate this to be, at that point, the beginning of
52   the end. I did expect it to be a poor diagnosis...And mother felt she was
53   really wrong, so it didn't surprise me when it turned out something was
54   really wrong.
55 WB: You and your dad confirmed that in the first call when you said "she's
56   never wrong, is she?"
57 Son: Never once, she never was.
58 Dad: Absolutely.
59 Son: She would know when it would be okay, and when it wouldn't. And she
60   would know when it was not what the doctors thought...She knew her
61   health. Probably, I guess, because it had always been problematic. She
62   was the best monitor and the doctors were not.
63   ...
64 WB: Do you remember any of those phone calls with the airline
65   representatives?
66 Son: Actually now I do. I vaguely remember making a number of phone calls
67   trying to track down plane tickets. I also, as I recall, had to figure out
68   somebody to take care of my dog.
69 WB: Yes.
70 Son: A couple other- I had just started dating a woman...and it seems to me I
71   talked to her in that mix as well...It was a flurry of uh things. I had to get
72   my classes covered.
73 Aunt: One of the arrangements where I had called, and said to you that I would
74   make sure that you go there. You were panicking about when to come.
75   And I said I will make sure, I will call you when you need to come. And I
76   remember making that call, and saying it is time for you to come home.
77   ...
78 WB: Aunt, did you make that call after talking with doctors?
79 Aunt: Oh yes...It was inevitable, it was doomed at that point. Probably a week,
80   we were given, maybe she would last a week.
81 Dad: The hospice people and the doctors at that point.
82 Aunt: And the doctors, yes.
83 WB: ...I think that's a common experience family members have, is trying to
84   figure out when to come and when not, if they're long distance.

85 Aunt: Exactly.

86 Son: The memorial was great for me, but not so good for my mother. I really
87   wanted to be able to be there to see her. So it's really easy to just wait til
88   someone passes away and then say okay, time to go. Since the moment is
89   always a guess, trying to time things was challenging.

90   ...

91 Son: The timing was astonishing. I got there, and I was there for one day. I
92   think she waited. Frankly, I am absolutely certain she waited until I got
93   home. And I went in, and sat down, and said okay I am here. It is okay
94   now. You know that night-

95 Aunt: It was a discussion that actually she and I had. And it was, you need to
96   hang on, your son is on his way.

97 WB: Yes.

98 Aunt: Now, did that actually work? I don't know, but it seemed that it worked.

99 Son: Yeah the timing, it might just be a magnificent coincidence, but I cannot
100   imagine my mother, with the strength of her will, she would have waited
101   if such a thing is possible. That is exactly what she did.

1 **Managing the Roller-Coaster of Cancer**

2 WB: ...At one point you asked your dad, how long? And he said he thought it
3   would be maybe a month. And indeed it was about another four or five
4   weeks before she died...At one point, your dad said to you "even doctors
5   only have educated crystal balls". So there is no way of knowing for sure
6   how long someone is going to live.

7   ...

8 WB: When that flux was occurring—she stabilized, no she's going to go quick,
9   and then she lives longer, but...it is a roller coaster—what would you say
10   to families to manage and cope with that 'living in flux'?

11 Aunt: Hold onto those who are standing next to you. Because that is the way
12   you have to do it. My brother-in-law held on to me, I held on to him.
13   And you just ride through it. There is no solution to it. It is part of this
14   journey. And any death remotely close to it, any other major disease that
15   is going to kill, and you just ride through it. You can't fall, but you can't
16   fix it, you can't change it.

17 WB: It strikes across the grain of the human need to control events, doesn't it?

18 Aunt: There is no control in any of this.

19 Dad: Yeah, it's frustrating from that standpoint. As aunt just said, you have no
20   control. You are just a victim of the circumstance I guess...But you lean on
21   others for moral support. One day one is up, one day the other one is up.
22   You hope somebody is up everyday, to pick up the ones that are down.
23   But the process just goes on until you reach an ultimate conclusion...

24   ...

25 Son: May I jump in here?

26 WB: Yeah, please.

27 Son: ...I have just, of course, gone through this again. When we were getting
28   information from doctors, relevant to my wife, she and I reacted to them
29   very differently. And I guess one of the things that I said to her was, she
30   would get a piece of good news and I wouldn't seem all that happy. And
31   then she would get a piece of bad news and I wouldn't seem all that sad.
32   And she would say what's up? And I would say that I had pretty much
33   learned that all this stuff, you just take with a grain of salt, because it is all
34   just the guess at the moment. And so I learned not to put too much faith,
35   good or bad, in any individual moment, or any individual data point...It

36   sounds really bad today, but tomorrow it might sound better. And it
37   might sound great today, but tomorrow it might sound terrible. And so I-
38   you just sort of try to step back and look at the whole picture, rather than
39   live in these little tiny moments, because that will give you whip lash.
40 WB: What you are suggesting would wear you out quicker.
41 Son: Exhausts you. If you constantly think well today I got a great diagnosis,
42   I'm cured, life is fine, everything is good, and I'm done. But then the next
43   day, when it comes back but oh yeah they forgot to tell you about this
44   other thing, then you set yourself up to fall so much further. And then the
45   same is true in reverse. You hear something and it sounds like a death
46   now, and ou just get down in these horrific pits of despair. And then the
47   next day someone says psych! …And then you feel this kind of, we used
48   the expression the roller coaster before. I think one of the lessons I got
49   from mom was, put all this stuff sort of in a buffer, and just don't ride each
50   individual data point to its extreme, because it makes you dizzy.
51 WB: …Your aunt told you on a phone call that it is similar to a "Russian
52   Roulette".
53 Son: It is.
54 Aunt: Yep.
55   …
56 WB: Living with uncertainty is a normal part of everyday life, and perhaps
57   (especially) in times of chronic or terminal illness, or other tragedies…
58   people don't always live with that amount of uncertainty, with that
59   intensity. But something like cancer can bring that on, especially with a
60   serious diagnosis.
61 Aunt: Well one of the things that I remember is the seemingly countless phone
62   calls from the doctors. And each call, and that's where the Russian
63   Roulette came in, was a life lesson because this call could be good, and the
64   next call would be not good, and they would be constantly back and forth.

1   **Assessing Medical Care**
2   WB: …Let's talk for a moment about doctors and nurses and medical care in
3   general. What memories do you have about things that went well, and
4   didn't go well, in terms of quality care for your mom…and life during that
5   cancer journey?
6   Aunt: Well, one of the problems…is that I have lost all of my family- I've lost
7   most of my family to medical illness. So I have a very difficult time with
8   looking at the medical profession and having any faith in it. My sister's
9   care, the primary doctor, was charming and inept. My sister had full faith
10   in this man, I did not. I was not the decision maker, therefore she
11   continued to go with him. It wasn't until I started losing my delightful
12   temper, and insisting that she do x y and z, that we found some kind of
13   care that was worthwhile. At least I thought it was. But again you walk
14   into this journey and there is truly- the outcome isn't going to be there, not
15   the one you want. And so finding someone, it doesn't matter.
16 WB: What's the relationship then, between a compassionate, caring, personal
17   doctor and someone that is less humane and (even) less technically
18   skilled?
19 Aunt: What you want, what I have learned, is that you want a doctor who is
20   completely passionate, caring, and who does not have all the answers.
21 WB: And is willing to share that with you?
22 Aunt: Oh absolutely…One of the things that I have learned over my life is that…
23   Was that when you have a doctor who doesn't know everything, that's

24		the one you want because that is the one that is going to find the answers.
25		When you have one that is full of them, that knows everything you are
26		signing-
27	Son:	They might get locking into a diagnosis, and you can't unlock them. Then
28		you say, well there is this one other thing. And instead of saying oh well,
29		maybe I was wrong, they say you're just imagining that one other thing.
30		Or it is just an anomaly, just ignore it.
31	Aunt:	One of the things I've learned to do when I locate a doctor, there is this
32		very serious issue that goes on and they don't realize it. I go in and sit
33		down in the examination room. The doctor walks in and says hello, my
34		name, my first name. They are now on a first name basis with me. They
35		do not have the title of doctor. The respect I am expecting is that I have
36		worked very hard for the title of "Mrs.", you're going to treat me the way
37		I treat you. If doctors aren't hesitant, you have a big problem because you
38		can't settle being right about you, and your body, or your family member
39		and how you feel or how they feel. You can't do it. Because their
40		arrogance gets in the way, they know everything.
41	WB:	So in your sister's case, did you eventually find someone you thought you
42		could work with?
43	Aunt:	Yes.
44	WB:	And that was a woman, as I recall.
45	Aunt:	Yes
46	WB:	Okay, and do you remember anything distinctly about the way she
47		handled the cancer as it progressed?
48	Aunt:	Yes, she was very upfront, and very clear. she would call me with
49		regularity and say I don't know. This is what I think we should do. That
50		in itself allowed me to realize that she was on the hunt, if nothing else.
51		She was looking for ways to do this, not assuming she had the only way.
52		And there were times where she would confer with other doctors, saying I
53		don't really know, what do you think?
54	WB:	Well, and again as I said earlier, the comment from one of the recordings
55		was she's only got "an educated crystal ball". So no matter what
56		biomedical education is going to teach, you cannot necessarily predict
57		something like the course of dying of a patient. There's so much that goes
58		into that.
59	Aunt:	Correct. And when the doctor knows that, when they fully understand
60		that in their practice, that is when they become great doctors. We go back
61		to the medical arrogance. When there is medical arrogance, you are at a
62		brick wall. And it has not failed me in my life time.
63		...

Short Sentences...We all Get It

2	WB:	Sometimes, in your talking with each other, you would get- one of you
3		would say "Shit", and the other would say "Yeah I know"...One of you
4		said "Its devastating", I believe aunt that was you, and the son says "It
5		sucks"...Another moment one of you said "Yuck huh", and the response is
6		"You're right, its yuck". So how would you describe those kinds of
7		moments?
8	Aunt:	They are moments of a family who understands short sentences.
9	Son:	Yeah, there really isn't any need to talk about it. You just need to say hey,
10		we all get it. And I think that if ever there's a nice way of just saying hey,
11		we're all in it, this is what the 'it' is. And it's shit, yeah it is.
12	Aunt:	You must remember that the nephew was also the godson. And the

13   brother-in-law has known me since I was ten.
14 WB: Yes.
15 Aunt: So we've already been through all the learning processes to words...
16   And we understand each other when we say hey, this sucks. This is shit.
17   Whatever, we get it. It doesn't need anymore...We understood each other.
18 WB: Yeah, you understood each other. Not a lot of words needed to be said,
19   and sometimes few words are enough.
20 Son: Yeah, I think it would be safe to say at those moments, a whole lot of
21   words would have, in fact, undermined the point.
22 Aunt: Yeah.
23   ...

1   **Comments About Cigarettes, Smoking, and Diagnosis**
2   WB: You told a lot of stories in these phone calls... What is it about cigarettes?
3   Could it have caused her cancer?...(Were you) frustrated that, here she is
4   in part dying of lung cancer, and of other tumors that had spread, but
5   (she is) still smoking? How would you comment on this issue of
6   cigarettes, and your frustration with it?
7   ...
8   WB: Dad, let's start with you. What was your frustration with (her) smoking
9   and use of cigarettes?
10 Dad: Well, I had smoked as a younger man and I had quit, and she never
11   would...
12   ...
13 Dad: It was something to blame for the situation I found myself in. I'm not sure
14   whether they do or don't. I mean obviously, it killed off three Marlboro
15   men now. They tell you right on the package the damn things will kill ya.
16   But I guess I'm of the belief people make decisions, and then are forced to
17   live with the result. If you want to smoke, that's your business. You're
18   the one that ultimately determines what the hell the outcome of that is.
19   And she chose to smoke. She said they kept her weight down, they made
20   her calmer, she liked smoking. And yeah, I resented them cuz they stink
21   and they give me headache. But we're talking about what she wanted, not
22   what necessarily what I wanted...Twenty five, fifty years ago cigarettes
23   killed my father. I'm sure they contributed to my mother-in-law's demise,
24   they contributed probably to my wife's demise...
25   ...
26 WB: Now son and aunt, any quick comments about cigarettes?
27   ...
28 Son: This is always the thing...you're liable to get different answers because
29   the aunt still smokes. You simply have the people who are scared of it,
30   and people who aren't. And clearly, I find the whole notion terrifying.
31   And there's nothing anybody's going to tell me, to this day, that's going to
32   change my mind that I think it was at least contributory.
33 Aunt: Yeah.
34 Son: Was it ultimately- this cancer can be traced back to (earlier) life treatment,
35   when my mother was sick...
36 Aunt: I know exactly what it was.
37 Son: I know, but the idea that all of medical science clearly says it's bad for
38   you. And then you think maybe it is not what caused it. But how likely is
39   it that it made things worse? Could we have gotten five more years out
40   her with out it? Could it have been spotted earlier, treated differently?...
41   And the answers, I don't know, but you know it is an easy target...Like

42   my father said. And whether or not it is a valid target, I think it is an
43   unknown. I don't think you can say it is, I don't think you can say it isn't.
44   Aunt: Well, it unfortunately is indeed an easy target and that was one of the
45   problems with the treatment of your mother. Is that the doctor
46   discovered, in fact the charming ones, knew that she smoked and
47   proceeded to treat her for lung cancer. One of the interns, that was a
48   young man in the hospital, came in and he also picked up the clipboard,
49   looked at all of it. And he was an endocrinologist and he said, oh why
50   haven't they treated her for metastasis from the shot? That was the part of
51   the medical arrogance that sent me into orbit, because I could never get
52   anyone to look at that. And the cancer that she had was absolutely in
53   direct line to where the shot was, where she originally had her thyroid
54   cancer. It was indeed a metastasis. But because she was a smoker, no one
55   would look further. That was the anger that I always had about it. Now
56   could her smoking have contributed? I'm sure it probably did. But it
57   wasn't the end of- it wasn't the original force…I don't mean she was
58   abused…I mean she was mistreated practically.
59   Son: She was treated incorrectly.
60   Aunt: She was treated incorrectly, and that goes back to the medical arrogance.
61   And it wasn't until I finally found the doctor- the woman doctor
62   who would look further, but the problem was it was already too late.

1   **The Importance of Play and Humor**
2   WB: There were a variety of moments…where you were obviously being
3   humorous and playing around.
4   Aunt: We do that a lot.
5   WB: Yes. And what would you say, for cancer patients and family members,
6   even medical experts, about the importance of play and humor?
7   Aunt: It's vital.
8   Dad: Oh yeah.
9   Aunt: It's vital to survival. Not only for the cancer patient but for the family. It
10   brings love and peace to an otherwise debilitating style of life. And you
11   have to have humor. I sit here, hasn't been that long ago since I lost my
12   husband, and I have had humor in that. Yes there's been many, many
13   rivers of tears, but the humor in it is what I've always called kind of a
14   macabre sense of humor…A sadistic little sense of humor…There have
15   been things that I've done, and others will look at and go holy smokes,
16   what's wrong with her? My family, the other two on the other end of the
17   phone, will look at it and say yup, right on…And it is one of my ways of
18   coping, is to use humor, almost a slight of hand.
19   Dad: I think it is a way to break tension.
20   Aunt: Oh yeah.
21   Dad: It isn't an even plane of morbidity, it is a downhill slide. And if you can
22   find some levity, something that gives you a little bit of uplift…
23   …
24   Dad: And you get a lift that says oh, okay, the world was all right at some
25   point, and it will be again. And this moment is only a passage of time…
26   And I think, as one or both of them have said, you got to have some kind
27   of levity to just preserve your sanity. Otherwise, you'll blow your brains
28   out. You'll say to hell with it, this is not going to work.
29   …
30   Son: I remember saying to my mother, at a point during that summer that I
31   was back in California, that it was her birthday coming up in September. I

32   was really kinda tickled with myself for being so clever. Because I was
33   going to get her a one year subscription to a magazine, and tell her it
34   was a life-time subscription. And she's laughing, just laughing at me. And we
35   did stuff like that like. I think it just sort of acknowledges the absurdity
36   and maybe say to it, screw you and the camel you road in on, a little bit.
37 WB: A little bright light in the darkness is never gonna hurt anyone.

1 "The Plaque"
2 Aunt: You have to have that. One of the things that I found very important,
3   and I will read it to you...This was spoken at my sister's memorial and she
4   had a way with these things. This has kept me moving throughout the
5   times she has been gone. It kept me moving at my husband's funeral, and
6   since he's been gone. And I have sent it to every single person I have ever
7   known that survived a death of a family or friend. And it's called "The
8   Plaque: Death is nothing at all. I have only slipped away into the next
9   room. I am I, and you are you. Whatever we were to each other, that we
10   still are. Call me by my old familiar name. Speak to me in the easy way
11   you always used. Put no difference in your tone, with no forced error of
12   polemity or sorrow. Laugh as we always laughed, at the little jokes we
13   enjoyed together. Pray, smile, think of me, pray for me. Let my name be
14   ever the household word that it always was. Let it be spoken, without
15   effect, without the trace of a shadow on it. Life means all that it ever
16   meant. It is the same as it ever was. There is unbroken continuity. Why
17   should I be out of mind, because I am out of sight? I am waiting for you,
18   for an interval. Somewhere there it is, just around the corner. All is
19   well"...I don't know where she found it, I will never know where she
20   found it. But it saved me then, and it has continued to walk with me
21   since.
22   ...

1 Reactions to "Unity is Strength, Knowledge is Power, and Attitude is Everything"
2 WB: I would like to ask a series of questions and bring it to a close.
3 Dad: Okay.
4 WB: Here's one of the questions. As you know, Lance Armstrong was
5   diagnosed with testicular cancer and it moved to his brain. And then, of
6   course, (he) then proceeded to win seven Tour de Frances.
7   ...
8 WB: He now has quite a prolific cancer foundation called the Lance Armstrong
9   Foundation. Their motto for the foundation is as follows. "Unity is
10   strength, knowledge is power, and attitude is everything". How would
11   you respond to that, given your experiences with the mom's cancer?
12 Aunt: Well, for me, unity is strength that is the family I am talking to currently.
13   Knowledge is power is the incredible task here that I tried to do. And
14   what was the last one?
15 WB: Attitude is everything.
16 Son: Sucks doesn't it?
17 Dad: Yeah.
18 Aunt: That's absolutely correct. Attitude is everything. Now (with) attitude,
19   one of the things I want to clearly say is that my dear sister was told many
20   times, by well known people in medicine, in psychology, in wellness
21   communities, etcetera... that if she just had positive attitude, she'd be
22   okay. I don't (think) anybody should ever say that to me, because that
23   sends me currently, and then, into orbit. That means if you feel bad,
24   you're going to die.

25	Dad:	And it's your fault.
26	Aunt:	And it's your fault. That is so wrong to say these things to people.
27		Because it gives them another guilt trip. And when you have been
28		diagnosed with these things, whatever it is, it takes no time at all for the
29		medical profession, or someone, to place guilt within the diagnosis.
30	WB:	How would you frame it in an alternative way then?
31	Aunt:	I don't think I can. Because you can't be positive everyday. You can't be
32		that way. You are in terror for your life.
33	WB:	Well perhaps that is the issue.
34	Son:	Let me jump in and say…to an extent it is going to depend, when they say
35		attitude is everything, the presumption is that we are talking about a very
36		particular attitude.
37	Aunt:	Right.
38	Son:	But I think just to say attitude is everything is correct. I think what is
39		incorrect is to say that you always have to have this artificially happy, up-
40		beat attitude…
41	Aunt:	That is often what is inferred.
42	Son:	Yes, I agree with that. And you just have to smile, and see yourself
43		through it, and everything will be okay. I think what you have to do is
44		recognize that the one thing you do have is attitude. And you do- you
45		have to live with it, with all of that. And everybody's got them, and they
46		change, and they're complicated, and they're messy, and they're in
47		discord with reality sometimes. And that's okay.
48	Aunt:	Well, and you're right. The thing that I take exception to with these
49		attitude things, is that it is too broad. It is too broad. It does infer. (One)
50		question though is who's attitude, and what attitude?
51	Dad:	Well, attitude is not an end all in itself. As far as I am concerned,
52		everybody is at a given point in time and attitude is, should certainly be a
53		contributor. But it depends on where science is, it depends on the
54		individual that's sick. My father's now been dead fifty years. If he'd
55		been around today, the minor problem that killed him could have been
56		fixed in two or three hours. He'd've been home in two days, and science
57		would have fixed him. They couldn't at that time. My wife thinks, given
58		all of the backlog of things that have happened to her, she did have a
59		wonderful attitude. But it is not an end all.
60	Aunt:	Correct.
61	Dad:	Life is terminal. I don't give a damn what we do with it. But in her case
62		she had been beaten down so badly, over so many years, you just literally —
63		attitude is nice, but it isn't the solution to everything. And in Lance
64		Armstrong's case, the power that he has, the opportunity, it is going to be
65		like the Michael J. Fox — it is going to be like the other people that now have
66		a goal they can pursue to help people…Maybe they help a lot of
67		somebodies. But to put the wholeness of your survival on your attitude, I
68		think is a little shortsided.
69	Son:	It is a little sound byte.
70		…
71	Dad:	And for him, marvelous. I wish him well. I hope he lives to two hundred.
72		But you know it is only a piece of the puzzle, and you've got to have the
73		other pieces. Some are luck, some are science, some are more points in
74		time. You know, hell, two hundred years ago, you'd've died of the flu
75		and scurvy and all kinds of things that we've fixed. Now we fix things
76		that cured Lance Armstrong. Two hundred years from now, they'll look

77   back and say what the hell were those damn fools dying for? We could've
78   given them a pill. But you know, that's not where you are in time...
79   Aunt: ...You can't just rely on attitude. I remember too many times, in the time
80   where my sister's diagnosis was just going on and on and on, and her—
81   how many countless people told her to just go home and meditate? And
82   she'd do that. I used to want to pummel them. And the wellness
83   community...that was their whole idea. That it had to be positive, every
84   thing had to be positive. Well that's great, but when you hear that the
85   cancer has metastasized into the brain, you only have a short time to live,
86   how are you going to be positive?
87   ...
88   Son: It seems so disingenuous. You know-
89   Aunt: It is, it is.
91   Son: At some point, this is a bad thing, so to be positive about it is to treat your
92   life fraudulently and unrealistically. And I—attitude of acceptance maybe,
93   but not attitude of oh everything is going to be okay.
94   ...
95   Aunt: She was told to visualize the cancer cells running out of her body.
96   ...

1   **Family Members as Cancer Survivors: Advice for Others' Journeys**
2   WB: One of the observations that can be made of any family that has
3   undergone cancer, is that you three are, each in your own way, cancer
4   survivors.
5   Aunt: Oh yeah.
6   WB: Not of an actual diagnosis, but clearly of a loved one's diagnosis. And the
7   journey through death, and now eighteen years since that death. As a
8   final question, what I would like to ask you (is could) you offer advice for
9   patients, or family members particularly, in terms of particular
10   communication skills for facing cancer as a family?...What comes to mind
11   that you could uh provide to others that may currently be...or will be
12   facing this in the future?
13   Aunt: Well, when it comes to dealing with the medical profession, make sure that
14   they are people who listen and don't know everything...because you need
15   that. When it comes to your family, hang onto them. This is not the time
16   for arguments, nor is it the time for fights. This is the time to hold on with
17   as much strength as you can. Levity is a part of it, and there needs to be
18   moments of being a smart alec.
19   Son: I would add remember the different ways of coping, maybe completely
20   paradoxical, but they're how people cope and you just have to let people
21   cope how they do it.
22   Aunt: Correct.
23   Son: And you also can actually sometimes remember that every approach to
24   problem solving, coping, whatever you want to call it, has good news and
25   bad news. And so learn how to take advantage of the unique strength
26   that each approach can provide you. If you need a detail person, if you
27   need a helicopter person, if you need somebody that can just go ahead
28   and weep, if you need somebody that can have a stiff upper lip. And
29   appreciate the fact that in most families, all those exist somewhere. And
30   instead of wondering why that person over there is always crying, or this
31   person over there doesn't seem to care, or whatever. Those are things that
32   you can draw strength from.
33   Aunt: One of the things that I've learned with the death of my family members

34		is that through all tragedy, there is a lesson to be learned that you cannot
35		have learned any other way. And it will come to you. That's life.
36	Dad:	And I think love, and compassion, and concern. And maybe a little bit of
37		what my son was alluding to was not forgiveness, but acceptance of all
38		the different ways you can move in the same direction. Because basically,
39		you have a patient here that you're all trying to help. And how to get to
40		that point may be varied, but the goal is to do that. Not conflict within
41		each other over minor things that are both counterproductive and hurtful.
42		Picking on each other doesn't solve the problem. If (you) hate the cancer,
43		then fine. But hating each other doesn't do the cancer any harm. So
44		fighting with each other accomplishes nothing. What you are trying to do
45		is get along and work towards the goal. And the other thing that probably
46		you don't think of as much, but after this is all over, you still should get
47		along. You have to say okay, not only to we have to protect each other
48		and help each other now to accomplish what we are attempting to do, but
49		after this is done we still need to get along. And if you waste all your time
50		and energy fighting among yourselves, when this is all said and done, you
51		are still in big trouble.
52	Aunt:	I think the thing that I always remember thinking is that we need to keep
53		circling the wagon and not throwing arrows. And this is—to me that is
54		paramount to any family. The other thing that is paramount to them, is
55		that when it is over, I don't think I've met anybody in my entire life that
56		did not have regret. But you cannot live in regret. Because you did what
57		you knew how to do at the time. And given the same circumstance and
58		the same knowledge, you would do it again. You can't look back and
59		regret I wish I had, whatever that may be.
60	Dad:	It is history at this point.
61	Aunt:	It destroys, it simply—regret simply continues the destruction. And my
62		goal has been to have my sister's name spoken, just as it says in "The
63		Plaque", and to keep her memory alive by making sure I say she was a
64		dummy, or whatever it was I needed to say at the time. I have walked
65		through my home and said where is she, I need her?…And so that levity,
66		that lack of regret. I have regrets, I know my brother-in-law does, I know
67		my nephew does. I have regrets from many things in my life. But I can't
68		fix them. I can only learn from those, and hopefully not do them again.
69	WB:	And son, we'll give the final word to you.
70	Son:	Oh gosh!…If I have the final word, my final word would be that even
71		though we are having a whole conversation about death and dying, and
72		cancer, that's not the final word. And there really isn't a final word. It is
73		something that brings one life to an end in one of its forms. But as my
74		aunt's poem says, it is just a shift in form. I don't go any length of time at
75		all with out thinking of my mother, talking about my mother. My children
76		talk about my mother, and so she just exists in a different form now. And
77		our family is different from how it was then. But what family isn't after
78		eighteen years? So it isn't a final word. It's just a movement to whatever
79		is the next word. And we've moved, as you would of course, with that
80		much time going by. And we've learned from things. And I hope we're
81		still learning from things.

REFERENCES

ABC News (2002). *Getting home soon: Finding the best bereavement fares*. Retrieved July 22, 2002, from http://abcnews.go.com/.

Ackerman, A., & Ackerman, A. (2002). *Our mom has cancer*. American Cancer Society.

Acocella Marchetto, M. (2006). *Cancer vixen: A true story*. New York: Random House.

Addington-Hall, J., & McCarthy, M. (1995). Dying from cancer: Results of a national population-based investigation. *Palliative Medicine, 9*, 295-305.

American Cancer Society (2006). *Cancer facts & figures 2006*. Retrieved January 13, 2006, from http:www.cancer.org.

American Cancer Society (2006). *Cancer facts & figures 2006*. Retrieved May 21, 2006, from http:www.cancer.org.

Arminen, I. (2004). Second stories: On the relevance of interpersonal communication in Alcoholics Anonymous. *Journal of Pragmatics, 36*, 319-347.

Atkinson, J.M. (1984). *Our master's voices: The language and body language of politics*. London: Methuen.

Atkinson, J.M., & Drew, P. (1979). *Order in court: The organisation of verbal interaction in judicial settings*. London: Macmillan.

Atkinson, J.M., & Heritage, J. (Eds.). (1984). *Structures of social action: Studies in conversation analysis*. Cambridge: Cambridge University Press.

Atkinson, P. (1984). Training for certainty. *Social Science & Medicine, 19*, 949-956.

Atkinson, P. (1995). *Medical talk and medical work*. London: Sage.

Babrow, A.S., Hines, S.C., & Kasch, C.R. (2000). Managing uncertainty in illness explanation: An application of problematic integration theory. In B.B. Whaley (Ed.), *Explaining illness: Research, theory, and application* (pp. 41-68). Mahwah, NJ: Erlbaum.

Babrow, A.S., Kasch, C.R., & Ford, L.A. (1998). The many meanings of *uncertainty* in illness: Toward a systematic accounting. *Health Communication, 10*, 1-23.

Babrow, A.S., & Kline, K.N. (2000). From "reducing" to "coping with" uncertainty: Reconceptualizing the central challenge in breast self-exams. *Social Science & Medicine, 51*, 1805-1816.

Baider, L., Cooper, C.L., & De-Nour, A.K. (Eds.). (1986). *Cancer and the family*. New York: Wiley.

Bailey, A.K. (1985). *Interactional patterns in families with breast cancer*. Doctoral dissertation, University of North Texas.

Baker, C., Emmison, M., & Firth, A. (2001). Discovering order in opening sequences in calls to a software helpline. In A. McHoul & M. Rapley (Eds.), *How to analyse talk in institutional settings*. London: Continuum.

Barbour, A. (1995). *Caring for patients: A critique of the medical model*. Stanford: Stanford University Press.

Barnhart, L.L., Fitzpatrick, V.D., Sidell, N.L., Adams, M.J., Gomez, S.J., & Shields, G.S. (1994). Perception of family need in pediatric oncology. *Child and Adolescent Social Work Journal, 11*, 137-149.

Barraclough, J. (1994). *Cancer and emotion: A practical guide to psycho-oncology*. Chichester, England: Wiley.

Bateson, G. (1971). Communication. In N.A. McQuown (Ed.), *The natural history of an interview* (pp. 1-40). Microfilm Collection of Manuscripts on Cultural Anthropology, 15th Series. Chicago: University of Chicago, Joseph Regenstein Library, Department of Photoduplication.

Bateson, G. (1996). Communication. In H. Mokros (Ed.), *Interaction and identity: Information and behavior* (Vol. 5, pp. 45-68). New Brunswick, NJ: Transaction.

Beach, D. (1993). Gerontological caregiving: An analysis of family experience. *Journal of Gerontological Nursing, 19*, 1-7.

Beach, W.A. (1985). Temporal density in courtroom interaction: Constraints on the recovery of past events in legal discourse. *Communication Monographs, 52*, 1-18.

Beach, W.A. (Ed.). (1989). Sequential organization of conversational activities. *Western Journal of Speech Communication, 53*, 85-246.

Beach, W.A. (1990a). Language as and in technology: Facilitating topic organization in a Videotex focus group meeting. In M.J. Medhurst, A. Gonzalez, & T.R. Peterson (Eds.), *Communication and the culture of technology* (pp. 197-220). Pullman: Washington State University Press.

Beach, W.A. (1990b). Orienting to the phenomenon. In J. Anderson (Ed.), *Communication yearbook 13* (pp. 216-244). Beverly Hills, CA: Sage. (Reprinted in *Building communication theories: A socio-cultural approach*, 133-163, by F.L. Casmir, Ed., 1994. Hillsdale, NJ: Erlbaum.

Beach, W.A. (1991). Avoiding ownership for alleged wrongdoings. *Research on Language and Social Interaction, 24*, 1-36.

Beach, W.A. (1993a). The delicacy of preoccupation. *Text and Performance Quarterly, 13*, 299-312.

Beach, W.A. (1993b). Transitional regularities for 'casual' "Okay" usages. *Journal of Pragmatics, 19*, 325-352.

Beach, W.A. (1995a). Conversation analysis: "Okay" as a clue for understanding consequentiality. In S.J. Sigman (Ed.), *The consequentiality of communication* (pp. 121-162). Hillsdale, NJ: Erlbaum.

Beach, W.A. (1995b). Preserving and constraining options: "Okays" and 'official' priorities in medical interviews. In G.H. Morris & R.J. Cheneil (Eds.), *The talk of the clinic: Explorations in the analysis of medical and therapeutic discourse* (pp. 259-289). Hillsdale, NJ: Erlbaum.

Beach, W.A. (1996). *Conversations about illness: Family preoccupations with bulimia*. Mahwah, NJ: Erlbaum.

Beach, W.A. (2000a). *Invoking the deity: Finding "God" in everyday conversation*. Manuscript.

Beach, W.A. (2000b). Inviting collaborations in stories about a woman. *Language in Society, 29*, 379-407.

Beach, W.A. (2001a). Introduction: Diagnosing lay diagnosis. *Text, 21*, 13-18.

Beach, W.A. (2001b). Stability and ambiguity: Managing uncertain moments when updating news about mom's cancer. *Text, 21*, 221-250.

Beach, WA (2002a). Between dad and son: Initiating, delivering, and assimilating bad cancer news. *Health Communication, 14*, 271-299.

Beach, W.A. (2002b). *When "okay" is not okay: Some prosodic displays of incongruity in interaction*. Manuscript.

Beach, W.A. (2002c). *Speaking like the "doctor": How family members report and understand cancer diagnosis and treatment options*. Manuscript.

Beach, W.A. (2003a). Managing optimism. In P. Glenn, C. LeBaron, & J. Mandelbaum (Eds.), *Studies in language and social interaction: In honor of Robert Hopper* (pp. 175-194). Mahwah, NJ: Erlbaum.

Beach, W.A. (2003b). Phone openings, 'gendered' talk, and conversations about illness. In P. Glenn, C. LeBaron, & J. Mandelbaum (Eds.), *Studies in language and social interaction: In honor of Robert Hopper* (pp. 573-587). Mahwah, NJ: Erlbaum.

Beach, W.A. (2003c). *When few words are enough: Assimilating bad news about cancer*. Unpublished manuscript.

Beach, W.A. (2005). Understanding how family members talk through cancer. In B. Whaley & W. Sampter (Eds.), *Advancements in communication theory & research*. Hillsdale, NJ: Erlbaum.

Beach, W.A. (2006). *Who are 'they'?: Speakers' practices for referring to known and unknown others*. Manuscript.

Beach, W.A. (2008). Conversation analysis. In W. Donsbach (Ed.), *The international encyclopedia of communication* (Vol. III, pp. 989-995). London: Blackwell.

Beach, W.A. (Ed.). (2009). *Handbook of patient-provider interactions: Raising and responding to concerns about life, illness, and disease.* Cresskill, NJ: Hampton Press.

Beach, W.A., & Andersen, J. (2003). Communication and cancer: The noticeable absence of interactional research. *Journal of Psychosocial Oncology, 21,* 1-23.

Beach, W.A., & Dixson, C.N. (2001). Revealing moments: Formulating understandings of adverse childhood experiences in a health appraisal interview. *Social Science & Medicine, 52,* 25-44.

Beach, W.A., & Dunning, D.G. (1982). Pre-indexing and conversational organization. *Quarterly Journal of Speech, 68,* 170-185.

Beach, W.A., Easter, D.E., Good, J.S., & Pigeron, E. (2004). Disclosing and responding to cancer "fears"during oncology interviews. *Social Science & Medicine, 60,* 893-910.

Beach, W.A., & Glenn, P. (2009). Inviting gender. In S. Speer & E. Stokoe (Eds.), *Gender and conversation.* Cambridge: Cambridge University Press.

Beach, W.A., & Good, J.S. (2004). Uncertain family trajectories: Interactional consequences of cancer diagnosis, treatment, and prognosis. *Journal of Social and Personal Relationships, 21,* 9-35.

Beach, W.A., & LeBaron, C. (2002). Body disclosures: Attending to personal problems and reported sexual abuse during a medical encounter. *Journal of Communication, 52,* 617-639.

Beach, W.A., & Lockwood, A. (2003). Making the case for airline compassion fares: The serial organization of problem narratives during a family crisis. *Research on Language and Social Interaction, 36,* 351-393.

Beach, W.A., & Mandelbaum, J. (2005). "My mom had a stroke": Understanding how patients raise and providers respond to psychosocial concerns. In L.H. Harter, P.M. Japp, & C.M. Beck (Eds.), *Narratives, health, and healing: Communication theory, research, and practice* (pp. 343-364). Mahwah, NJ: Erlbaum.

Beach, W.A., & Metzger, T.R. (1997). Claiming insufficient knowledge. *Human Communication Research, 23,* 562-588.

Benjamin, H.H. (1987). *From victim to victor: The Wellness Community guide to fighting for recovery for cancer patients and their families.* New York: St. Martin's.

Bennett, M., & Alison, D. (1995). Discussing the diagnosis and prognosis with cancer patients. *Postgraduate Medical Journal, 72,* 25-29.

Bennett, W.L., & Feldman, M.S. (1981). *Reconstructing reality in the courtroom: Justice and judgment in American culture.* New Brunswick, NJ: Rutgers University Press.

Benzein, E., Norber, A., & Saveman, B.I. (2001). The meaning of the lived experience of hope in patients with cancer in palliative home care. *Palliative Care, 15,* 117-126.

Bergman, J. (1992). Veiled morality: Notes on discretion in psychiatry. In P. Drew & J. Heritage (Eds.), *Talk at work: Interaction in institutional settings* (pp. 137-162). Cambridge: Cambridge University Press.

Bergman, J. (1993) *Discreet indiscretions: The social organization of gossip.* New York: Aldine De Gruyter.

Bergman, J., & Linnell, P. (Eds.). (1998). Morality in discourse. Special issue of *Research on Language and Social Interaction, 31*(3/4).

Bertolone, S.J., & Scott, P. (1990). The cancer educator as role model: A means of initiating attitude change. In A. Blitzer et al. (Eds.), *Communicating with cancer patients and their families* (pp. 56-59). Philadelphia, PA: The Charles Press.

Bigel, D.E., Sales, E., & Schulz, R. (1991). *Family caregiving in chronic illness: Alzheimer's disease, cancer, heart disease, mental illness, and stroke.* Newbury Park, CA: Sage.

Blachman, L. (2006). *Another morning: Voices of truth and hope from mothers with cancer.* Emeryville, CA: Seal Press.

Blackhall, L.J., Murphy, S.T., Frank, G., Michel, V., & Azen, S. (1995). Ethnicity and attitudes toward patient autonomy. *The Journal of the American Medical Association, 74,* 820-826.

Blanchard, C.G., Ruckdeschel, J.C., & Albrecht, T.L. (1996). Patient-family communication with physicians. In L. Baider, C.L. Cooper, & A Kaplan De-Nour (Eds.), *Cancer and the family* (pp. 369-387). New York: Wiley.

Blitzer, A., Kutscher, A.H., Klagsbrun, S.C., DeBellis, R., Selder, F.E., Seeland, I.B., & Siegel, M-E. (Eds.). (1990). *Communicating with cancer patients and their families.* Philadelphia, PA: The Charles Press.

Bloom, J.R. (1996). Social support of the cancer patient and the role of the family. In L. Baider, C.L. Cooper, & A. Kaplan De-Nour (Eds.), *Cancer and the family* (pp. 53-70). Chichester, UK: Wiley.

Bloom, J.R. (2000). The role of family support in cancer control. In L. Baider, C.L. Cooper, & A. Kaplan De-Nour (Eds.), *Cancer and the family* (2nd ed., pp. 55-71). Chichester, UK: Wiley.

Bloom, J.R., Kang, S.H., & Romano, P. (1991). Cancer and stress: The effects of social support as a resource. In C.L. Cooper & M. Watson (Eds.), *Cancer and stress: Psychological, biological and coping studies* (pp. 95-124). Chichester, UK: Wiley.

Borneman, T., Stahl, C., Ferrell, B.R., & Smith, D. (2002). The concept of hope in family caregiviers of cancer patients at home. *Journal of Hospice and Palliative Nursing, 4*, 21-33.

Brabner, J., Perkar, H., & Stack, F. (1994). *Our cancer year.* New York: Four Walls Eight Windows.

Broccolo, A. (1997). My father's hands. *The Journal of the American Medical Association, 277*, 1809.

Brookes, T. (1997). *Signs of life: A memoir of dying and discovery.* New York: Times Books.

Brown, P., & Levinson, S.C. (1987). *Politeness.* Cambridge: Cambridge University Press.

Bunston, T., Mings, D., Mackie, A., & Jones, D. (1995). Facilitating hopefulness: The determinants of hope. *Journal of Psychosocial Oncology, 13*, 79-104.

Butow, P.N., Kazemi, J.N., Beeney, L.J., Griffin, A.-M., Dunn, S.M., & Tattersall, M.H.N. (1996). When the diagnosis is cancer: Patient communication experiences and preferences. *Cancer, 77*, 2630-2637.

Buttny, R. (1997). Reported speech in talking race on campus. *Human Communication Research, 23*, 475-504.

Buttny, R. (1998). Putting prior talk into context: Reported speech and the reporting context. *Research on Language and Social Interaction, 31*, 45-58.

Button, G. (1987). Moving out of closings. In G. Button & J.R.E. Lee (Eds.), *Talk and social organization* (pp. 101-151). Clevedon, UK: Multilingual Matters.

Button, G. (1984). Generating topic: The use of topic initial elicitors. In J.M. Atkinson & J. Heritage (Eds.), *Structures of social action: Studies in conversation analysis* (pp. 167-190). Cambridge: Cambridge University Press.

Button, G. (1990). On varieties of closings. In G. Psathas (Ed.), *Interaction competence* (pp. 93-148). Lanham, MD: University Press of America.

Button, G., & Casey, N. (1985). Topic nomination and pursuit. *Human Studies 8*, 3-55.

Button, G., & Casey, N. (1988-1989). Topic initiation: Business-at-hand. *Research on Language and Social Interaction, 22*, 61-91.

Byock, I. (1997). *Dying well: The prospect for growth at the end of life.* New York: Riverhead Books.

Calman, K.C. (1987). Definitions and dimensions of quality of life. In N.K. Aaronson & J. Beckman (Eds.), *The quality of life of cancer patients* (pp. 1-9). New York: Raven Press.

Cancer causes relationship changes (research on terminally ill and their familial relationships). (1994). *USA Today, 123*, p. 9.

Capps, L., & Ochs, E. (1995). *Constructing panic: The discourse of agoraphobia.* Cambridge, MA: Harvard University Press.

Cassell, E.J. (1985). *Talking with patients: Volumes I & II.* Cambridge, MA: MIT Press.

Chapman, K. (1994). When the prognosis isn't as good. *RN, 57*, 55-57.

Chesler, M.A., & Barbarin, O.A. (1987). *Childhood cancer and the family: Meeting the challenge of stress and support.* New York: Brunner/Mazel.

Clayman, S. E. (1992). Footing in the achievement of neutrality: The case of news interview discourse. In P. Drew & J. Heritage (Eds.), *Talk at work: Interaction in institutional settings* (pp. 163-198). Cambridge: Cambridge University Press.

Clayman, S., & Heritage, J. (2002a). *The news interview: Journalists and public figures on the air.* Cambridge: Cambridge University Press.

Clayman, S.E. & Heritage, J. (2002b). Questioning presidents: Journalistic deference and adversarialness in the press conferences of U.S. Presidents Eisenhower and Reagan. *Journal of Communication, 52*, 749-775.

Clifford, C. (2003). *Not now...I'm having a no hair day.* Minneapolis: University of Minnesota Press.

Clifford, C., & Palmer, A. (2002). *Cancer has its privileges: Stories of hope and laughter.* New York: The Berkeley Publishing Group.

Comaroff, J., & Maguire, P. (1986). Ambiguity and the search for meaning: Childhood leukemia in the modern clinical context. In P. Conrad & R. Kern (Eds.), *The sociology of health and illness* (pp. 100-109). New York: St. Martin's.

Conrad, P. (1987). The experience of illness: Recent and new directions. In J.A. Roth & P. Conrad (Eds.), *Research in the sociology of health care Vol. 6: The experience and management of chronic illness* (pp. 1-31). Greenwich, CT: JAI Press.

Coulter, J. (1979). *The social construction of mind: Studies in ethnomethodology and linguistic philosophy.* Totowa, NJ: Rowman & Littlefield.

Couper-Kuhlen, E., & Selting, M. (1996). Towards an interactional perspective on prosody and a prosodic perspective on interaction. In E. Cooper-Kuhlen & M. Selting (Eds.). *Prosody in conversation: Interactional studies* (pp. 11-56). Cambridge: Cambridge University Press.

Cournos, F. (1990). Psychosocial interventions with cancer patients and their families. In A. Blitzer et al. (Eds.), *Communicating with cancer patients and their families* (pp. 45-48). Philadelphia, PA: The Charles Press.

Crase, A.E. (2003). *The social construction of hope and optimism in family interactions about cancer.* Unpublished masters thesis. San Diego State University.

Creagan, E.T. (1993). Psychosocial issues in oncologic practice. *Mayo Clinic Proceedings, 68,* 161-167.

Crosson, K. (1998). The informational needs of patients with cancer and their families. *Cancer Practice, 6,* 39-46.

Davis, F. (1963). *Passage through crisis: Polio victims and their families.* Indianapolis, IN: Bobbs-Merrill.

Di Giacomo, F. (2003). *I'd rather do chemo than clean out the garage: Choosing laughter over tears.* Dallas: Brown Books.

Drew, P. (1984). Speakers' reportings in invitation sequences. In J. M. Atkinson & J. Heritage (Eds.), *Structures of social action: Studies in conversation analysis* (pp. 129-151). Cambridge: Cambridge University Press.

Drew, P. (1987). Po-faced receipts of tears. *Linguistics, 25,* 219-253.

Drew, P. (2002). Out of context: An intersection between domestic life and the workplace, as contexts for (business) talk. *Language and Communication, 22,* 477-494

Drew, P. (2003). Comparative analysis of talk-in-interaction in different institutional settings: A sketch. In P. Glenn, C. LeBaron, & J. Mandelbaum (Eds.), *Studies in language and social interaction: In honor or Robert Hopper* (pp. 293-308). Mahwah, NJ: Erlbaum.

Drew, P., & Heritage, J. (Eds.). (1992). *Talk at work: Interaction in institutional settings.* Cambridge: Cambridge University Press.

Drew, P., & Holt, E. (1988). Complainable matters: The use of idiomatic expressions in making social complaints. *Social Problems, 35,* 398-417.

Drew, P., & Holt, E. (1998). Figures of speech: Figurative expressions and the management of topic transition in conversation. *Language in Society, 27,* 495-522.

Drew, P., & Wootton, A. (Eds.). (1988). *Erving Goffman: Exploring the interaction order.* Boston: Northeastern University Press.

Dunkel-Schetter, C., & Wortman, C.B. (1982). The interpersonal dynamics of cancer: Problems in social relationships and their impact on the patient. In H. S. Freidman & M. R. DiMatteo (Eds.), *Interpersonal issues in health care* (pp. 69-100). New York: Academic Press.

Eden, O.B., Black, I., & Emery, A.E.H. (1993). The use of taped parental interviews to improve communication with childhood cancer families. *Pediatric Hematology and Oncology, 10,* 157-162.

Eden, O.B., Black, I., & MacKinlay, G.A. (1994). Communication with parents of children with cancer. *Palliative Medicine, 8,* 105-114.

Edwards, B.K., Howe, H.L., Ries, L.A., Thun, M.J., Rosenberg, H.M., Yancik, R., Wingo, P.A., Jemal, A., & Feigal, E.G. (2002). Annual report to the nation on the status of cancer, 1973-1999, featuring implications of age and aging on U.S. cancer burden. *Cancer, 94,* 2766-2792.

Edwards, D. (2000). Extreme case formulations: Softeners, investment, and doing nonliteral. *Research on Language and Social Interaction, 33,* 347-373.

Ellis, C. (1993). "There are survivors": Telling a story of sudden death. *The Sociological Quarterly, 34,* 711-730.

Engel, G.L. (1977). The need for a new medical model: A challenge for biomedicine. *Science, 196,* 129-136.

Engelberg, M. (1995). *Cancer made me a shallower person: A memoir in comics.* New York: HarperCollins.

Engle, V.F., Fox-Hill, E., & Graney, M.J. (1998). The experience of living and dying in a nursing home: Self reports of black and white older adults. *Journal of the American Geriatrics Society*, *46*, 1091-1096.

Epstein, R.M., & Street, R.L., Jr. (2007). *Patient-centered communication in cancer care: Promoting healing and reducing suffering* (NIH Publication No. 07-6225). Bethesda, MD: National Cancer Institute.

Farran, C.J., Herth, K.A., & Popovich, J.M. (1995). *Hope and hopelessness: Critical and clinical constructs*. Thousand Oaks, CA: Sage.

Farran, C.J., Wilken, C., & Popovich, J.M. (1992). Clinical assessment of hope. *Issues in Mental Health Nursing*, *13*, 129-138.

Farrow, J.M., Cash, D.K., & Simmons, G. (1990). Communication with cancer patients and their families. In A. Blitzer, A. H. Kutscher, S. C. Klagsbrun, R. DeBellis, F. E. Selder, I. B. Seeland, & M. Siegel (Eds.), *Communicating with cancer patients and their families* (pp. 1-17). Philadelphia: The Charles Press.

Fies, B. (2006). *Mom's cancer*. New York: Abrams.

Finlay, I.G., Stott, N.C.H., & Kinnersley, P. (1995). The assessment of communication skills in palliative medicine: A comparison of the scores of examiners and simulated patients. *Medical Education*, *29*, 424-429.

Fitzgerald, M. (1994). Adults' anticipation of the loss of their parents. *Qualitative Health Research*, *4*, 463-479.

Fitzsimmons, E. (1994). One man's death: His family's ethnography. *Omega*, *30*, 23-29.

Fobair, P.A., & Zabora, J.R. (1995). Family functioning as a resource variable in psychosocial cancer research. *Journal of Psychosocial Research*, *13*, 97-122.

Foley, G.V. (1993). Enhancing child-family-health team communication. *Cancer* (Supplement), *71*, 3281-3289.

Foote, A.W., Piazza, D., Holcombe, J., Paul, P., & Daffin, P. (1990). Hope, self-esteem and social support in persons with multiple sclerosis. *Journal of Neuroscience Nursing*, *22*, 155-159.

Ford, L.A., Babrow, A.S., & Stohl, C. (1996). Social support messages and the management of uncertainty in the experience of breast cancer: An application of problematic integration theory. *Communication Monographs*, *63*, 189-207.

Frank, A.W. (1991). *At the will of the body*. Boston: Houghton Mifflin.

Frank, A.W. (1995). *The wounded storyteller: Body, illness, and ethics*. Chicago: The University of Chicago Press.

Frankel, R.M. (1989). "I wz wondering—uhm could *Raid* uhm effect the brain permanently d'y know?": Some observations on the intersection of speaking and writing in calls to a poison control center. *Western Journal of Speech Communication*, *53*, 195-226.

Frankel, R. (1995). Some answers about questions in clinical interviews. In G.H. Morris & R. Cheneil (Eds.), *The talk of the clinic: Explorations in the analysis of medical and therapeutic discourse* (pp. 233-258). Hillsdale, NJ: Erlbaum.

Freeman, M. (1996). WNET clears 5 prime-time hours for health special (Cancer: A Family Matter). *Mediaweek*, *6*, 37.

Freese, J., & Maynard, D.W. (1998). Prosodic features of bad news and good news in conversation. *Language in Society*, *27*, 195-219.

Friedenbergs, I., Gordon, W., Hibbard, M., Levine, L., Wolf, C., & Diller, L. (1982). Psychosocial aspects of living with cancer: A review of the literature. *International Journal of Psychiatric Medicine*, *11*, 303-329.

Friedman, H.S., & DiMatteo, M.R. (1982). Relations with others, social support, and the health care system. In H.S. Friedman & M.R. DiMatteo (Eds.), *Interpersonal issues in health care* (pp. 3-8). New York: Academic.

Friedrich, W.N., Jowarski, T.M., Copeland, D., & Pendergrass, T. (1994). Pediatric cancer: Predicting sibling adjustment. *Journal of Clinical Psychology*, *50*, 303-320.

Fuller, S., & Swensen, C.H. (1992). Marital quality and quality of life among cancer patients and their spouses. *Journal of Psychosocial Oncology*, *10*, 41-56.

Gabb, J. (1996). Narratives on pain and comfort: Casey's story. *Journal of Law, Medicine, and Ethics*, *24*, 292-293.

Gaskins, S. (1995). The meaning of hope: Implications for nursing practice and research. *Journal of Genontological Nursing, 21*, 17-24.

Gill, V.T. (1998). Doing attributions in medical interaction: Patients' explanations for illness and doctor's responses. *Social Psychological Quarterly, 61*, 342-360.

Gill. V.T., Halkowski, T., & Roberts, F. (2001). Accomplishing a request without making one: A single case analysis of a primary care visit. *Text, 21*, 13-268.

Gill, V.T., & Maynard, D.W. (1995). On "labeling" in actual interaction: Delivering and receiving diagnoses of developmental disabilities. *Social Problems, 42*, 11-31.

Gill, V.T., & Maynard, D. (2006). Explaining illness: Patients' proposals and physicians' responses. In J. Heritage & D. Maynard (Eds.), *Practicing medicine: Structure and process in primary care consultations* (pp. 115-150). Cambridge: Cambridge University Press.

Glaser, B.G., & Strauss, A.L. (1965). *Awareness of dying*. Chicago: Aldine De Gruyter.

Glenn, P. (1995). Laughing *at* and laughing *with*: Negotiations of participant alignments through conversational laughter. In Paul ten Have & George Psathas (Eds.), *Situated order: Studies in the organization of talk and embodied activities* (pp. 43-56). Washington, DC: University Press of America.

Glenn, P. (2003). *Laughter in interaction*. Cambridge: Cambridge University Press.

Glenn, P.J., & Knapp, M.L. (1987). The interactive framing of play in adult conversations. *Communication Quarterly, 35*, 48-66.

Glenn, P., LeBaron, C., & Mendelbaum, J. (2003). *Studies in language and social interaction: In honor of Robert Hopper*. Hillsdale, NJ: Erlbaum.

Glimeus, B., Birgegard, G., Hoffman, K., & Kvale, G. (1995). Information to and communication with cancer patients: Improvements and psychosocial correlates in a comprehensive care program for patients and their relatives. *Patient Education & Counseling, 25*, 171-182.

Goffman, E. (1961). *Encounters*. Indianapolis: Bobbs-Merrill.

Goffman, E. (1963). *Behavior in public places: Notes on the social organization of gatherings*. Glencoe: The Free Press.

Goffman, E. (1971). *Relations in public: Microstudies of the public order*. New York: Basic Books.

Goffman, E. (1981). Footing. In *Forms of talk* (pp. 124-159). Philadelphia: University of Pennsylvania Press.

Good, J.S., & Beach, W.A. (2005). Opening up gift-openings: Birthday parties as situated activity systems. *Text, 25*, 565-594.

Goodell, E. (1992). Cancer and family members. *Journal of Health Care Chaplaincy, 4*, 73-85.

Goodwin, C. (1987). Forgetfulness as an interactive resource. *Social Psychology Quarterly, 50*, 115-130.

Goodwin, C. (1996). Transparent vision. In E. Ochs, E.A. Schegloff, & S.A. Thompson (Eds.), *Interaction and grammar* (pp. 370-404). Cambridge: Cambridge University Press.

Goodwin, C., & Duranti, A. (1992). *Rethinking context: Language as an interactive phenomenon*. Cambridge: Cambridge University Press.

Goodwin, M. (1990). *He-said-she-said: Talk as social organization among black children*. Bloomington: Indiana University Press.

Goodwin, M. H., & Goodwin, C. (2000). Emotion within situated activity. In N. Budwig, I.C. Uzgiris, & J.V. Wertsch (Eds.), *Communication: An arena of development* (pp. 33-54). Stamford, CT: Ablex.

Gotay, C.C. (1984). The experience of cancer during early and advanced stages: The views of patients and their mates. *Social Science & Medicine, 18*, 605-613.

Gotcher, J.M. (1992). Interpersonal communication and psychosocial adjustment. *Journal of Psychosocial Oncology, 10*, 21-39.

Gotcher, J.M. (1993). The effects of family communication on psychosocial adjustment of cancer patients. *Journal of Applied Communication Research, 21*, 176-188.

Gotcher, J.M. (1995). Well-adjusted and maladjusted cancer patients: An examination of communication variables. *Health Communication, 7*, 21-33.

Gotcher, J.M., & Edwards, R. (1990). Coping strategies of cancer patients: Actual communication and imagined interactions. *Health Communication, 2*, 255-266.

Groopman, J. (2004). *The anatomy of hope: How people prevail in the face of illness*. New York: Random House.

Gubrium, J.F., & Holstein, J.A. (1990). *What is family?* Mountain View, CA: Mayfield.

Haakana, M. (2001). Laughter as a patient's resource: Dealing with delicate aspects of medical inter-action. *Text, 21,* 187-220.

Haber, S. (1995). Specialization in psychotherapy: From psychotherapist to psychooncologist. *Professional Psychology, Research and Practice, 26,* 427-433.

Halkowski, T. (2000). *Patients' alcohol counts and accounts.* Paper presented at the annual conference of the National Communication Association, Seattle, WA.

Halkowski, T. (2006). Realizing the illness: Patients' narratives of symptom discovery. In J. Heritage & D. Maynard (Eds.), *Practicing medicine: Structure and process in primary care consultations* (pp. 86-114). Cambridge: Cambridge University Press.

Hanks, W. (1992). The indexical ground of deictic reference. In A. Duranti & C. Goodwin (Eds.), *Rethinking context, Language as an interactive phenomenon* (pp. 43-77). Cambridge: Cambridge University Press.

Heath, C. (1988). Embarrassment and interactional organization. In P. Drew & A. Wootton (Eds.), *Erving Goffman: Exploring the interaction order* (pp. 136-160). Boston: Northeastern University Press.

Heath, C. (1992). The delivery and reception of prognosis in the general-practice consultation. In P. Drew & J. Heritage (Eds.), *Talk at work: Interaction in institutional settings* (pp. 235-267). Cambridge: Cambridge University Press.

Heath, C. (1986). *Body movement and speech in medical interaction.* Cambridge: Cambridge University Press.

Heath, C. (2002). Demonstrable suffering: The gestural (re)embodiment of symptoms. *Journal of Communication, 52,* 597-616.

Heath, S. (1996a). Childhood cancer—a family crisis 1: The impact of diagnosis. *British Journal of Nursing, 5,* 744-748.

Heath, S. (1996b). Childhood cancer—a family crisis 2: Coping with diagnosis. *British Journal of Nursing, 5,* 790-793.

Heinrich, R.L., Schag, C.C., & Ganz, P A. (1984). Living with cancer: The cancer inventory of prob-lem situations. *Journal of Clinical Psychology, 40,* 972-980.

Hensel, W.A. (1997). Bea's legacy. *Journal of the American Medical Association, 277,* 1913-1914.

Hepburn, A. (2004). Crying: Notes on description, transcription, and interaction. *Research on Language and Social Interaction, 37,* 251-290.

Heritage, J. (1984a). A change-of-state token and aspects of its sequential placement. In J.M. Atkinson & J. Heritage (Eds.), *Structures of social action: Studies in conversation analysis* (pp. 229-345). Cambridge: Cambridge University Press.

Heritage, J. (1984b). *Garfinkel and ethnomethodology.* Cambridge and New York: Polity Press.

Heritage, J. (1998). Oh-prefaced responses to inquiry. *Language in Society, 27,* 291-334.

Heritage, J. (2002). *Oh*-prefaced responses to assessments: A method of modifying agreement/dis-agreement. In C.E. Ford, B.A. Fox, & S.A. Thompson (Eds.), *The language of turn and sequence* (pp. 196-224). Oxford: Oxford University Press.

Heritage, J., & Atkinson, J.M. (1984). Introduction. In *Structures of social action: Studies in conver-sation analysis* (1-16). Cambridge: Cambridge University Press.

Heritage, J., & Drew, P. (1992). Analyzing talk at work: An introduction. In P. Drew & J. Heritage (Eds.), *Talk at work: Interactions in institutional settings* (pp. 3-65). Cambridge: Cambridge University Press.

Heritage, J., & Lindstrom, A. (1998). Motherhood, medicine, and morality: Scenes from a medical encounter. *Research on Language and Social Interaction, 31,* 397-438.

Heritage, J., & Maynard, D. (Eds.). (2006). *Communication in medical care: Structure and process in primary care consultations.* Cambridge: Cambridge University Press.

Heritage, J., & Raymond, G. (2005). The terms of agreement: Indexing epistemic authority and sub-ordination in assessment sequences. *Social Psychology Quarterly, 68,* 15-38.

Heritage, J.H., & Robinson, J.D. (2006). Accounting for the visit: Giving reasons for seeking medical care. In J. Heritage & D. Maynard (Eds.), *Communication in medical care: Interaction between primary care physicians and patients* (pp. 48-87). Cambridge: Cambridge University Press.

Heritage, J., & Sefi, S. (1992). Dilemmas of advice: Aspects of the delivery and reception of advice in interactions between health visitors and first-time mothers. In P. Drew & J. Heritage (Eds.), *Talk at work: Interaction in institutional settings* (pp. 359-417). Cambridge: Cambridge University Press.

Heritage, J., & Sorjonen, M.L. (1994). Constituting and maintaining activities across sequences: *And*-prefacing as a feature of question design. *Language in Society, 23*, 1-29.

Heritage, J., & Stivers, T. (1999). Online commentary in acute medical visits: A method of shaping patient expectations. *Social Science & Medicine, 49*, 1501-1517.

Heritage, J.C., & Watson, D.R. (1979). Formulations as conversational objects. In G. Psathas (Ed.), *Everyday language: Studies in ethnomethodology* (pp. 123-162). New York: Irvington.

Heritage, J.C., & Watson, D.R., (1980). Aspects of the properties of formulations in natural conversations: Some instances analyzed. *Semiotica, 30*, 245-262.

Hermann, J.F., Wojtkowiak, S.L., Houts, P.S., & Kahn, S.B. (1988). *Helping people cope: A guide for families facing cancer.* Pennsylvania Department of Health.

Herth, K. (1990). Fostering hope in terminally ill people. *Journal of Advanced Nursing,* 1250-1259.

Herth, K. (1991). Development and refinement of an instrument to measure hope. *Scholarly Inquiry for Nursing Practice: An International Journal, 5*, 39-51.

Herth, K. (1992). Abbreviated instrument to measure hope: Development and psychometric evaluation. *Journal of Advanced Nursing, 17*, 1251-1259.

Herth, K. (1993). Hope in the family caregiver of terminally ill people. *Journal of Advanced Nursing, 18*, 538-548.

Herth, K. (2000). Enhancing hope in people with a first recurrence of cancer. *Journal of Advanced Nursing, 32*, 1431-1441.

Heusinkveld, K.B. (1972). Cues to communication with the terminal cancer patient. *Nursing Forum, 11*, 105-113.

Hilton, B.A. (1994). Family communication patterns in coping with early breast cancer. *Western Journal of Nursing Research, 16*, 366-391.

Hinds, C. (1992). Suffering: A relatively unexplored phenomenon among family caregivers of non-institutionalized patients with cancer. *Journal of Advanced Nursing, 17*, 918-925.

Hinds, P., & Gattuso, J.S. (1991). Measuring hopefulness in adolescents. *Journal of Pediatric Oncology Nursing, 8*, 92-94.

Hinds, P.A., Quargnenti, A., Fairclough, D., Bush, A.J., Betcher, D., Rissmiller, G., Pratt, C.B., & Gilchrist, G.S. (1999). Hopefulness and its characteristics in adolescents with cancer. *Western Journal of Nursing Research, 21*, 600-620.

Hinton, J. (1998). An assessment of open communication between people with terminal cancer, caring relatives, and others during home care. *Journal of Palliative Care, 14*, 15-23.

Holt, E. (1993). The structure of death announcements: Looking on the bright side of death. *Text, 13*, 189-212.

Holt, E. (1996). Reporting on talk: The use of direct reported speech in conversation. *Research on Language and Social Interaction, 29*, 219-245.

Holt, E. (1999). Just gassing: An analysis of direct reported speech in a conversation between two employees of a gas supply company. *Text, 19*, 505-537.

Holt, E. (2000). Reporting and reacting: Concurrent responses to reported speech. *Research on Language and Social Interaction, 33*, 425-454.

Holt, E., & Clift, R. (2006). "I'm eyeing your chop up mind": Reporting and enacting. In *Reporting talk: Reported speech in interaction* (pp. 47-80). Cambridge: Cambridge University Press.

Holt, E., & Drew, P. (2005). Figurative pivots: The use of figurative expressions in pivotal topic transitions. *Research on Language and Social Interaction, 38*, 35-61.

Hopper, R. (1989). Speech in telephone openings: Emergent interaction v. routines. *Western Journal of Speech Communication, 53*, 240-252.

Hopper, R. (1992). *Telephone conversation.* Bloomington: Indiana University Press.

Hopper, R. (1995). Episode trajectory in conversational play. In P. ten Have & G. Psathas (Eds.), *Situated order: Studies in the social organization of talk and embodied activities* (pp. 57-72). Washington, DC: University Press of America.

Hopper, R., & Drummond, K. (1992). Accomplishing interpersonal relationship: The telephone openings of strangers and intimates. *Western Journal of Communication, 56*, 185-199.

Hopper, R., & Glenn, P. (1994). Repetition and play in conversation. In B. Johnstone (Ed.), *Perspectives on repetition* (Vol. 2, pp. 29-40). Norwood, NJ: Ablex.

Hoskins, C.N. (1995). Adjustment to breast cancer in couples. *Psychological Reports, 77*, 435-454.

Hunt, M. (1991). Being friendly and informal: Reflected in nurses', terminally ill patients' and relatives' conversations at home. *Journal of Advanced Nursing, 16*, 929-938.

Hyde, M. (2001). *The call of conscience: Heideggar and Levinas, rhetoric and the euthanasia debate.* Columbia: University of South Carolina Press.

Illich, I. (1975). *Medical nemesis: The expropriation of health.* Oxford: Calder & Byers, Publishers.

Independent Traveler.com (2002). *Emergency reservations.* Retrieved July 21, 2002, from http://www.independenttraveler.com/.

Iocovozzi, D. D. S. (1991). We're ready now; by being honest with a dying patient, this nurse helped him be honest with his family. *Nursing, 21*, 77.

Jefferson, G. (1972). Side sequences. In D.N. Sudnow (Ed.), *Studies in social interaction* (pp. 294-338). New York: Free Press.

Jefferson, G. (1973). A case of precision timing in ordinary conversation: Overlapped tag-positioned address terms in closing sequences. *Semiotica, 9*, 47-96.

Jefferson, G. (1977). *On the poetics of ordinary talk.* Lecture presented at the International Conference on Ethnomethodology and Conversation Analysis, Boston.

Jefferson, G. (1978). Sequential aspects of storytelling in conversation. In J. Schenkein (Ed.), *Studies in the organization of conversational interaction* (pp. 219-247). New York: Academic Press.

Jefferson, G. (1979). A technique for inviting laughter and its subsequent acceptance declination. In G. Psathas (Ed.), *Everyday language: Studies in ethnomethodology* (pp. 79-96). New York: Irvington.

Jefferson, G. (1980a). *The analysis of conversations in which "troubles" and "anxieties" are expressed.* Final report for the (British) Social Science Research Council: Report nos. HR 4805/1-2.

Jefferson, G. (1980b). On 'trouble premonitory' response to inquiry. *Sociological Inquiry, 50*, 153-185.

Jefferson, G. (1981). *Caveat speaker: A preliminary exploration of shift implicative recipiency in the articulation of topic.* Final Report, Social Science Research Council, The Netherlands (mimeo).

Jefferson, G. (1984a). On the organization of laughter in talk about troubles. In J.M. Atkinson & J. Heritage (Eds.), *Structures of social action: Studies in conversation analysis* (pp. 347-369). Cambridge: Cambridge University Press.

Jefferson, G. (1984b). On stepwise transition from talk about a trouble to inappropriately next-positioned matters. In J.M. Atkinson & J. Heritage (Eds.), *Structures of social action: Studies in conversational analysis* (pp. 191-222). Cambridge: Cambridge University Press.

Jefferson, G. (1988). On the sequential organization of troubles talk in ordinary conversation. *Social Problems 35*, 418-441.

Jefferson, G. (1990). List construction as a task and resource. In G. Psathas (Ed.), *Interaction competence* (pp. 63-92). Lanham, MD: University Press of America.

Jefferson, G. (1993). Caveat speaker: Preliminary notes on recipient topic-shift implicature. *Research on Langue and Social Interaction, 26*, 1-30.

Jefferson, G. (1996). On the poetics of ordinary talk. *Text and Performance Quarterly, 16*, 1-61.

Jefferson, G. (2004a). A note on laughter in 'male-female' interaction. *Discourse Studies, 6*, 117-133.

Jefferson, G. (2004b). 'At first I thought': A normalizing device for extraordinary events. In G.H. Lerner (Ed.), *Conversation analysis: Studies from the first generation* (pp. 131-167). Philadelphia: John Benjamins.

Jefferson, G., & Lee, J.R.E. (1981/1992). The rejection of advice: Managing the problematic convergence of a "troubles-telling" and a "service encounter." In P. Drew & J. Heritage (Eds.), *Talk at work: Interaction in institutional settings* (pp. 521-548). Cambridge: Cambridge University Press.

Jefferson, G., Sacks, H., & Schegloff, E.A. (1987). On laughter in the pursuit of intimacy. In G. Button & J.R.E. Lee (Eds.), *Talk and social organization* (pp. 152-205). Clevedon, UK: Multilingual Matters.

Jefferson, G., & Schegloff, E.A. (1975). *Sketch: Some orderly aspects of overlap in conversation.* Paper presented at meetings for the American Anthropological Association.

Jeffrey, N. (2000, Sept. 17). Bereavement fares can often be beaten with a little searching. *San Diego Union Tribune.*

Jones, C. M. (1997). "That's a good sign": Encouraging assessments as a form of social support in medically related encounters. *Health Communication, 9*, 119-153.

Jones, C.M. (2005a). *Displays of reluctance in talk about cancer: Lay expressions of fear and professional expressions of sensitivity*. Manuscript.

Jones, C.M. (2005b). *The self-concept of cancer patients: Its reconstruction in interaction*. Manuscript.

Jones, C.M., & Beach, W.A. (2005). "I just wanna know *why*": Patients' attempts and physicians' responses to premature solicitation of diagnostic information. In J.F. Duchan & D. Kovarsky (Eds.), *Diagnosis as cultural practice* (pp. 103-136). New York: Mouton de Gruyter Publishers.

Jones, S.E., & LeBaron, C. (Eds.). (2002). Special issue on relationships between verbal and nonverbal communication. *Journal of Communication, 52*.

Joseph, S. (1992). One of the family. *Nursing, 22*, 92.

Jospe, M. (1989). *The role of family communication patterns in a child's adjustment to cancer*. Doctoral dissertation, California School of Professional Psychology, Los Angeles.

Kaiser Permanente (1999). *I've never died before*. San Diego, CA. Department of Preventive Medicine/Health Appraisal.

Karp, D.A. (1992). Illness ambiguity and the search for meaning. *Journal of Contemporary Ethnography, 21,* 139-170.

Keller, M., Henrich, G., Sellschopp, A., & Beutel, M. (1996). Between distress and support: Spouses of cancer patients. In L. Baider, C.L. Cooper & A.K. De-Nour (Eds.), *Cancer and the family* (pp. 187-223). New York: Wiley.

Keitel, M.A., Cramer, S.H., & Zevon, M.A. (1990). Spouses of cancer patients: A review of the literature. *Journal of Counseling and Development, 69*, 163-167.

Kendon, A. (1990). *Conducting interaction: Patterns of behavior in focused encounters*. Cambridge: Cambridge University Press.

Kinnell, A.M., & Maynard, D.W. (1996). The delivery and receipt of safer sex advice in pre-test counseling sessions for HIV and AIDS. *Journal of Contemporary Ethnography, 35*, 405-437.

Komp, D. M. (1992). A mystery story: Children, cancer, and covenant. *Theology Today, 49*, 68-75.

Kowalczyk, R.S. (1995). Breast cancer: A family survival guide. *Choice, 33*, 498.

Kreps, G., & Kunimoto, E.N. (1994). *Effective communication in multicultural health care settings*. Thousand Oaks, CA: Sage.

Kristjanson, L.J., & Ashcroft, T. (1994). The family's cancer journey: A literature review. *Cancer Nursing, 17,* 1-17.

Kubler-Ross, E. (1969a). Preface, On the fear of death, & attitudes towards death and dying (pp. 1-37.). In *On death and dying*. New York: Macmillan.

Kubler-Ross, E. (1969b). *On death and dying*. New York: MacMillan.

Kubler-Ross, E. (1974). *Questions and answers on death and dying*. New York: Macmillan.

Kumar, P.J., & Clark, M.L. (1990). *Clinical medicine*. London: Bailliere Tindall.

Kutner, N.G. (1987). Social worlds and identity in end-stage renal disease (ESRD). In J.A. Roth & P. Conrad (Eds.), *Research in the sociology of health care: The experience and management of chronic illness* (Vol. 6). Greenwich, CT: JAI Press.

Lamm, M. (1997). *The power of hope: The one essential of life and love*. New York: Fireside.

Leeds-Hurwitz, W. (1987). The social history of *The Natural History of an Interview*: A multidisciplinary investigation of social communication. *Research on Language and Social Interaction, 20*, 1-51.

Leeds-Hurwitz, W. (2005). The natural history approach: A Bateson legacy. *Cybernetics and Human Knowing, 12*, 137-146.

Leiber, L., Plumb, M.M., Gerstenzang, M.L., & Holland, J. (1976). The communication of affection between cancer patients and their spouses. *Psychosomatic Medicine, 38*, 379-389.

Lerner, G.H. (1987). *Collaborative turn sequences: Sentence construction and social action*. Doctoral dissertation, University of California, Irvine.

Lerner, G. H. (1989). Notes on overlap management in conversation: The case of delayed completion. *Western Journal of Speech Communication, 53*, 167-177.

Lerner, G.H. (2003). Selecting next speaker: The context-sensitive operation of a context free organization. *Language in Society, 32*, 177-201.

Lerner, G.H. (2004). On the place of linguistic resources in the organization of talk-in-interaction: Grammar as action in prompting a speaker to elaborate. *Research on Language and Social Interaction, 37*, 151-184.

Lewis, F.M., & Hammond, M.A. (1996). The father's, mother's, and adolescent's functioning with breast cancer. *Family Relations, 45,* 456-466.

Lewis, M., Pearson, V., Corcoran-Perry, S., & Narayan, S. (1997). Decision-making by elderly patients with cancer and their caregivers. *Cancer Nursing, 20,* 389-397.

Lichter, I. (1987). *Communication in cancer care.* New York: Churchill Livingstone.

Lichtman, R.R., & Taylor, S.E. (1986). Close relationships and the female cancer patient. In B.L. Andersen (Ed.), *Women with cancer: Psychological perspectives* (pp. 233-256). New York: Springer-Verlag.

Litman, T.J. (1974). The family as a basic unit in health and medical care: A social-behavioral overview. *Social Science & Medicine, 8,* 495-519.

Local, J. (1996). Conversational phonetics: Some aspects of news receipts in everyday talk. In E. Couper-Kuhlen & M. Setling (Eds.), *Prosody in conversation: Interactional studies* (pp. 177-230). Cambridge: Cambridge University Press.

Lockwood, L. (2002). *Communication and cancer: Creating a play script from family conversations.* Unpublished masters thesis, San Diego State University.

Lomax, B. (1997, April 23). Learning to understand patient's silence. *Nursing Times, 93,* 48-49.

Lutfey, K., & Maynard, D.W. (1998). Bad news in oncology: How physician and patient talk about death and dying without using those words. *Social Psychology Quarterly, 61,* 321-341.

Lyons, R.F., & Meade, D. (1995). Painting a new face on relationships: Relationship remodeling in response to chronic illness. In S. Duck & J.T. Wood (Eds.), *Confronting relationship challenges: Understanding relationship processes series, Vol. 5.* Thousand Oaks, CA: Sage.

Ma, J.L.C. (1996). Desired and perceived social support from family, friends, and health professionals: A panel study in Hong Kong of patients with nasopharyngeal carcinoma. *Journal of Psychosocial Oncology, 14,* 47-68.

MacDonald, N. (1996). The interface between oncology and palliative medicine. In D. Doyle, G.W.C. Hanks, & N. MacDonald (Eds.), *Oxford textbook of palliative medicine* (pp. 11-17). Oxford: Oxford University Press.

Mandelbaum, J. (1987). Couples sharing stories. *Communication Quarterly,* 144-171.

Mandelbaum, J. (1989). Interpersonal activities in conversational storytelling. *Western Journal of Communication, 53,* 114-126.

Mandelbaum, J. (1991). Conversational noncooperation: An exploration of disattended complaints. *Research on Language and Social Interaction, 25,* 97-138.

Mandelbaum, J. (1993). Assigning responsibility in conversational storytelling: The interactional construction of reality. *Text, 13,* 247-266.

Martinson, I.M., McClowry, S.G., Davies, B., & Kuhlenkamp, E.J. (1994). Changes over time: A study of family bereavement following childhood cancer. *Journal of Palliative Care, 10,* 19-25.

Maynard, D.W. (1988). Language, interaction, and social problems. *Social Problems, 35,* 311-334.

Maynard, D.W. (1989). Perspective-display sequences in conversation. *Western Journal of Speech Communication, 53,* 91-113.

Maynard, D.W. (1991). Perspective-display sequences and the delivery and receipt of diagnostic news. In D. Boden & D. Zimmerman (Eds.), *Talk and social structure* (pp. 164-192). Cambridge: Polity Press.

Maynard, D.W. (1992). On co-implicating recipients in the delivery of diagnostic news. In P. Drew & J. Heritage (Eds.), *Talk at work: Interactions in institutional settings* (pp. 331-358). Cambridge: Cambridge University Press.

Maynard, D.W. (1996). On "realization" in everyday life: The forecasting of bad news as a social relation. *American Sociological Review, 61,* 109-131.

Maynard, D.W. (1997). The news delivery sequence: Bad news and good news in conversational interaction. *Research on Language and Social Interaction, 30,* 93-130.

Maynard, D.W. (2003). *Good news, bad news: Conversational order in everyday talk and clinical settings.* Chicago: The University of Chicago Press.

Maynard, D.W., & Frankel, R.M. (2006). On diagnostic rationality: Bad news, good news, and the symptom residue. In J. Heritage & D.W. Maynard (Eds.), *Communication in medical care: Interaction between primary care physicians and patients* (pp. 248-278). Cambridge: Cambridge University Press.

Maynard, D.W., Houtkoop-Stenstra, H., Schaeffer, N.C., & van der Zouwene, J. (Eds.). (2002). *Standardization and tacit knowledge: Interaction and practice in the survey interview*. New York: Wiley.

Maynard, D.W., & Schaeffer, N.C. (1997). Keeping the gate: Declinations of the request to participate in a telephone survey interview. *Sociological Methods and Research, 30*, 323-370.

Maynard, D.W., & Schaeffer, N.C. (2002a). Opening and closing the gate: The work of optimism in recruiting survey respondents. In D. W. Maynard, H. Houtkoop-Stenstra, N.C. Schaeffer, & J. van der Zouwene (Eds.), *Standardization and tacit knowledge: Interaction and practice in the survey interview* (pp. 179-204). New York:Wiley.

Maynard, D.W., & Schaeffer, N.C. (2002b). Refusal conversion and tailoring. In D.W. Maynard, H. Houtkoop-Stenstra, N.C. Schaeffer, & J. van der Zouwene (Eds.), *Standardization and tacit knowledge: Interaction and practice in the survey interview* (pp. 219-239). New York: Wiley.

Mazeland, H., Huisman, M., & Schasfoort, M. (1995). Negotiating categories in travel agency calls. In A. Firth (Ed.), *The discourse of negotiation: Studies of language in the workplace* (pp. 271-297). Oxford: Elsevier Science.

Mesters, I., Van Den Borne, H., McCormick, L., Pruyn, J., De Boer, M., & Imbos, T. (1997). Openness to discuss cancer in the nuclear family: Scale, development, and validation. *Psychosomatic Medicine, 59*, 269-279.

Metzger, T.R., & Beach, W.A. (1996). Preserving alternative versions: Interactional techniques for organizing courtroom cross-examination. *Communication Research, 23*, 749-765.

Meyer, M., & Rao, L. (1997). How top cancer docs beat (their own) cancer: What they learned could save your life. *Prevention, 49*, 85-94.

McGuire, M.B., & Kantor, D.J. (1987). Belief systems and illness experiences: The case of non-medical healing groups. In J. A. Roth & P. Conrad (Eds.), *Research in the sociology of health care. Vol. 6: The experience and management of chronic illness* (pp. 221-248). Greenwich, CT: JAI Press.

Mireault, G.C., & Compas, B.E. (1996). A prospective study of coping and adjustment before and after a parent's death from cancer. *Journal of Psychosocial Oncology, 14*, 1-18.

Miller, B.D. (1988). *The role of family communication patterns in a child's adjustment to cancer*. Doctoral dissertation, California School of Professional Psychology—Los Angeles.

Miller, J.F., & Powers, M.J. (1988). Development of an instrument to measure hope. *Nursing Research, 2*, 23-29.

Milton, E. (1996). Thinking about Houdini. *Michigan Quarterly Review, 35*, 460-469.

Mokros, H. (1996). *Interaction and identity: Information and behavior.* (Vol. 5.) New Brunswick, NJ: Transaction.

Montazeri, A., Milroy, R., Gillis, C.R., & McEwen, J. (1996). Interviewing cancer patients in a research setting: The role of effective communication. *Support Care Cancer, 4*, 447-454.

Morris, G.H., & Cheneil, R.J. (Eds). (1995). *The talk of the clinic: Explorations in the analysis of medical and therapeutic discourse* (pp. 259-289). Hillsdale, NJ: Erlbaum.

Morse, J.M., & Johnson, J.L. (Eds.). (1991). *The illness experience: Dimensions of suffering.* Newbury Park: Sage.

Mott, K. (1996). Cancer and the Internet: When I became physically isolated by illness, my computer brought family and friends to me. *Newsweek, 128*, 19.

Mulcahey, A.L., & Young, M.A. (1995). A bereavement support group for children. *Cancer Practice, 3*, 150-156.

Naber, S. J., Halstead, L. K., Broome, M., & Rehwaldt, M. (1995). Communication and control: Parent, child and health care professional interactions during painful procedures. *Issues in Comprehensive Pediatric Nursing, 18*, 79-90.

Nekolaichuk, C.L., Jevne, R.F., & Maguire, T.O. (1999). Structuring the meaning of hope in health and illness. *Social Science & Medicine, 48*, 591-605.

Norrick, N.R. (1997). Twice-told tales: Collaborative narration of familiar stories. *Language in Society, 26*, 199-220.

Norrick, N.R. (1998). Retelling stories in spontaneous conversation. *Discourse Processes, 25*, 75-97.

Norrick, N.R. (2000). *Conversational narrative: Storytelling in everyday talk*. Amsterdam: Benjamins.

Northouse, L.L. (1994). Breast cancer in younger women: Effects on interpersonal and family relations. *Journal of the National Cancer Institute Monographs, 16*, 183-190.

Northouse, P.G., & Northouse, L.L. (1987). Communication and cancer: Issues confronting patients, health professionals, and family members. *Journal of Psychosocial Oncology, 5*, 17-46.

Nowotny, M.L. (1989). Assessment of hope in patients with cancer: Development of an instrument. *Oncology Nursing Forum, 16*, 57-61.

Nunn, K.P., Lewin, T.J., Walton, J.M., & Carr, V.J. (1996). The construction and characteristics of an instrument to measure personal hopefulness. *Psychological Medicine, 26*, 531-545.

Obayuwana, A.O., Collines, J.L., Carter, A.L., Rao, M.S., Mathura, C.C., & Wilson, S.B. (1982). Hope index scale: An instrument for the objective assessment of hope. *Journal of the National Medical Association, 74*, 761-765.

Ochs, E., Schegloff, E.A., & Thompson, S.A. (Eds.). (1996). *Interaction and grammar.* Cambridge: Cambridge University Press.

Ong, C. (2001). Abandon all hope, all ye who enter here. *The Journal of Alternative Complementary Medicine, 7*, 289-294.

O'Hair, D., Kreps, G., & Sparks, L. (2007). *Handbook of communication and cancer care.* Cresskill, NJ: Hampton Press.

Ott, J.K. (1999). *Emotional experiences embraced: Communicating identity and illness survivorship.* Unpublished master's thesis, San Diego State University.

Ott, J., Beach, W.A., & Dixson, C.N. (2000). *Communication and terminal cancer care.* Manuscript.

Pace, K. (1993, February). Communicating with cancer patients and families. *Caring, 72*, 77.

Packer, J. I. (1973). *Knowing God.* Downer's Grove, IL: Intervarsity Press.

Packo, J.E. (1991). *Coping with cancer and other chronic life-threatening diseases.* Camp Hill, PA: Christian Publications.

Parisi, S.B. (1996). Nothing to fear. *Nursing, 26*, 80.

Parle, M., Maguire, P., & Heaven, C. (1997). The development of a training model to improve health professionals' skills, self-efficacy and outcome expectancies when communicating with cancer patients. *Social Science Medicine, 44*, 231-240.

Parsons, T. (2002). *Getting home soon: Finding the best bereavement fares.* Retrieved July 22, 2002, from http://abcnews.90.com/sections/travel/economyclass/bereavfares.html.

Paternoster, J. (1990). The caring process and the cancer patient. In A. Blitzer et al. (Eds.), *Communicating with cancer patients and their families* (pp. 18-25). Philadelphia, PA: The Charles Press.

Pearcey, N. (2004). *Total truth: Liberating Christianity from its cultural captivity.* Wheaton, IL: Crossway Books.

Penrod, J., & Morse, J.M. (1997). Strategies for assessing and fostering hope: The hope assessment guide. *Oncology Nursing Forum, 24*, 1055-1063.

Peräkylä, A. (1991). Hope work in the care of seriously ill patients. *Qualitative Health Research, 1*, 407-433.

Peräkylä, A. (1993). Invoking a hostile world: Discussing the patient's future in AIDS counseling. *Text, 13*, 302-338.

Peräkylä, A. (1995). *AIDS counselling: Institutional interaction and clinical practice.* Cambridge: Cambridge University Press.

Pillet-Shore, D. (2003). Doing "okay": On the multiple metrics of an assessment. *Research on Language and Social Interaction, 36*, 285-319.

Pistrang, N., Barker, C., & Rutter, C. (1997). Social support as conversation: Analysing breast cancer patients' interactions with their partners. *Social Science and Medicine, 5*, 773-782.

Pomerantz, A. (1978). Compliment responses: Notes on the cooperation of multiple constraints. In J.N. Schenkein (Ed.), *Studies in the organization of conversational interaction* (pp. 79-112). New York: Academic Press.

Pomerantz, A. (1980). Telling my side: "Limited access" as a "fishing" device. *Sociological Inquiry, 50*, 186-198.

Pomerantz, A. (1984a). Agreeing and disagreeing with assessments: Some features of preferred/dispreferred turn shapes. In J.M. Atkinson & J. Heritage (Eds.), *Structures of social action: Studies in conversation analysis* (57-101). Cambridge University Press.

Pomerantz, A. (1984b). Pursuing a response. In J.M. Atkinson & J. Heritage (Eds.), *Structures of social action: Studies in conversation analysis* (pp. 152-163). Cambridge: Cambridge University Press.

Pomerantz, A. (1986). Extreme case formulations: A way of legitimizing claims. *Human Studies, 9,* 219-229.

Pomerantz, A. (1990). Conversation analytic claims. *Communication Monographs,* 57, 231-249.

Ptacek, J.T., & Eberhardt, T.L. (1996). Breaking bad news: A review of the literature. *Journal of the American Medical Association, 276,* 496-502.

Pudlinski, C. (1998). Giving advice on a consumer-run warm line: Implicit and dilemmatic practices. *Communication Studies, 49,* 323-341.

Quill, T.E. (1991). Death and dignity: A case of individualized decision making. *The New England Journal of Medicine, 324,* 691-695.

Rait, D., & Lederberg, M. (1990). The family of the cancer patient. In J.C. Holland & J.H. Rowland (Eds.), *Handbook of psychooncology: Psychological care of the patient with cancer* (pp. 585-597). New York: Oxford.

Raleigh, E.D.H. (1992). Sources of hope in chronic illness. *Oncology Nursing Forum, 19,* 443-448.

Raymond, G. (2000). *The structure of responding: Conforming and nonconforming response to yes/no type interrogatives.* Dissertation, University of California, Los Angeles.

Raymond, G. (2004). Prompting action: The stand-alone 'so' in sequences of talk-in-interaction. *Research on Language and Social Interaction, 37,* 185-218.

Raymond, G., & Heritage, J. (2006). The epistemics of social relationships: Owning grandchildren. *Language in Society, 35,* 677-705.

Razavi, D., & Delvaux, N. (1995). The psychiatrist's perspective on quality of life and quality of care in oncology: Concepts, symptom management, communication issues. *European Journal of Cancer, 31A*(Suppl 6), 25-29.

Renz, M.C. (1994). Room full of love. *Nursing, 24,* 104.

Rittenberg, C.N. (1996). Helping children cope when a family member has cancer. *Support Care Cancer, 4,* 196-199.

Robinson, C.A. (1993). Managing life with a chronic condition: The story of normalization. *Qualitative Health Research, 3,* 6-28.

Robinson, J.D. (2001). Asymmetry in action: Sequential resources in the negotiation of a prescription request. *Text, 21,* 19-54.

Robinson, J.D. (2003). An interactional structure of medical activities during acute visits and its implications for patients' participation. *Health Communication, 15,* 27-59.

Robinson, J.D. (2004). The sequential organization of 'explicit' apologies in naturally occurring English. *Research on Language and Social Interaction, 37.*

Robinson, J.D. (2006). Managing trouble responsibility and relationships during conversational repair. *Communication Monographs, 73,* 137-161.

Rootman, I., & Hershfield, L. (1994). Health communication research: Broadening the scope. *Health Communication, 6,* 69-72.

Rose, J.H. (1990). Social support and cancer: Adult patient's desire for support from family, friends, and health professionals. *American Journal of Community Psychology, 18,* 439-465.

Rowland, J.H. (1990a). Developmental stage and adaptation: Adult model. In J.C. Holland & J.H. Rowland (Eds.), *Handbook of psychooncology: Psychological care of the patient with cancer* (pp. 25-43). New York: Oxford.

Rowland, J.H. (1990b). Interpersonal resources: Social support. In J.C. Holland & J.H. Rowland (Eds.), *Handbook of psychooncology: Psychological care of the patient with cancer* (pp. 58-71). New York: Oxford.

Ryave, A.L. (1978). On the achievement of a series of stories. In J. Schenkein (Ed.), *Studies in the organization of conversational interaction* (pp. 113-132). New York: Academic Press.

Sacks, H. (1984a). Notes on methodology. In J.M. Atkinson & J. Heritage (Eds.), *Structures of social action: Studies in conversation analysis* (pp. 21-27). Cambridge: Cambridge University Press.

Sacks, H. (1984b). On doing-being ordinary. In J.M. Atkinson & J. Heritage (Eds.), *Structures of social action: Studies in conversation analysis* (pp. 347-369). Cambridge: Cambridge University Press.

Sacks, H. (1992). *Lectures on conversation: Volumes I & II* (G. Jefferson, Ed.). Oxford: Blackwell.

Sacks, H., & Schegloff, E. (1979). Two preferences in the organization of reference to persons in conversation and their interaction. In G. Psathas (Ed.), *Everyday language: Studies in ethnomethodology* (pp. 15-21). New York: Irvington.

Sacks, H., Schegloff, E.A., & Jefferson, G. (1974). A simplest systematics for the organization of turn-taking for conversation. *Language, 50,* 696-735.

Scheflen, A.E. (1971). Natural history method in psychotherapy: Communicational research. In A.R. Mahrer & L. Pearson (Eds.), *Creative developments in psychotherapy* (pp. 393-422). Cleveland, OH: Case Western Reserve University Press. (Original work published 1966)

Scheflen, A.E. (1973). *Communicational structure: Analysis of a psychotherapy transaction.* Bloomington: Indiana University Press.

Schegloff, E.A. (1968). Sequencing in conversational openings. *American Anthropologist, 70,* 1075-1095.

Schegloff, E.A. (1972). Notes on a conversational practice: Formulating place. In D.N. Sudnow (Ed.), *Studies in social interaction* (pp. 75-119). New York: MacMillan, The Free Press.

Schegloff, E.A. (1979). Identification and recognition in telephone conversation openings. In G. Psathas (Ed.), *Everyday language: Studies in ethnomethodology* (pp. 23-78). New York: Irvington.

Schegloff, E.A. (1980). Preliminaries to preliminaries: 'Can I ask you a question? *Sociological Inquiry, 50,* 104-152.

Schegloff, E.A. (1986). The routine as achievement. *Human Studies, 9,* 111-152.

Schegloff, E.A. (1987). Analyzing single episodes of interaction: An exercise in conversation analysis. *Social Psychology Quarterly, 50,* 101-114.

Schegloff, E.A. (1988). Presequences and indirection: Applying speech act theory to ordinary conversation. *Journal of Pragmatics, 12,* 55-62.

Schegloff, E.A. (1991). Reflections on talk and social structure. In D. Boden & D.H. Zimmerman (Eds.), *Talk and social structure* (pp. 44-70). Cambridge: Polity Press.

Schegloff, E.A. (1992). Repair after next turn: The last structurally provided defense of intersubjectivity in conversation. *American Journal of Sociology, 97,* 1295-1345.

Schegloff, E.A. (1996a). Confirming allusions: Toward an empirical account of action. *American Journal of Sociology, 102,* 161-216.

Schegloff, E.A. (1996b). Issues of relevance for discourse analysis: Contingency in action, interaction and co-participant context. In E. H. Hovy & D. Scott (Eds.), *Computational and conversational discourse: Burning issues—An interdisciplinary account* (pp. 3-38). Heidelberg: Springer-Verlag.

Schegloff, E.A. (1996c). Some practices for referring to persons in talk-in-interaction: A partial sketch of a systematics. In B. Fox (Ed.), *Studies in anaphora* (pp. 437-485). Amsterdam: John Benjamins.

Schegloff, E.A. (1997). Whose text? Whose context? *Discourse & Society, 8,* 165-187.

Schegloff, E.A. (1998). Reflections on studying prosody in talk-in-interaction. *Language and Speech, 41,* 235-263.

Schegloff, E.A. (1998). *Word repeat at turn end.* Paper presented to the National Communication Association, San Diego.

Schegloff, E.A. (2000). Overlapping talk and the organization of turn-taking for conversation. *Language in Society, 29,* 1-63.

Schegloff, E.A. (2004). On dispensability. *Research on Language and Social Interaction,* 95-149.

Schegloff, E.A. (2006). *Sequence organization in interaction: A primer in conversation analysis.* Cambridge: Cambridge University Press.

Schegloff, E.A., Jefferson, G., & Sacks, H (1977). The preference for self-correction in the organization of repair in conversation. *Language, 53,* 361-382.

Schegloff, E.A., & Sacks, H. (1973). Opening up closings. *Semiotica, 8,* 298-327.

Scherz, J.W., Edwards, H.T., & Kallail, K.J. (1995). Communicative effectiveness of doctor-patient interactions. *Health Communication, 7,* 163-177.

Schulz, K.H., Schulz, H., Schulz, O., & von Kerekjarto, M. (1996). Family structure and psychosocial stress in families of cancer patients. In L. Baider, C.L. Cooper, & A.K. De-Nour (Eds.), *Cancer and the family* (pp. 225-255). New York: Wiley.

Seaburn, D.B., Lorenz, A., Campbell, T.L., & Winfield, M.A. (1996). A mother's death: Family stories of illness, loss, and healing. *Families, System & Health, 14,* 207-221.

Seale, C. (1991). Communication and awareness about death: A study of a random sample of dying people. *Social Science and Medicine, 32,* 943-952.

Shapiro, J., & Shumaker, S. (1987). Differences in emotional well-being and communication styles between mothers and fathers of pediatric cancer patients. *Journal of Psychosocial Oncology, 5,* 121-131.

Shields, G., Schondel, C., Barnhart, L., Fitzpatrick, V., Sidell, N., Adams, P., Fertig, B., & Gomez, S. (1995). Social work in pediatric oncology: A family needs assessment. *Social Work in Health Care, 21,* 39-54.

Shields, P. (1984). Communication: A supportive bridge between cancer patient, family, and health care staff. *Nursing Forum, 21,* 31-36.

Sigman, S.J. (Ed.). (1995). *The consequentiality of communication.* Hillsdale, NJ: Erlbaum.

Skorupka, P., & Bohnet, N. (1982). Primary caregivers' perceptions of nursing behaviors that best meet their needs in a home care hospice setting. *Cancer Nursing, 5,* 371-374.

Sloper, P., & While, D. (1996). Risk factors in the adjustment of siblings of children with cancer. *Journal of Child Psychology and Psychiatry and Allied Disciplines, 37,* 597-608.

Spears, J.B. (1990). Until death do us part. *Nursing, 20,* 45.

Spiro, H. (1998). *The power of hope: A doctor's perspective.* New Haven, CT: Yale University Press.

Sternberg, E. (2000). *The balance within: The science connecting health and emotions.* New York: Freeman.

Stevenson, B.S. (1985). Cancer in the family: Roles of the clergy. *The Christian Century, 102,* 419-421.

Stewart, D., & Sullivan, T. (1982). Illness behavior and the sick role in chronic disease: The case of multiple sclerosis. *Social Science and Medicine, 16,* 1397-1404.

Stivers, T. (1998). Pre-diagnostic commentary in verterinarian-client interaction. *Research on Language and Social Interaction, 31,* 241-277.

Stivers, T. (2002). Participating in decisions about treatment: Overt parent pressure for antibiotic medication in pediatric encounters. *Social Science & Medicine, 54,* 1111-1130.

Stivers, T. (2005). Modified repeats: One method for asserting primary rights from second position. *Research on Language and Social Interaction, 38,* 131-158.

Stivers, T. (2007). *Prescribing under pressure: Parent-physician conversations and antibiotics.* New York: Oxford.

Stivers, T., & Heritage, J. (2001). Breaking the sequential mold: Answering "more than the question" during comprehensive history taking. *Text, 21,* 151-186.

Streeck, J. (1980). Speech acts in interaction: A critique of Searle. *Discourse Processes, 3,* 133-154.

Stuber, M.L. (1995). Stress responses to pediatric cancer: A family phenomenon. *Family Systems Medicine, 13,* 163-172.

Suchman, A., Markakis, K., Beckman, H.B., & Frankel, R. (1997). A model of empathic communication in the medical interview. *Journal of the American Medical Association, 277,* 678-682.

Sudnow, D. (1967). *Passing on: The social organization of dying.* Englewood Cliffs, NJ: Prentice-Hall.

Sullivan, I. (1990). Cancer: A situational problem. In A. Blitzer et al. (Eds.), *Communicating with cancer patients and their families* (pp. 60-76). Philadelphia, PA: The Charles Press.

Surbone, A. (1996). The patient-doctor-family relationship: At the core of medical ethics. In L. Baider, C.L. Cooper, & A.K. De-Nour (Eds.), *Cancer and the family* (pp. 389-405). New York: Wiley.

Surbone, A., & Zwitter, M. (Eds.). (1997). *Communication with the cancer patient: Information and truth.* New York: New York Academy of Sciences.

ten Have, P. (1999). *Doing conversation analysis: A practical guide.* London: Sage.

Terasaki, A.K. (1976). *Pre-announcement sequences in interaction.* (Social Science Working Paper 99). Irvine: University of California.

Time Magazine (2002, July 15). Chevy Trailblazer advertisement.

Torode, B. (1995). Negotiating "advice" in a call to a consumer helpline. In A. Firth (Ed.), *The discourse of negotiation: Studies of language in the workplace* (pp. 345-372). Oxford: Elsevier Science.

Tracy, K. (1997). Interactional trouble in emergency service requests: A problem of frames. *Research on Language and Social Interaction, 4,* 315-343.

Tracy, K., & Tracy, S.J. (1998). Rudeness at 911: Reconceptualizing face and face attack. *Human Communication Research, 25,* 225-251.

Tracy, S.J. (2002). When questioning turns to face threat: An interactional sensitivity in 911 call-taking. *Western Journal of Communication, 66,* 129-157.

Tracy, S.J., & Tracy, K. (1998). Emotion labor at 911: A case study and theoretical critique. *Journal of Applied Communication Research, 26,* 390-411.

USA Today (1994). Cancer causes relationship changes (research on terminally ill and their familial relationships), *123,* 9.

Veach, T.A., Nicholas, D.R., & Barton, M.A. (2002). *Cancer and the family life cycle.* New York: Brunner-Routledge.

Vess, J.D., Moreland, J.R., & Schwebel, A.I. (1985). A follow-up study of role functioning and the psychological environment of families of cancer patients. *Journal of Psychosocial Oncology, 3,* 1-14.

Wakin, M.A., & Zimmerman, D.H. (1999). Reduction and specialization in emergency and directory assistance calls. *Research on Language and Social Interaction, 32*, 409-437.

Walsh-Burke, K.E. (1990). *Family communication and coping with cancer.* Doctoral dissertation, Boston College.

Watson, M. (1994). Psychological care for cancer patients and their families. *Journal of Mental Health, 3*, 457-465.

Waxler-Morrison, N., Doll, R., & Hislop, T.G. (1995). The use of qualitative methods to strengthen psychosocial research on cancer. *Journal of Psychosocial Research, 13*, 177-191.

Weihs, K., & Reiss, D. (1996). Family reorganization in response to cancer: A developmental perspective. In L. Baider, C.L. Cooper & A.K. De-Nour (Eds.), *Cancer and the family* (pp. 3-29). New York: Wiley.

Weissman, D.E. (1997). Consultation in palliative medicine. *Archives of Internal Medicine, 157*, 733-737.

Wellisch, D.K., Hoffman, A., & Gritz, E. (1996). Psychological concerns and care of daughters of breast cancer patients. In L. Baider, C.L. Cooper, & A.K. De-Nour (Eds.), *Cancer and the family* (pp. 289-304). New York: Wiley.

Westburg, N.G. (1999). Hope and humor: Using the hope scale in outcome studies. *Psychological Reports, 84*, 1014-1020.

Westman, A.S., Lewandowski, L.M., & Procter, S.J. (1993). A preliminary list to identify attitudes toward different conditions for discussing possible termination or refusal of medical treatment except for pain relief. *Psychological Reports, 72*, 279-284.

Whalen, J. (1990). *Ordinary talk in extraordinary situations: The social organization of interrogation in calls for help.* Unpublished doctoral dissertation, University of California, Santa Barbara.

Whalen, J., & Zimmerman, D.H. (1998). Observations on the display and management of emotion in naturally occurring activities: The case of "hysteria" in calls to 9-1-1. *Social Psychology Quarterly, 61*, 141-159.

Whalen, M., & Zimmerman, D.H. (1987). Sequential and institutional contexts in calls for help. *Social Psychological Quarterly, 50*, 172-185.

Whalen, M.R., & Zimmerman, D.H. (1990). Describing trouble: Practical epistemology in citizen calls to the police. *Language in Society, 19*, 465-492.

Whalen, M.A., & Zimmerman, D.H. (1999). Reduction and specialization in emergency and directory assistance calls. *Research on Language and Social Interaction, 32*, 409-437.

Whalen, J., Zimmerman, D.H., & Whalen, M.R. (1988). When words fail: A single case analysis. *Social Problems, 35*, 335-362.

Wilkinson, S., & Kitzinger, C. (2006). Surprise as an interactional achievement: Reaction tokens in conversation. *Social Psychology Quarterly, 69*, 150-182.

Williamson, G.M., & Schulz, R. (1995). Caring for a family member with cancer: Past communal behavior and affective reactions. *Journal of Applied Social Psychology, 25*, 93-117.

Wittgenstein, L. (1958). *Philosophical investigations* (2nd ed.). Oxford: Basil Blackwell.

Wittgenstein, L. (1969). *The blue and brown books* (2nd ed.). Oxford: Basil Blackwell.

Wootton, A.J. (1988). Remarks on the methodology of conversation analysis. In D. Roger & P. Bull (Eds.), *Conversation: An interdisciplinary perspective* (pp. 238-258). Clevedon, England: Multilingual Matters.

Wortman, C., & Dunkel-Schetter, C. (1979). Interpersonal relationships and cancer. *Journal of Social Issues, 35*, 120-155.

Wu, R. (2004). *Stance in talk: A conversation analysis of Mandarin final particles.* Amsterdam: Benjamins.

Yancik, R., Edwards, B.K., & Yates, J.W. (1989). Assessing the quality of life of cancer patients: Practical issues in study implementation. *Journal of Psychosocial Oncology, 7*, 59-74.

Zerwekh, J.V. (1984). Understanding the patient experience. In A.G. Blues & J.V. Zerwekh (Eds.), *Hospice and palliative nursing care* (pp. 29-44). Orlando, FL: Grune & Stratto.

Zimmerman, D.H. (1988). On conversation: The conversation analytic perspective. In J.A. Anderson (Ed.), *Communication yearbook 11* (pp. 406-432). Newbury Park, CA: Sage.

Zimmerman, D.H. (1992). The interactional organization of calls for emergency assistance. In P. Drew & J. Heritage (Eds.), *Talk at work: Interaction in institutional settings* (pp. 359-417). Cambridge: Cambridge University Press.

AUTHOR INDEX

SUBJECT INDEX

CPSIA information can be obtained
at www.ICGtesting.com
Printed in the USA
FSOW02n1736170118
43279FS